OUR PARENTS, OU

Our Parents, Ourselves

How American Health Care Imperils

Middle Age and Beyond

DISCARD

Judith Steinberg Turiel

UNIVERSITY OF CALIFORNIA PRESS   Berkeley   Los Angeles   London

University of California Press
Berkeley and Los Angeles, California

University of California Press, Ltd.
London, England

Library of Congress Cataloging-in-Publication Data

Turiel, Judith Steinberg, 1948–.
   Our parents, ourselves : how American health care
imperils middle age and beyond / Judith Steinberg
Turiel.
      p.   cm.
   Includes bibliographical references and index.
   ISBN 0–520–23276–3 (cloth : alk. paper).—
ISBN 0–520–24524–5 (pbk. : alk. paper)
      1. Older people—Medical care—United
States. [DNLM: 1. Aging—United States.   2. Activities
of Daily Living—Aged—United States.   3. Health Pol-
icy—Aged—United States.   4. Health Services Accessi-
bility—Aged—United States.   5. Quality of Life—
Aged—United States.]   I. Title.
RA564.8.T87   2005
362.6′0973—dc22   2005002628

Manufactured in the United States of America

14   13   12   11   10   09   08   07   06   05
10 9 8 7 6 5 4 3 2 1

Printed on Ecobook 50 containing a minimum 50%
post-consumer waste, processed chlorine free. The balance contains virgin pulp, including 25% Forest Stew-
ardship Council Certified for no old growth tree cutting, processed either TCF or ECF. The sheet is acid-free
and meets the minimum requirements of ANSI/NISO
Z39.48–1992 (R 1997) (Permanence of Paper).

Contents

Figures

Acknowledgments

At the outset I did not envisage the labor of love *Our Parents, Ourselves* would become. Every chapter stands as an appreciation of the book's main personalities: my parents, Edith and Seymour Steinberg, my mother-in-law, Mathilde Turiel, and my friend Lillian Rabinowitz. Less observable, but involved deeply in much the book describes, are my husband and son, Elliot and Joshua Turiel, each so very loving and patient. Throughout several of Joshua's middle and high school years, extraordinary daily care of aged grandparents became his main extracurricular activity, including on nights and weekends. These activities grew to include not only marketing with his grandmother, cooking and serving dinner each night (along with other household tasks), but also organizing their many daily medications into weekly pillboxes and refilling prescriptions, bandaging and rebandaging a continuous array of skin wounds, and managing each night his grandfather's catheter (then guiding him upstairs to bed)—leading visiting nurses and paid caregivers to call him Dr. Josh. To the nurses, aides, and doctors my deepest thanks, with special affection to the main paid caregivers, Connie Parker, Vladimir Tkachenko, Mahnaz Tayarani, Joe Barrett, and my mother-in-law's companion, Yolanda Flores.

Less obviously, *Our Parents, Ourselves* is also a labor of love directed toward Lifelong Medical Care, a network of health clinics that includes the Over 60 Health Center and provides high-quality health and social services for the least privileged of our community. This essential mission, and the excellence of the clinics' accomplishments each day, defy the boundaries of space available here. However, I want to thank especially fellow members of Lifelong's board of directors, the organization's administrators, and the staff at each clinic who continue to educate me about comprehensive and humane care for people of all ages. A particular thank-you to Marty Lynch, executive director initially of the Over 60 Health Center and, after it merged with other clinics, of Lifelong Medical Care—not only for his consistent commitment and exceptional guidance, but also for the many conversations we continue to have about issues discussed in this book.

Fortunate to be a neighbor of the University of California, Berkeley, I have learned much about American health care from two professors emeriti in the School of Public Health—elder statesmen of public health (and physicians) with a long view of the health-care crisis so apparent now. Early in my thinking about problems for people trying to obtain good care, Dr. Henrik Blum, a health economist and longtime Over 60 board member, provided invaluable perspective on the country's bigger health-care picture and its impact on local communities. Dr. Sheldon Margen, founding editor of the *Wellness Letter,* among his myriad accomplishments (and an even closer neighbor, a few houses up the street), generously shared his knowledge and experience, commented on early stages of *Our Parents, Ourselves,* and encouraged my efforts to convey in writing concerns of critical importance to health professionals and the public. Sadly, he died before seeing the book and this thank-you in print. Both Drs. Blum and Margen have voiced for decades a goal that remains elusive in this country: a health-care system in which everyone maintains the same basic right to high-quality care, sharing mutual responsibility among all members of society by spreading fairly the benefits and costs. I can well imagine the frustration and disappointment they have felt viewing the state of American health care.

Also at the university I found much needed, valuable support from a small group of women and men responsible for their aged relatives' care and intimately aware of the exhausting logistics and complicated emotions of family caregiving. My thanks to the individuals, who enjoy our times of contentment and never feel burdened by tales of woe, and to the group's coordinator, Emanuelle Gomez, who radiates concern and support for us all.

As to the actual writing of *Our Parents, Ourselves,* my great appreciation, first, to Naomi Schneider, my University of California Press editor, who saw a book at the core of rather sprawling initial ideas, and who patiently read drafts, pruning away unnecessary tangents while sharpening what should stay. Careful and kind attention from senior project editor Dore Brown and copyeditor Edith Gladstone contributed greatly to the book's final polished form. Thank-you to Dr. Andrew Leavitt, a friend from childhood and more recently (and significantly) a geriatrician, for his thoughtful comments. And my boundless gratitude to Richard Hill, another friend from junior and senior high school, as well as undergraduate Berkeley days (which neither of us believes was several decades ago). He offered to read the entire manuscript, and I took him up on it, never expecting the stream of typed pages—an insightful critique, chapter-by-chapter, raising essential questions, finding weak points and suggesting changes, saving me the embarrassment of incorrect metaphors (as well as excessive semicolons). I thank him also for remaining constant in his encouragement throughout my writing and rewriting.

And a final acknowledgment about the book's title, especially for readers who missed the 1960s and 1970s women's health movement. *Our Bodies, Ourselves,* a comprehensive and detailed self-care book, became a women's health bible of sorts, followed by several revised editions and new variations, all written by the ongoing Boston Women's Health Book Collective. The books and the collective inspired many young women like me to become active, informed, and critical participants in matters of our own health and well-being, and to apply our education and skills within a broad consumer health effort. The books and collective also conveyed in no uncertain terms serious concern, and at times anguish, about the state of our health care and of American society as a whole.

Introduction
People and Their Environment

Vibrant, focused, engaged, and engaging, Lillian Rabinowitz was the picture of independence when I first met her. Divorced many years, she lived alone in a home purchased decades earlier when young families, many connected to the university, could afford a modest bungalow in the Berkeley hills. She was immersed in her work on aging, especially on improving health care for older people. The calendar beside her phone displayed a full schedule of meetings, presentations to public health or medical students, trips to Sacramento, California's capital, to lobby for statewide legislation. Everyone involved with aging—professors, doctors, lawyers, community organizers, and politicians—seemed to know Lillian, the Bay Area's activist-authority on needs of the elderly.

In the early 1970s, after retiring from teaching elementary school, Lillian had become the moving force behind a local Gray Panther chapter focused on the needs of older people. The fledgling core group, initially a handful of Berkeley women, soon identified its uppermost priority: finding solutions to the serious problems people face in obtaining high-quality health care as they grow older, especially people with limited economic means. Horrified by what they saw when investigating the fate of residents in some of Berkeley's nursing homes, and barely satisfied with the better facilities, these women concluded that what old

1

people most need is health care that will help keep them out of such places. The Gray Panthers forged ahead with their new mission of establishing a health clinic, controlled by members of the community, to provide primary and preventive health care, as well as social services, designed specifically for older women and men. For the country's first community health clinic specializing in geriatric care, they had one overarching goal: to enable people to remain in their own homes, living as independently as possible.

The organization's initial accomplishment came in 1976, when the Over 60 Health Center opened its doors in a small storefront located in the Berkeley flatlands, a primarily low-income, minority neighborhood dotted with small groceries, liquor stores, functional apartment buildings, and tidy homes, many with windows barred against the potential burglar. In little more than a decade the clinic had outgrown this and its next site, and by the summer of 1998 groundbreaking ceremonies marked a major step toward its larger and more ambitious third incarnation, a building that would include an adult day-care program and housing for frail, low-income elders.

By spring 1999 Lillian was the lone survivor of Over 60's half-dozen "founding mothers." During that winter Lillian's memory and concentration began to wane noticeably, her ability to maintain a conversation faltered. Her only sibling, a sister in New York, suffered a debilitating stroke. Lillian worried increasingly about her own health and, especially, whether she could continue to live by herself.

"Maybe living to eighty-eight is too long?" she remarked one day, in a statement that ended as a question. Of all people, even this activist for elders, matriarch of the local Gray Panthers and an enlarging health-care center, faced the same difficulties of aging and health care experienced by so many others in this country—difficulties she had identified and worked to remedy long before reaching this point.

Lillian reflected the country's demographics. A member of the fastest growing age group, the category called oldest old, she was living on a fixed middle-class income. She lived alone, as do approximately 75 percent of Americans over the age of seventy-five.[1] And being female, she was one of the disproportionate number of the oldest old. Women outlive men by about five years, according to the Older Women's League; 80 percent of the approximately 9 million older adults living alone in 2000 were women.[2] Only one of Lillian's three children, an unmarried son, lived nearby; although daughters (and daughters-in-law) generally provide what family care elders receive, hers lived on the other side of the country.

I met Lillian in the early 1990s, when I joined the Over 60 board of directors. She was often the person who asked pointed questions about the topics at hand, zeroing in on the concerns of old people. I learned that Lillian had pressured her own health-care provider (Kaiser Permanente) to introduce consultations with geriatric specialists and to establish a committee of members and doctors focusing on senior care. She had played a key role in developing county programs for older adults who could live at home but needed facilities that provide daytime care and activities.

One day, to my surprise, she telephoned to ask if I could help her for a few evenings. She had recently fallen, injuring a wrist. Though she had arranged adequate help for daytime needs, bedtime remained a problem. With one arm in a sling, she could not quite manage changing into a nightgown and, especially, cleaning her dentures. Since we lived quite near each other, perhaps I could stop by in the evenings. A few years passed before Lillian asked me to help again—this time changing bandages on an infected toe. By then she had sold her house and moved to an apartment in a cooperative building for seniors. No longer comfortable with driving, she had sold her car as well. I became her usual driver for board meetings and other Over 60 events, giving Lillian and me more opportunities to chat, learn snippets of each other's lives, and become friends.

At the same time I was watching my parents grow old before my eyes. Living near them, a physical proximity unusual in this day and age, I saw them navigate illnesses and surgeries, the loss of friends and siblings, elimination of work and recreational activities, the deterioration of body and mind. As they survived beyond eighty-five years of age, I felt anxiety, for them and for myself, finally convinced that I would turn around one day and find myself old.

As a baby boomer with a then young child and old parents, I also reflected the demographics. Except for friends whose parents had died too early, everyone I knew seemed to face decisions about a mother and/or father too ill, fragile, or forgetful. It is hard to watch parents weaken. To see my mother's body so diminished, her once broad shoulders now hunched, back humped, made me wince. My mother's sturdy frame, with acclaimed tennis backhand, appeared to melt year by year, taken over by chronic pain, leaving this thin wisp of a frail old woman with tissue-paper skin. Suddenly, it seemed, my father's feet shuffled as he barely managed to stay on them, even with the newly accepted cane and then the walker. Legally blind from macular degeneration, a progressive loss of eyesight becoming common now that more people are living more years, he was no longer able to drive, even with my mother as copilot. Forced to surrender his driver's license, he lost a primary means of independence and activity. He could no longer read the newspaper, long a daily pleasure, or his magazines, which still arrived week after week in the mail. He felt embarrassed, he told me, by the confused disarray of bills and checks and correspondence on his once meticulous desk. A retired lawyer, expert in crafting succinct contractual phrases throughout his career, he smiled ruefully now at words, entire sentences, that would not come. "I'm not well," he stated frequently, shaking his head, fully aware that his mind was not operating as it should, as it used to, that thoughts or memories came and went with no apparent reason.

I had touched old age in my grandmothers, each widowed long before my birth. However, I could summon only veiled memories, and their last years held for me certain mysteries. One grandmother suffered a late-life depression, but I never knew her symptoms; the other lived out her last years, following a stroke, in a nursing home where my parents would never take me, not wanting me to see her that way. Now the topic, aging, is everywhere, encompassing far more than the very old. You need only observe newspapers and television to grasp a major population shift, as the largest bulge moves inexorably toward later decades of the life span. The media know their audience. Today's news reflects well the interests and concerns of the country's most lucrative market, the 78 million Americans born between the end of World War II and the mid-1960s. Stories focus commonly on menopause or Medicare, and on prospects for living longer, whether owing to lifestyle choices or longevity genes.

Commercial messages increasingly target the market of aging baby boomers, as well as our parents. On television, in magazines, in our mailboxes (electronic and otherwise), advertisements promote moisture cream for "wonderful" and always attractive women older than fifty. Hot flashes join the announced array of problems a touted product can solve. For men, the message has progressed from hair coloring to Viagra: a silver-haired man in blue jeans, the contemporary matured Marlboro man, knowingly hugs his wife, or perhaps lover (wedding bands are visible in some versions, not others). Ads peddle memory aids, nutritional boosts, and other manner of life-extenders.

"AS LONG AS YOU'VE GOT YOUR HEALTH"

The commercial onslaught that aging has engendered can erase neither face wrinkles nor serious health concerns as people grow older. The baby boom's leading edge, people moving through their fifties, may feel they are handling a three-ring medical circus. Caring for their children and parents, as the caught-between women and men commonly known as the sandwich generation, they increasingly face health problems related to their own advancing age. My generation dealt with our children's pediatrician even as news reports warned of society's need for geriatricians, doctors specially trained to care for aging baby boomers in years to come. In fact, the most common belief people hold about living a long life may be the crucial importance of good health. At the least, they want to live their older years free of debilitating or painful health problems.

As if growing old were not challenge enough, with questions of meaning and purpose, as well as of physical and mental well-being, an additional dimension complicates the process of aging in the United States: dissatisfaction with the health-care system. By the twentieth century's close, the paradox characterizing American health care, from birth through old age, was striking. The country could claim the best in modern medicine, with highly trained physicians and nurses, well-equipped hospitals, sophisticated diagnostic and treatment methods, and scientific research promising always further breakthroughs in technology and biology. Yet throughout the country, Americans were disturbed and angered by recent experiences at a doctor's office or hospital. In many instances, enrolling in a health insurance plan, most commonly through an employer, meant leaving a doctor known and liked over many years, even disrupting midstream an ongoing medical treatment. Many health plans limited the choice of doctors patients could see. The primary doctor, selected from a health-plan list, served as gatekeeper, the patients' entrée to diagnostic and treatment procedures and to specialists, also selected from a restricted list. However people chose a doctor, appointments felt more rushed. Doctors squeezed more patients and paperwork into a managed-care hour, sixty minutes of lowered insurance reimbursement to doctors for each patient seen, leading doctors, in turn, to schedule more patients. In hospitals, patients complained that nurses took longer to respond and, when they finally appeared, seemed frazzled. Mistakes became more common. All the while, health-plan premiums and co-payments increased while services declined.

Doctors and nurses were unhappy as well. Beyond diminishing fees, managed-care plans created too many forms and rules and ways of interfering. Insurance company requirements—for example, that medical procedures must receive prior authorization—wasted endless time. Even more disturbing, medical decisions, the very core of a doctor-patient relationship, were consigned to insurance company employees who could veto the doctor's orders. Concern for fiscal bottom lines, insisted doctors and nurses, meant that hospitals were downsizing staff below safe levels, cutting medical corners too frequently and severely.

During the late 1990s state legislatures began passing laws to curb the most flagrant abuses arising within managed-care health plans. Among the most notorious practices were exceedingly brief hospital stays, including what critics called drive-through births or mastectomies, and refusals to authorize or reimburse care in an emergency room. Congress debated a patient's bill of rights for members of health maintenance organizations (HMOs), legislation sideswiped initially by the politics and process of impeaching President Clinton. Even doctor shows on television dramatized HMO laments. Although the Clinton administration's original reform proposal for universal health insurance suffered a spectacular collapse in 1994, people perceived severe problems with the path taken instead—market competition among insurers, physicians, and hospitals, all shaped by managed-care rules. Inadequacies plagued not only the uninsured or underinsured, whose ranks continued to grow, but also a broad swath of the population—people in acute or chronic need of health care, as well as the people providing that care.

Yet unprecedented prosperity filled the mass media's image of America as the new century began. *Newsweek*'s April 2000 cover story proclaimed "A New Middle Age," presenting first of all "A Boomer's Guide to Health, Wealth and Happiness."[3] Although the *Newsweek* report declared that today's middle-aged would redefine growing old, with their good health and wealth, nearly two-thirds of those it surveyed were concerned about taking care of elderly parents, and a similar proportion worried that they would not be able to afford needed health care if a family member became ill.

The 2000 presidential election did give voice to health-care concerns. At least temporarily, the campaign revived talk of a bill of rights for

HMO members (a prospect that ignores the increasing numbers of people with no medical insurance at all). Candidates debated Medicare's overall financial health for the years ahead and its more specific, immediate failure to provide older Americans with affordable prescription drugs, the mainstay of most elders' health care. Eons removed from universal health insurance, George W. Bush offered such free market proposals as individual medical savings accounts and tax incentives for purchasing private insurance, and prescription drug discount cards for low-income Medicare recipients.

For people sharing my demographic niche, the new century's constellation of circumstances—relatives and friends who are old; dissatisfactions with health care; scientific and public attention to aging and longevity, including its commercialization and even glamorization—only heighten concerns about how we will be treated after we pass through middle age. How we will be treated not only in a strictly medical sense, but in ways that more generally affect how we grow old and, simply put, whether we can enjoy doing so. Seeing my parents, and Lillian, and other individuals involved with the Over 60 Health Center raises persistent questions: If I live to their age, will I remember my past, and what someone just said? Will I be in pain, all over and always? Will I be able to see and hear, take walks, drive a car? Will I live longer than I want, my abilities, desires, and my health too diminished? Or, by then, will I see it all differently?

Answers to these intensely personal questions depend on an inescapable public policy side as well: How will this country manage when the baby boom generation swells its population of the old, then of the oldest old? Will social and health-care policies meet our needs more adequately than do policies currently affecting older Americans? Will the politics of health care move the country beyond commercial exploitation of the expanded market, allowing baby boomers to define differently our own aging? Will our generation fulfill the upbeat media themes, truly reshaping the concept of aging in the twenty-first century?

The chapters that follow address both the personal experience of aging and the health-care issues and policies that surround individuals. Through this dual focus, I try to convey the flavor of people's lives, while weaving in information from medical literature and media reports, along with discussion of political developments that affect greatly how Americans grow old. In general terms, the information and policy considerations involve independent living, social and medical support, the quality of life and of life endings, and the role of families and institutions and politics. Naturally, the country's Medicare program comes into play, as do its major gaps—especially, its forty-year lack of prescription drug coverage and the newly legislated benefit starting in 2006, and the absence of coverage for daily care if an individual can no longer live independently.

Throughout the book I maintain another dual focus. I discuss healthcare concerns central to the lives of people who are presently old and, perhaps of even more profound impact over time, to the greater numbers of women and men now at midlife, people witnessing and often caring for an aged relative or friend, their own old age still at some remove. Although *Our Parents, Ourselves* does not provide practical advice about daily care at home or detailed information on care in a residential institution, it does identify crucial issues for the course through later years of life. Ideally, this approach can help readers stay at least one step ahead of problems and decisions facing them, rather than playing catch-up, a pattern all too common for the parents' generations.[4]

OVERVIEW

While writing this book I, along with my husband and son, became immersed in the care of my parents. That immersion not only swallowed time, day and night, but also rendered even basic concepts less clear-cut, uncertainties and complexities more pronounced. Until recent years my life felt pulled along through fairly predictable, anticipated phases—college, work, marriage, a child—with daily life shaped pretty much by my own choosing. I did not anticipate that care for aged parents would fill a sizable segment of my middle age, at times sapping my energy and spirits. The task tired me in a new way, absent the invigorating thrill of nurturing an infant, the joy of watching a loved one blossom. And so this book slowed and diverged, because writing it was more difficult than expected, and there was so little time.

That said, I present below the overview of what *Our Parents, Ourselves* turned out to be, its framework consisting of people in a place and time.

THE PEOPLE

To explore aging and health care, I describe the experiences of people I know, especially in the book's first section. Chapter 1 focuses on people's basic goal of independence as they age, illustrating how tightly intertwined with independence is the health care they receive. Chapter 2 discusses vulnerabilities of the old that can threaten their ability to live independently. I write in these chapters about Lillian, a woman who spent her later decades working to improve very concrete aspects of aging but in her last years had no choice for herself other than a skilled nursing facility. I write about my parents because I know their story best and, like many women and men my age, I am part of it. For reasons of privacy, there are many questions I did not ask and personal specifics I chose not to include in this book; and because I am not yet old, there is much I cannot yet know to ask. Both chapters 1 and 2 discuss basic concerns and information I wish I had better understood before backing into the care of aging parents.[5] And these chapters suggest an ironic twist: health professionals committed to a low-income clientele, seen within community health clinics such as the Over 60 Health Center, have developed more adequate programs of care for aging patients and others with chronic conditions than have their counterparts in the private medical realm, serving the predominantly white middle-class, people well able to afford the health-care extras money can buy.

Chapters 3 through 5 take up components of health care that are central to the way people age: prescription drugs, implicit and explicit health-care rationing, end-of-life decisions and care. Each of these chapters highlights key issues that are critical for all of us who live into our seventies, eighties, and beyond. As individuals alone, we cannot improve the quality of aging in America. Rather, needed change requires action on the broader social policy context that creates the larger health-care picture. The book's final chapter pulls together the various dimensions of that picture as it presently affects older adults' health and well-being—for better or worse—and points the way toward changes that could improve the prospects for those of us reaching old age, however redefined, in years to come.

Another group of people informed my thoughts as I wrote this book: over several years I participated in a support group for university faculty and staff who, in addition to their day job, carry responsibilities for an aged family member (I was the one faculty spouse; most members were daughters, with a sprinkling of nieces and sons). Overall, about twenty-five individuals joined as care demands filled more attention and time or left if work demands grew too large or a parent died. Though not visible on the pages that follow, this welcoming cadre of individuals—sharing worries and decisions, emotional ups and downs, as well as information—kept before me, through their individual stories, a much fuller array of experiences than my own.[6]

Among the group's members, those not living with or near their aged relative attempt to organize care across the state or country. Some are an only child, others have siblings, helpful or not. Many find themselves financially squeezed because a parent is still alive, using up savings, pensions, Social Security budgeted carefully to cover fewer years and fewer disabilities. Perhaps the most strained are single women handling it all, the crises and day-to-day care, on their own. Immediate and chronic problems of the members' relatives include Parkinson's disease and diabetes, heart and lung disease, cancers, dementias and depression, alcoholism, repeated falls, a parent in declining health considering suicide and asking his daughter to help. Other difficult and troubling questions rest in participants' hands. A son, for example, visits his mother frequently in a nursing home, vigilantly watching over her care; with severe dementia, unable to recognize him, physically frail and bed-bound, she again develops an infection, this time pneumonia, and he must again provide consent for the medical response. He relates previous episodes involving illness or bedsores, nutrition, and dehydration, finally verbalizing his question: "Why," he asks, "am I trying so hard to keep her healthy?" At times, individuals in the group express resentment that their substantial care efforts go unappreciated; at other times they feel guilt about not doing more. Most commonly felt is fatigue, and grief spread over time, long before a death.

THE ENVIRONMENT

Though Berkeley, California, might never be characterized as a typical American city, it does reflect well, at times in stark relief, significant realities of health care in the United States, including as it affects people growing old. Despite Berkeley's reputation for progressive policies, it is a city of troubling social and economic disparities. You see them most obviously in its geography and neighborhoods, the flatlands of racial and ethnic diversity rising along with income to hills of woodsy meandering roads boasting architect-designed homes and spectacular bay views, enjoyed by primarily white professionals and professors. Within the city's one public high school, its teenagers, thrown together, quickly separate and reassemble not only into daily social clusters but into distinct streams of academic success or failure. The pattern persists into the university, which struggles with the contentious question of who will be admitted to gain further education in its lecture halls and classrooms, libraries, and research laboratories.

Berkeley's health disparities are undeniable. The disparities begin at birth: African American residents of the flats suffer significantly higher rates of disease and shorter length of life than the Caucasians in the hills. Many of Berkeley's 103,000 residents are likely unaware of the city's health department report for the year 2000 that left officials shaken. The report quantified the grim inequities through low birth weight, high chronic illness rates, and reduced life expectancy for African Americans.[7] These statistics materialize within the city's one hospital emergency room, the women and men and teenagers waiting hours at a time, as I have done several times with one parent or the other. And the ER dramatizes another undeniable fact: health care for all segments of society in Berkeley as throughout the United States is ultimately intertwined in practice and outcomes—care for the poor; the uninsured; middle-class members of a health maintenance organization, preferred provider organization (PPO), or any other managed-care acronym; children; and people who have reached the age for Medicare.

My work on this book was broken up in September 2001. The questions I was pursuing gained a new edge. Suddenly, beyond vast personal loss suffered by so many people, much of what anyone assumed about their future collapsed in doubt. For at least a few collective moments, there was some sense that everyone is in this—this horrific event, this life—together, sharing responsibility for the welfare of one another, and that a government's role is to ensure adequate and equitable distribution of needed resources. Even Secretary of Treasury Paul O'Neill supported in public comments a concept not commonly promoted within the Bush administration: the country would need to "socialize" its response to security needs, he said (the issue was airport security), spreading resources across the entire society, with direct government participation and oversight. This sense of shared social responsibility and support did not long survive within an administration committed to private rather than government enterprise whenever possible (nor did that secretary of treasury). Moreover, the concept has never held much sway within the arena of health-care needs. Only Medicare embodies partially, and only for older or disabled Americans, the concept that people have a right to health care, and that a government-insured, publicly funded system is most fair and humane, a principle that holds for people of any age throughout Canada, western Europe, Australia, and New Zealand.

The September 11 attack, by defining the Bush administration and shaping dynamics of the 2004 presidential campaign, appears to have dimmed immediate prospects for moving toward such a system. Indeed, George Bush's second administration, claiming a mandate and freed from constraints of a next election, could throw American health care more forcefully into reverse. The concluding chapter will return to prospects for change and especially to questions of fairness and human needs. During the last decade's health-care battles a principle of shared responsibility did not prevail, even in the distorted, poorly devised form of the Clintons' universal health insurance plan. Beyond its flaws and the onslaught of private insurance and pharmaceutical and other commercial health-care-related corporations, the plan's unpopularity reflects a society that seems not to accept the socialization of risks and resources as a value underlying the response to such fundamental needs as care for people's health. And so, by marshaling evidence on the universal process of aging and its inescapable effects on health, *Our Parents, Ourselves* will emphasize a different principle: self-interest. Individuals at any age can be certain of high-quality health care that meets predictable as well as unforeseen needs only if such care is available for all.

The evidence begins with a personal experience.

. . .

Our Friday night dinners have been a tradition. A routine. My mother used to wash and bake the chickens each week, but now I buy them already cooked. This rainy Friday evening starts the same—my mother wakened from her long afternoon nap, the table set, chicken warmed, vegetables ready. But two hours later I am dialing 911; for the second time during dinner she has drifted away, not answering when we ask if she is okay. "Nonresponsive," the paramedics who swoop into the house will call what I describe. By then she is better, but they detect an irregular heartbeat. We are headed for the emergency room, and not for the first time.

This night in the ER takes nearly seven hours, starting with my mother on a gurney against a wall waiting for a bed in a curtain-partitioned room. The nurses and technicians move through the hallways and rooms nonstop; a doctor appears within the curtained space, examines my mother, asks questions, and orders tests. It is 1 A.M. when a nurse jabs my mother's arm and hooks her up to intravenous antibiotics, a blood test having revealed the highly elevated white blood cell count of infection—some kind, somewhere. Old people don't always

show the same symptoms, the nurse tells me—no fever or chills, no particular pains. At 2:30 the doctor reappears and to my surprise, and despite my hesitations, sends my mother home, a fragile, septic eighty-five-
year-old woman on a cold wet night, her intravenous medications just
completed. There will be no overnight stay, no nurse who can monitor
her condition, no doctor available if need arises.

We leave with a prescription and a set of confusing, not completely
accurate written instructions. ER care will not include follow-up on the
case. No one inquires whether there is anyone in her home to care for
her, observe her response to the medication, watch in case she again becomes nonresponsive or experiences other reactions to the infection, no
one to obtain the oral antibiotics needed first thing in the morning and
see that she takes them properly. Surely not her then ninety-year-old,
cognitively impaired, legally blind husband. And in fact not until Monday, when I call her regular physician and he calls the hospital laboratory for Friday night's additional test results, will the antibiotic be
changed, her infection unaffected by the one prescribed.

1

Independence in Daily Life
Aging In-Place or Elsewhere

We have all seen them. Tanned, smiling, silver-haired women and men, golf clubs in hand. They appear in glossy magazine advertisements for retirement communities, or in newspaper supplements bearing such titles as "Primetime," or on health insurance brochures that arrive unsolicited in the mail offering, for example, "Secure Horizons." These women and men are obviously enjoying golden years filled with recreation and companionship, free of worries, certainly not dependent on their grown children or anyone else for that matter.

Yet how many older adults look, let alone live, like that? Enjoying country-clublike retirement requires not only ample finances but also relatively good health. Ironically, good health is sometimes necessary to purchase the private health insurance plan a brochure promotes to substitute for Medicare (certain for-profit-Medicare HMOs), or to fill some of Medicare's coverage gaps (a Medi-gap policy). Furthermore, most people will not live their later years as a couple. Rather, women who are widowed, divorced, or who never married outlive and outnumber men.

This chapter takes as a starting point the desire of older Americans to live independently, able physically and mentally to accomplish everyday tasks, to socialize with family and friends, and to enjoy the comfort of being at home. It also explores a prominent concern of aging—long-term care, a concept and an array of personal, financial, and residential arrangements confronting anyone who lives long enough or is involved in decisions about an aged person's daily life. The discussion of living options not only introduces residential institutions that care for the old; it also addresses the reality that remaining at home does not necessarily mean living independently.

For most people, the topic of long-term care hovers peripherally until it bursts onto center stage, sometime in their fifties, when the health of an aged parent, other relative, or friend requires a change in living arrangements, perhaps immediately. As they weather decisions now for those who are older, moreover, today's middle-aged face questions about their own later years. As they think ahead, these individuals need to recognize two core themes highlighted in this chapter: the lifelong importance of social contact and the extent to which aging becomes a women's issue. They need also to appreciate one basic fact of life that shapes everyone's passage into older age: the unavoidable influence of uncertainty and chance in delineating life circumstances and needs. Plan as we might, personal finances can decline dramatically, as can the country's economy. So, too, unexpected illness or disability can strike suddenly or sneak up insidiously, too long unnoticed.

LIVING WITH NEEDS FOR CARE

Nobody can count on breezing through later years of life without considerable support, including health care that does not center solely, or even predominantly, on medical diagnoses and treatments. People face potential obstacles, beyond the financial, to living as they want. Close to 90 percent of women and men sixty-five and older live with at least one chronic health problem, 70 percent with more than one.[1] Arthritis is the most common, but it could be heart disease, diabetes, high blood pressure, failing eyesight or hearing, or dementia. Their years will be punctuated by acute illness (a respiratory infection, influenza), less commonly by a sudden heart attack or stroke, a debilitating accident, or a cancer (though certain cancers are increasingly treated as chronic conditions managed medically over many years). Individuals commonly experience ups and downs in overall health. The good news is that most nondisabled older adults can recover from health setbacks, regaining former abilities. As they age further, the bad news is that doctors may not be providing appropriate monitoring, follow-up care, and preventive measures that can minimize adverse effects and decline from recurrent acute episodes.[2]

Most people in their seventies and beyond need health care that manages chronic and acute conditions in ways that best support independent living, avoiding the most disabling symptoms and complications, slowing an overall deterioration. Medical care, however, focuses overwhelmingly on treatment of acute illness, a limitation particularly problematic for older adults whose health is most vulnerable. One study, based on interviews with such patients, suggests poor quality of care for chronic disease and for preventive or follow-up care. While treatment of acute illness and general adult disease appeared to be adequate, the quality of care was particularly low for falls and other mobility problems, urinary incontinence, pressure sores, cognitive decline and dementia, depression, and end-of-life care.[3] Physicians were not following, and were not educated to provide, a primary care approach best suited to frail patients with multiple health problems and a decline in functional abilities. Nor does Medicare currently reimburse many aspects of the needed approach. That approach includes evaluation and treatment of geriatric conditions by a multidisciplinary health-care team, coordination of care from different health professionals in various settings (office, hospital, home), and careful attention to hospitalizations (e.g., patient disorientation and delirium, medication changes, discharge plans, and follow-up care).[4]

In support of such an approach, recent data on Veterans' Administration patients suggest that reduced hospitalization, intensive-care unit days, and emergency room treatments do not result in worse health outcomes for older patients with serious chronic illness *if* a corresponding emphasis on primary and preventive care prevails.[5] Efforts aimed at preventing illness and injury will range more broadly than standard doctor's office ministrations. Beyond flu and pneumonia vaccinations, comprehensive preventive care includes help with nutrition and exercise regimens, home safety information and visits, interventions to stop smoking and other substance abuse, and social support for living safely and well at home. In sum, older people need care that is generally low-tech, though it does require time—time for doctors and other health professionals to know individual patients, to hear what patients are saying about symptoms they are experiencing, to learn about the impact of medical interventions on their lives, and to talk with them about wishes regarding their own health. Less dazzling or heroic than cutting-edge medical cures, health care responsive to aging requires comprehensiveness and continuity. That is, individuals see the same familiar doctors and nurses over time, including when they're in a hospital or other facility; a continuum of care services escalates in tandem with people's enlarging needs. Indeed, individuals' health and changes in it, and availability of care that supports as much independence in daily life as possible, are intimately entwined with decisions about where to live.

AN INDEPENDENT APARTMENT

When the time came for Lillian to sell her house and move to an apartment with low maintenance, away from narrow winding hill roads, she had foresight. She wanted two bedrooms, because at some point down the line she thought she might need a companion living with her, someone to help an older Lillian cook and shop, get to doctor's appointments and take her medications, go out for walks. With a little luck, this move—the packed boxes, winnowed possessions, new surroundings to learn—could be her last.

Lillian found an apartment in Berkeley's only cooperatively owned building for older adults. To live there requires health and mobility good enough to use the building's elevator, to prepare meals, to manage in case of earthquake or fire. With occupancy full, it also helps to know a resident who will soon be moving out, usually to an assisted living facility, or know that a resident recently died.

Lillian qualified on all counts. From her corner location, she enjoyed sweeping views not only of the hills where she had lived, but also of the university, the San Francisco Bay, and two bridges. Her in-building neighbors included Gray Panther friends who kept the lobby's bulletin board filled with notices of political rallies, organization meetings, an occasional birthday celebration in the building's first-floor meeting/living room space. The neighborhood outside buzzed with college students walking or bicycling to or from the campus, the disabled in wheelchairs maneuvering Berkeley's accommodating sidewalks, and people heading for nearby book or record stores, the market or bakery. On Sundays, whatever was the year's current music escaping from dormitory windows found harmony with organ chords arising from deep within churches, an ecumenical array that claim numerous blocks along the campus edge, tending to the spiritual needs of this famously irreverent community.

During the first years of apartment life Lillian maintained her active schedule, including occasional visits to her sister and to plays, museums, concerts in New York. Then, little by little, she began cutting back. No longer driving, she depended on friends to take her to the market or a movie, on members of the same organizations to bring her to meetings. She began to waver about our monthly board of directors meetings, explaining that she could not hear, even with her hearing aid. She would comment as we drove about the amount of material we had to read for each meeting, the financial and program reports, Medicare and MediCal information, plans for the new Over 60 building. She had trouble following discussions of reimbursements, foundation grants, staff morale and turnover, relationships with hospitals and labor unions, the pressures of managed care, and the competition from HMOs. Soon I was driving to meetings alone.

From a friend I learned that Lillian had asked to have a doctor test her for Alzheimer's disease—another example of her foresight and determination to face rather than avoid difficulties of aging, I thought, with not the slightest notion of how profound were the request's implications. I never heard the results. Now, I saw Lillian mostly at her apartment. Not only did I see her age further; through photographs and the stories they sparked in her, I encountered Lillian as a child growing up poor, then a young woman with dark, thick, long braided hair, a secretary needing to earn money rather than attend college. I saw Lillian two times a wife, three times a mother, on family vacations happy and not. Then, in color, Lillian the retired teacher and newly forged activist appeared more matronly and familiar, her grayed hair cut short and hugging the thinned face like a soft, curly cap. Reviewing her photographs, pulled each visit from one drawer or another, seemed Lillian's most enjoyable activity, a magnet for her attention and conversation. The photographs spanned czarist Russia, with stories of her mother, European travels with her sister and brother-in-law, and solo summer studies in Cuernavaca. Local politicians posed honoring Lillian for her work on aging. And fondly she showed me her friend and colleague Maggie Kuhn, the founder of the national Gray Panthers, painfully frail on her last trip to California at an Over 60 party that celebrated Lillian's eightieth birthday.

Lillian's physical health and abilities generally remained strong. However, her efforts to *age-in-place*—as social scientists describe growing old in a familiar home and community, not needing to move, finally, to institutional care—faltered at one obstacle she could not foresee. By the time she needed a companion living in the apartment's second bedroom, to assure that she was safe living in her apartment and in the outside world, Lillian rejected the available candidates. She seemed no longer to perceive her original plan as an acceptable living arrangement.

Already my conversations with Lillian had become difficult, her train of thought halting before a sentence's end. "Not tracking," another of Lillian's friends, a professor who studies aging, described it, using a term I would hear later from my own cousin about our fathers. Already I had noticed Lillian not recognizing people. "Do I know you?" she responded to acquaintances greeting her at a memorial service for a dear friend. And there was her upset beyond proportion, a feeling of panic it seemed, returning home that day, standing outside her building fishing through every pocket and her handbag for keys. Frequently now there was uncertainty in her voice over small decisions such as where we would go for lunch and did this sweater match, a passivity and dependence surprising to me in this activist woman. Most strikingly, the photographs became a guessing game. "Do you know who this is?" she would ask about a snapshot shown many times before, a contest for her as much as me. Then Lillian became a third-person character. "That man is interested in her, but she thinks not," Lillian explained about a photograph of herself and a man in conversation, sitting on the ground outdoors among redwood trees at a mountain conference site. And the portrait in Lillian's bedroom of a blond three-year-old girl became her daughter and sister at once.

It was during this time that Lillian first showed me brochures from assisted living facilities. Her family was strongly urging a move—trying to take over, in Lillian's view—so that she would receive the needed care. Friends were taking her to visit one or the other, and Lillian was not pleased. One choice seemed too far away; people might not be able to visit. Moreover, what clearly struck Lillian as unimaginable, her room would have no shower or bath. She could bathe down the hallway, only three times a week and only at set times of the day. The expense of any such place, Lillian insisted, restacking several brochures on the coffee table, was well beyond her means.

From Lillian's friends I heard an urgency. The time for her to move was now. I heard the same from her sister when she visited Berkeley. Of all the family members Lillian spoke about, she seemed closest to her sister, now a wealthy widow who told me the expense of assisted living was not an obstacle for Lillian.

OPTIONS WITHIN THE LONG-TERM WORLD

"It's 10 P.M. . . . Do you know where your parents are?" The question dominates a local newspaper advertisement for a "senior living community," framing the photograph of a well-dressed elderly couple who stand, the man using a cane, gazing at each other. The creators of this marketing theme, like their target baby boom audience, doubtless hear an echo and appreciate the twist: in our youth a public service television announcement asked each night, "It's 10 P.M. . . . Do you know where your children are?" The children were adolescent, often testing their independence from parents about whom they now worry. Today, it is the parents whose independence is precarious. As marketers of long-term care well know, it's the adult children who often wonder and then decide where and how aging parents or other relatives will pass their nights and days as living on their own grows difficult and dangerous. And so a "life care village" advertisement features one contented resident who declares, "I don't know who's *happier* about my life at Spring Lake Village—*me* or *my children*" (original emphasis). An agency providing personal elder care and case coordination assures offspring in a nationally distributed magazine, "You can't always be there for MOM & DAD in FLORIDA . . . but we can!"

As advertisements and solicitations began arriving in my parents' mail, I began learning the lay of the long-term land. Promise of creative independence or compassionate care, a homelike atmosphere or restaurant-quality meals, social activities, companionship, just plain fun and peace of mind barely hint at essential considerations for individuals and families. Indeed, the spate of marketing targeted to offspring raises first questions: Who will make decisions about care for an individual's later years? And when is the time to decide?

Ideally, people make choices about the course of their own lives at a time when they can understand, compare, and think about the options, not during a health crisis or after substantial cognitive decline (which I discuss in chapter 2). Presently, many of the old have not planned for their own changing needs, and it is adult offspring who are realizing their parents can neither live safely in their current place, even with additional help, nor decide on their own where to move. At the broadest level, today's options fall within a realm called senior housing, though most commonly the choice narrows to housing with some form of care.

RETIREMENT COMMUNITIES These age-restricted housing developments initially attracted older women and men—usually married couples, their children grown—who bought their own downsized, low-maintenance home in order to enjoy a job-free, child-free life. Prototypes built during the 1960s, the Leisure Worlds and Sun Cities, typically clustered along a golf course in a region known for warm desert air or a cool ocean breeze. Residents were generally healthy and active, white and middle class, in their late sixties and seventies; the community provided no medical or personal care. More recent versions include some activities and meals, and a health clinic might be available on-site. Adult communities of the twenty-first century, aiming for a somewhat younger and wealthier clientele, emphasize resortlike features—pools, spas, gyms, tennis, and various other options—near existing suburbs for the impending surge of midlife baby boomers, retired or not. In 2001, prices advertised in the San Francisco Bay area ranged from "the high $150,000s" to nearly $2,000,000.

Since the 1960s, the enlarging population of older and more disabled old has created a need for residential facilities that fill a spectrum that stretches between golf course retirement and late life nursing-home care. The label "retirement community" now frequently attaches to gradations in the balance of independence and help. For people who cannot or do not want to live in their own or a relative's home, available options differ along two basic dimensions: the level or type of care provided, and the facility's size. Type of care is crucial not only for matching an individual's needs but also for determining whether government insurance (Medicaid) will pay. Whatever the category of care, a facility's size figures significantly in its overall atmosphere and services. An often related and always important characteristic is the number of residents under each staff person's care, a resident-staff ratio that greatly affects an individual's social interactions, activities, and direct daily care.

ASSISTED LIVING FACILITIES For a monthly fee, assisted living facilities provide residents with housing and housekeeping, meals, and help with such daily activities as dressing, bathing, and taking medications. Residents must generally be able to get themselves in and out of bed, to the bathroom, and to meals, and must require no more than two hours daily personal care (whether residents actually receive these two hours is a basic quality question, with variable answers). To varying degrees, and often at added cost, the package includes social activities, recreation, planned excursions, transportation, and other services. Following a period of great expansion and marketing, such facilities numbered about 10,000 by this century's start, 90 percent of them built during the 1990s. Much of the newer assisted living facilities consist of small apartments in buildings and settings that range from basic functional to luxurious, for twenty to more than a hundred residents.

A decidedly different atmosphere prevails in single-family homes that are licensed by the state to provide similar daily assistance, a bedroom, meals, and activities for the handful of residents a house can accommodate. In California 85 percent of licensed facilities have fewer than sixteen beds, and many have only five or six. Usually located in a residential neighborhood, these board-and-care homes tend to be less expensive than larger facilities.

Nationwide, the average monthly cost for assisted living as the century began was $1,800 for basic services but ranged as high as $5,000; many facilities charge extra for additional hours of assistance or certain personal supplies.[6] What assisted living cannot do is provide skilled nursing care for medical needs, from registered or licensed nurses available twenty-four hours, or the additional daily help very frail and disabled elders need.

SKILLED NURSING FACILITIES   Skilled nursing facilities, or SNFs, fit generally the public's image of nursing homes, where the oldest old, the badly disabled stroke victims, sufferers of dementia, and the semiconscious wait out their last months or years. These institutions are licensed by states to provide round-the-clock, physician-ordered care from nurses (e.g., injections, intravenous medications and nutrition, monitoring of respirators, wound care), as well as additional care to help with eating, drinking, bathing, taking oral medications, using a toilet or bedpan, using a walker or wheelchair, moving out of and into bed, even turning over if bed-bound. The average monthly cost in 2000 was about $5,000.

According to some estimates, up to 90 percent of SNF residents experience mental illness and cognitive impairment.[7] However, appropriate care for these conditions is commonly lacking. More generally, as the public glimpses from time to time, care provided residents in these institutions too often amounts to shameful neglect and abuse. A recent California report stated that the responsible state agency "has been unable to ensure high-quality nursing facility care." During a two-year period, one-third of California's nursing facilities received citations "for harming or seriously jeopardizing the lives of their residents."[8] A report from the Department of Health and Human Services (DHHS) published in 2000 linked poor-quality care nationwide to inadequate staffing. Investigators found that nearly all of the country's nursing homes (over 90 percent of approximately 17,000 facilities) function with too few staff, especially the most highly trained registered nurses as well as licensed nurses and aides. Residents receive neither the type nor the amount of daily care they require, including relatively simple help with eating, moving to a bathroom or bedpan, showering, exercising, or turning in bed. The result: festering bedsores and other serious infections, malnutrition, weight loss, dehydration, pneumonia, and loss of even minimal mobility. The report, ordered by the Clinton administration, brought some prospect of increased government regulation and oversight; it recommended, for instance, setting federal requirements for minimal levels of staffing and care.[9] When the final report emerged two years later from a Bush administration DHHS, the basic findings remained the same: substandard care endangering residents in 90 percent of the country's nursing homes because of unsafe staff-resident ratios. However, the report's recommendations had changed. No federal requirements should be imposed, given the cost of such quality improvement to the nursing-home industry. Attaining minimal levels of care must rely instead on market forces, shaped by informed consumer demand. In theory, with consumers choosing a SNF—say, for a parent—based on available information about services and quality, competing facilities would increase the productivity of existing staff (by having the too few people work harder) as well as enlarge the number of nurses and aides (not likely with a nationwide nurses' shortage and economic recession).[10] In other words, in a tradeoff between controlling cost for facility owners and/or investors and improving quality of care—for instance, by establishing and enforcing federal staffing requirements, increasing inspection frequency and scope—quality lost. The following year the Bush administration loosened requirements for staff helping nursing-home residents who cannot feed themselves. In place of more highly skilled employees, newly designated "feeding assistants" could, with eight hours of training, perform this task and likely be drafted to perform other tasks, such as lifting and bathing residents, for which they had no training at all.[11]

Although an advertisement may describe a SNF as providing skilled nursing and rehabilitation, following a stroke or hip fracture for instance, approximately three out of four facilities are custodial, with minimal rehabilitative services, if any.[12] In many cities, subacute-care units do treat illness or injury that does not require full hospitalization. Or a SNF might specialize in neurological and/or physical rehabilitation. In contrast to custodial care, these facilities, often associated with a hospital, are intended to be transitional between a patient's hospitalization and return home (including to assisted living). Receiving such rehabilitative therapy can make all the difference in an individual's recovery, while custodial care remains truly a last resort.

At both the assisted living and skilled nursing level, specialized facilities, within a larger institution or free-standing, are increasingly being designed for Alzheimer's disease or more general dementia care. Ideally, these residences incorporate enlarging knowledge about the behavioral and physical needs of individuals at varying stages of dementia. Through architecture, interior and outdoor design, staff ratios and training, as well as programs and policies, the best of these facilities create a therapeutic physical and social environment that most successfully meets those needs.[13]

CONTINUING CARE RETIREMENT COMMUNITIES   Another recent trend is toward continuing care retirement communities, or CCRCs (often called Life Care), which offer a continuum of care. Residents can initially live in an apartment quite independently (with meals provided in a communal dining room, for instance); later, they will receive daily assistance and, if needed, skilled nursing and/or dementia care. The great attraction is that people need not move away as the level of care they require changes—that is, they can age-in-place. This Cadillac of long-term care is costly. For a substantial entry fee, residents essentially purchase an apartment and membership in the community for the rest of their lives; they are entitled to use all recreational and other common areas and, if they wish, to participate in social, cultural, and recreational programs. An additional monthly fee covers meals, housekeeping, building maintenance, and, most importantly, their own maintenance—health and personal care at whatever level is needed, including doctor's visits, daily assistance, skilled nursing, and hospitalization (residents must have

Medicare coverage)—guaranteed for life. Marketing messages appeal to retired professionals, professors, businesspeople, individuals, or couples able to finance their own in-place insurance policy, their own comprehensive long-term care.[14]

For less affluent older Americans, financing determines their choice of residence and care throughout the final years of their lives. Medicare will not pay for assisted living or for the custodial care most nursing home residents receive. State-administered Medicaid insurance covers certain types of institutional long-term care for people below a designated poverty level, but individuals who do not (yet) qualify as poor must first become poor by using up, in a process known as "spending down," nearly all their financial assets. Several states cover only skilled nursing, a policy that pushes into nursing homes people who could live more independently if they could afford help at home or the cost of an assisted living residence. Even in states that do pay for some assisted living costs, many facilities refuse such residents because of the government's low reimbursement rates.

Whatever the type of residential care, quality can vary dramatically. Many residential facilities are for-profit enterprises, a characteristic influencing the balance of cost and quality concerns. For-profit institutions include national and regional chains (for instance, the Marriot and Hyatt hotel corporations now run life-care communities, as do more strictly senior housing/health-care corporations) that need to maintain financial gain for their investors. Nonprofits often bring religious, ethnic, or fraternal organization ties. Recent years have seen an increase of group residences within immigrant communities economically strong enough to sustain such settings. For these ethnic elders, traditional patterns of care, such as living with a grown son or daughter, cannot fit into their offspring's Americanized, two-career and/or geographically distant nuclear family.

All levels of long-term care suffer chronic problems with staffing: too few people, and they receive too little pay and training. Staff turnover rates can exceed 100 percent each year. Though federal and state regulations on skilled nursing facilities exist, monitoring and enforcement are notoriously poor. Assisted living lacks federal regulation altogether, and this level of care facility is beginning to accumulate its own stories of abuse and neglect.[15] Assisted living generally allows greater independence, more social activities, and a cheerier atmosphere than a skilled nursing facility. However, the assistance may not be adequate for a resident who develops an acute illness, such as a respiratory or urinary tract or intestinal infection, or for the more frail members of an assisted living population.

A CLOSER LOOK

I took Lillian to visit an assisted living facility in an Oakland neighborhood quite far from her Berkeley apartment. This residence towers surprisingly high above an equally surprising four acres, described in brochures as a "campus." Crowded city blocks surround these acres, and the store signs here are predominantly Spanish. In the high-rise shadow, tucked beside a large parking lot, sits a separate single-story annex of hospital-like rooms for residents requiring more than assistance with daily living—the acutely ill, the more seriously disabled who need twenty-four-hour skilled nursing care. Small and unassuming, its inclusion on this campus is an institutional plus, filling out a care continuum; the proximity of this annex may reassure tower residents likely someday to need it. Yet I could not help sensing a whisper of the end-of-the-line.

We were now well into the world of long-term care, with its varying terrain of health and social services, residences, transportation, and other programs designed for people unable to live on their own. Inevitably, perhaps, wheelchairs and walkers dominated first impressions as Lillian and I toured the assisted living high-rise. Also evident was the preponderance of women: both among residents, many bent by osteoporosis, and among the uniformed staff, predominantly African American, Hispanic, Filipino, who waited at the elevator, pushed a wheelchair, steadied a resident's walk. Our escort showed us sitting areas, the dining room with tables set, the choice of rooms presently available for Lillian. She pointed out one unusual feature of this residence—a dog, this shared pet resting its head on a man's lap, receiving and providing lavish affection. There were unobtrusive signs of the facility's Catholic sponsor, the Sisters of Mercy: a crucifix on a wall, a nun barely noticeable in modernized attire, a chapel.

Neither of us knew what in particular to look for during this first brief, rather half-hearted visit—the number of staff helping residents during meals, for instance, fresh fruits and vegetables on the plates, water pitchers and juices accessible to residents near sitting areas and bedrooms, measures taken to protect residents' privacy and individualize their daily routine. Nor did we talk with residents or family members about the assistance provided, or whether advertised social activities do happen, or if they like the meals or, simply, if they enjoy living here. Aside from asking our guide a few basic questions, Lillian remained quiet, noncommittal, as we moved from floor to floor or stood in the lobby where a small group of residents gathered for a scheduled outing to a museum, perhaps, or downtown shopping. She said nothing as we exited the basement level past a small beauty parlor and store, past cavernous spaces for building maintenance and institutional laundry.

We emerged into the sunny outdoors and drove several city blocks before Lillian asked what I thought; but I deferred a response, making her go first. Generally, our reactions were similar: group living all of a sudden, reminiscent of a college dormitory, but at a time of life when that lifestyle is not appealing. She disliked the thought of coming downstairs at fixed hours for all her meals. And what Lillian called the "culture" did not feel familiar or homey for even a nonobservant Jew. The social activism so central to Lillian's life the past decades was nowhere evident—no political meeting schedules, discussion groups, certainly no announcements of protest demonstrations. I imagine neither Lillian nor I could see her living here. Yet I knew this facility must be among the better ones: not-for-profit, offering a continuum of care, placed on Lillian's list by friends who work in the gerontology field and know well the perils and possibilities, the needs.

Neither of us could foresee the changes in Lillian that would so alter her needs. But in early spring 2000 Lillian's family did move her into an assisted living facility created from a former motel. Her world no longer included a sweeping view of hills and bay. Her small, spare room felt conventlike, even more so than the rooms sponsored by the Sisters of Mercy. She had her bed, one chair, her dresser with a few neat stacks of clothing in its drawers and the one child's portrait on top. The window of this "so-called apartment," as Lillian referred to it, looked out on a tar-papered roof and air conditioning equipment for the level below. The sound of rain hitting metal, she told me, drove her crazy. But Lillian could wander the hallways here. Along the way she would find doors of other residents' rooms open. Often a television would be on, with or without someone watching. In many rooms, a walker stood parked in a corner and in many a commode was beside the bed. Near the lobby Lillian might find a small group of residents eating ice cream or popcorn, perhaps watching a movie video. Between mealtimes she might see a board game in progress spread across several dining room tables. If her wandering appeared too aimless for too long, a staff person might stop and ask, "Lillian, do you need help finding your room?" or tell her "Lillian, it's time for lunch."

At lunch or dinnertime, a slow migration of white haired women appeared, as if pulled by a magnet through the hallway toward the dining room. Whatever the dinner menu posted on the wall, and no matter how nicely set the tables, there was the smell of large batches of food cooked and served, again the college dormitory feel, a certain odor that clung as far as the lobby, into the outside world.

With each phone call Lillian spoke less coherently, with each visit she appeared a bit more disheveled. Perhaps the move accelerated Lillian's decline. Had she remained with a companion in the apartment she might have been less disoriented, with fewer spells of agitation. Or perhaps she was lucky. Perhaps the family had moved her just in time, keeping a step ahead of what I gradually, belatedly, knew was an inexorable dementia. It was not terrible, Lillian's current existence and where she found herself. The place felt clean, with efforts taken to make the environment pleasant. There were activities and people, and she was still living in the heart of Berkeley. It's just not what we might most want at the end of our lives: feeling unhappy and dislocated, no longer dwelling in our home surroundings, homes so familiar we barely notice, in rooms as comfortable as our oldest, softest faded sweatshirt and jeans. Yes, this assisted living staff seemed competent and friendly, but they were not neighbors and friends, not family.

By the spring of 2001 I was visiting Lillian in her fourth residence since we met: a skilled nursing facility, tucked into a quiet Berkeley cul-de-sac, flanked by small stucco homes and wooden cottages. Here the front door is locked; residents like Lillian, who might wander out, wear on one wrist a device that sets off an alarm if they come too near an exit. These hallways fill with wheelchairs, their occupants gnarled by a stroke, felled by a broken bone or by more broadly immobilizing disability. A glance into a room may well catch a gaunt, unmoving body, a tiny old person lying on a hospital bed, perhaps connected to intravenous tubes or an oxygen tank.

Unlike with assisted living, a nursing station is central here, a partitioned swab of busy space kept bright under fluorescent ceiling lights, with clipboards, binders, and hanging stethoscopes, a medicine cart, and nurses in white jackets. This station is a hub for the daily routine of care, and for sudden disruptions—for instance, a nurse rushing outside with blood pressure cuff and wheelchair to the garden where a resident has fallen. This area seems also a focal point where residents sit, many in wheelchairs, to pass certain times of the day. Often I find Lillian sitting here in one of the armchairs lining the wall. As we chat she points, one by one, to others nearby, telling me a sentence or two about their past or present lives, although her facts are not always confirmed by those able to talk. Lillian's sentences, their tone sounding like a completed thought, are increasingly laden with nonsense words, what one researcher describes as "word soup."[16] A man walks by asking repeatedly for a glass of water and later for something to eat. Lillian points to a resident so old, with a body so very twisted. She is making a gargling noise, which Lillian imitates, not seeming to react, not seeming disturbed, as I feel.

Some of the residents can tell their own story. On a sunny day in summer I circle with Lillian around the garden path, then rest in a small gazebo. We share the bench with a neatly coifed woman, her hair as soft and pale as her eyes and skin. She is ninety-two, born and raised in Berkeley, something of a rarity in this city of people who come to the university or to visit, then never leave. In fact, she tells us, her parents moved across the bay from San Francisco after the great 1906 earthquake, hoping for more solid ground. She has always lived in Berkeley, working several decades as a hairdresser in what was nominally a downtown department store. She retired on her fifty-ninth birthday, she says with some pride, which I quickly figure must be a good three decades before the store, its merchandise as dowdy and dwindling as its clientele, finally closed its heavy wooden doors. A longtime widow, this woman lived in an apartment by herself until two years ago, when she fell down the stairs leading to her building's laundry room, breaking her hip. After leaving the hospital, she moved here. And here she stays. She has a son, a retired fireman, and a daughter; they live in nearby towns. The daughter, who suffers from diabetes and its complications, can't visit; she too lives in a nursing home.

This Berkeley native's memory of the past seems sharp. She is eager to talk and is skilled at ignoring other residents' digressions and non sequiturs. Perhaps this ability helps her live here, surrounded by people in such poor condition. Though I feel certain I do not ever want to find myself living in even the best of nursing homes and quite certain I would not do so pleasantly, what if I am the one who falls and breaks a hip, or the one commenting in non sequiturs? The man who wanted a glass of water and something to eat, one of the few men I see, comes outside asking, "Can someone tell me where we are?" It is a question my father might someday ask, sitting in his living room chair. The woman barely misses a beat before resuming her story as the man returns indoors unanswered, saying he is hungry.

Many of the residents here neither talk nor walk. I see them wheeled to the facility's living room and placed in a semicircle where a physical therapist tosses a plastic ball to one and then another, or they wait for a piano player scheduled for the next hour or for visiting dogs they can pet, or they sit in front of a large-screen television staring at a travel video on the wonders of the Nile.

As Lillian settles into the rhythm of nursing-home life, I learn that offering her a change, such as a picnic on a rare hot day before the fog rolls in, can cause her greater anxiety than pleasure. Instead at times I join Lillian in the dining room, pulling an extra chair up to the table where she and four other women eat lunch. Mealtime has its own rhythm: residents are pushed or self-propelled in wheelchairs, a few walking to their place; metal carts arrive in succession from the kitchen laden with cold drinks, main course, dessert, coffee, and tea; an aide circulates from one table to another helping diners eat; the forks or spoons or cups are raised slowly to mouths, then lowered. Lillian talks to others at her table, seeming unperturbed by no response. Usually, when all are well, the same women appear, a small card at each place noting her dietary needs or strong dislikes. Then one week the woman to Lillian's left is gone, replaced by someone new. She reaches silently for the plastic cup with a straw in front of her, a slow, painstaking effort like my father reaching for a word. She rests, tries again, but her curled, spastic hand misses by a fraction of an inch. Unsure if I should offer, or if she can even understand, I ask if I can help. She nods and, with the cup moved to her hand, lifts it to her mouth.

One lunchtime Lillian is holding a watercolor she says she just painted, two pastel streaks and two words, one in English, one in no recognizable language. She reads me both words several times, as she reads signs on the wall as we walk to her room. There, I discover a stack of watercolors she had painted years before, perhaps retrieved from some carton by her son. They are beautiful and lush, mostly scenes from her travels. I never knew Lillian painted, and I had learned only recently that she spoke German. More and more often she would comment or break into song—if not in gibberish, then in German, a language that may reach back to her childhood. When she demonstrates for me her Spanish, studied as an adult during summers in Mexico, it comes out German.

Mixed into the stack of watercolors is a month-old letter from Lillian's sister. After visiting Berkeley more than a year before, she had suffered a disabling stroke. She writes that she is better except for her speech, and that she longs to hear from Lillian. Lillian reads matter-of-factly, without comment or explanation or emotion. She seems not to know what this letter could be.

I leave my visits with Lillian now feeling a surprising ambivalence. Of course, she has lost much, just as friends and family have lost the Lillian they knew. Pursuing a conversation is no longer possible, but sharing time certainly is. On the first warm day after a spell of cold and dreary rain, her first winter at the skilled nursing facility, Lillian's enjoyment of the garden is contagious. She repeats how beautiful is the blue of the sky and notes, like a painter, an enveloping green of surrounding trees, a row of multicolored flowers, the redness of tomatoes ripening on a vine. She exclaims again and again how amazing are two rambunctious squirrels chasing jittery birds across high branches, each time seen as if the first time. If Lillian has cranky, unhappy times now, I don't see them. I no longer sense the anxiety of recent years, simmering close to the surface and frequently bubbling through. I have heard no complaints, no worries about next decisions, no anger with her nearby son or distant daughters. Lillian appears calm, even content. Staff people who walk by, she tells me, are so sweet, and they say the same of her. Perhaps she still becomes irritable or upset with her son when he arrives or when he leaves. Perhaps with time she has adjusted. More likely, her particular dementia has progressed enough beyond previous awareness that she feels secure in this smaller place, comfortable with its more limited routine, relaxed by the freedom from deciding what to do. Perhaps she has forgotten her last apartment, as the family hoped, along with much that went before. Her reaction to her present surroundings seems blessedly agreeable, mercifully not the same as mine.

AGING AT HOME

Perhaps my involvement with Lillian and the Over 60 Health Center contributed to my determination to keep my parents in their home, as they wished, bolstered by whatever help their independent living required. Long-term care, I had learned, is a concept defined largely by questions: How long a term? What manner of care? Initially, my parents were fortunate and atypical. They had each other, one propping up the other through days, nights, and years of old age; between the two of them, they managed for a long time to live in their house essentially on their own. They pieced together the necessary tasks, their activities of daily life, with one's deficiencies covered by the other's abilities, just as they handled far too long my father's driving, with my partially deaf mother warning of pedestrians and stoplights while my not yet legally blind father listened for honking horns and sirens. And they had help, which became increasingly necessary to enable them to stay in their home. They had family, close in relationship and location, and they could afford paid, or formal, help.

For years, a Berkeley version of formal help solved the maintenance problems of a house barely younger than my parents, in its own stage of disrepair. A handyman-gardener with advanced college degrees, a scraggly ponytail, rumored stint in the navy, and consistent disavowal of monetary gain, Joe worked at several houses on our block, but every Tuesday morning was my parents' turn. At the stroke of 9:00 he peddled his bicycle up the hill to recycle their newspapers, sweep slippery pine needles from the walkway, and keep their small garden from being overrun by the weeds my mother picked at when the weather and she felt fine. Most weeks Joe fixed something, inside or out.

Eventually, when my father returned home from a weeklong hospitalization, Joe solved another immediate problem for us all. By then I was backing into the realization that my father's behavior and thoughts reflected an enlarging dementia. Although a neurological evaluation did not suggest Alzheimer's disease, the specialist's summary did note, rather vaguely, cognitive deficits that would progress. Maintaining as much independence as possible, said this report, would require increasing support. While in the hospital, my father had grown noticeably disoriented, as is common among patients who are old, especially those already suffering mental impairments. He was unable to see, let alone understand, a sign on the wall saying, "Call, don't fall." His attempts to climb out of bed night and day resulted in straps tying him into bed or chair, a policy apparently discussed among the nurses, who reached the decision I could barely stand to see.[17] Now home, he was unable to mount stairs to the bedroom. My mother could not hear him call or fall, nor was she strong enough to help in either event. Joe became his night shift, both of them sleeping downstairs in the living room. For my father we brought up a bed from the basement. Joe declined a second extra bed, preferring to sleep as he does at his home, on the floor. Joe was ideal. The two of them, each uncomfortable with conversation, enjoyed a mutually positive relationship, not an easy or frequent development for my father or, I would guess, for Joe. And Joe was not the least flustered that his roommate thought they were in the army. To my father's late-night questions about bivouacking more troops there, Joe responded simply, "They don't do that anymore."

During that hospitalization my parents' doctor asked me for the first time, over the phone, whether home was the best place for my father to live. When I said we wanted him to be at home, he mentioned a nursing facility as transition temporarily between hospital and home. I declined, knowing this stopgap often grows unintentionally permanent. But clearly, my parents needed more help. Already we had escalated our daily checks on them, most recently after the morning several months earlier, when I had let myself in and found the downstairs filling with dark, fetid smoke. In the kitchen, a coffee pot, the old-fashioned percolator from my childhood, sat empty on the burner, a healthy blue flame underneath, black smoke spewing from the spout. The standing electric space heater warmed an empty breakfast nook. My parents, upstairs as usual after breakfast, were oblivious. They smelled nothing, could not say exactly why they had used the old percolator or who had left the burner on. Apparently, smoke had not yet gathered in sufficient density near the downstairs smoke detector to trigger its alarm. They would probably not have heard it anyway.

They remained in place, though barely. Now my parents were struggling through each day at home, even with a hired health aide. When nights became too sleepless and difficult for Joe, we hired an aide for those dark hours as well. Now it was my father who described himself as miserable, tired of his life. I used to see Lillian as the unhappy one with no options, forced by circumstances to live in a way she had never wanted, ultimately in a residential-care institution. Late in her own life, Lillian was experiencing the fate she had worked so diligently to help old people avoid. Now the irony was my parents. Fortunate enough to enjoy, theoretically, ideal circumstances—able to remain together in their own home with family actively involved—they were living as if trapped within each difficult day, two too old people facing always some threat to what was until recently their comfortable routine. Now when I caught myself thinking people should not live their last years unhappy or in pain, I saw not Lillian but my own parents.

Did I think it would be easy, my parents aging-in-place? Or if not easy, certainly not unhappy? Logistically, I had the great advantage of knowing whom to ask about good home health-care agencies, eliminating difficult preliminary inquiries, interviews, and decisions. Still, there was the piecing together and keeping track of who was coming when, to do what, from which agency. Which were the short-term posthospital visits Medicare covered, which were the people we had hired to assist for the longer haul? There were instructions and advice from a succession of nurses, physical and occupational therapists, a social worker, and my father's doctors, whose instructions and advice did not always coincide with the nurses' or others'. There was my father's agitation with what seemed to him an unending stream of intrusions by nearly faceless strangers, when all he wanted was to be left alone. At times I even found myself fending off assistance, such as the morning I encountered by chance the Medicare aide arriving to bathe my father at 7:45, as if he were still in the hospital—before he would be awake, longer still before he would be somewhat less confused and cranky, not to mention during weeks when he was determined not to bathe at all rather than allow anyone to help. Other mornings I chose to have no substitute when Connie, the private agency health aide—finally familiar, accepted, and available for the long term—had a day off or a sick child at home. I would spend the hours with him myself to avoid having yet another unfamiliar person appear or, worse, a substitute my father already disliked for whatever reason and had already tried to fire, a woman who I guess would be called a bad match for this client.

Some people would have an easier time aging at home. For instance, my mother-in-law in New York—a sociable, talkative woman who gradually lost all memory as her dementia advanced—resisted adamantly the idea of a companion staying in her apartment with her. However, once the idea was a fait accompli, she enjoyed the company of the woman she called her guest; she seemed less anxious, relieved of the pressure of trying to manage alone. Here in Berkeley, as in many American cities, senior centers and privately run programs offer classes, lunch, and recreation—providing social contact and physical activity for generally healthy individuals (some programs include early dementia care). For people with more severe physical and/or cognitive impairments—the very frail and disabled who might otherwise be moved to a skilled nursing facility—adult day health care offers more comprehensive programs aimed at slowing participants' further deterioration, at the same time providing respite for family caregivers during the day. The goal is to avert or delay placement in a residential institution. Adult day health care supports people's ability to live at home by providing medical consultations, nursing, rehabilitation (physical, occupational, and speech therapies), and

1. DOES AN INDIVIDUAL NEED ADULT DAY CARE AND/OR MORE HELP AT HOME?

Needs help with at least one of the following: bathing, dressing, and other personal grooming; walking; using toilet; eating

Needs ongoing treatment and/or monitoring for a chronic health condition

Needs rehabilitation from a recent stroke or other illness

Seems unstable when walking, has fallen, needs constant supervision

Can no longer drive safely or manage public transportation (e.g., problems with vision, mobility, judgment, or memory)

Misses or forgets meals; finds food too difficult to prepare

Can no longer do grocery shopping, laundry, keep home adequately cleaned

Has recently had dangerous kitchen accidents

Confuses medications; misses or takes wrong doses

Has frequent memory lapses, including for recent conversations; needs help making appointments or other arrangements by phone, remembering, and getting to scheduled activities

Has trouble managing money and personal finances

If adequate help for living safely at home—with a day-care program, for some individuals—is *not* available, a good residential facility may be a better option.

other health-related services (see figure 1). Many programs include transportation to and from home. Most participants live with an adult child or a spouse and on average attend the day-care program for two years.[18] In some states Medicaid insurance will pay for eligible recipients to attend regularly a licensed adult day health-care program several days a week, several hours a day, in order to remain living at home. Individuals with higher income and assets than Medicaid allows pay privately for such programs. Even so, 26 percent of adult day health-care centers have been open only since the late 1990s, and most areas of the country lack enough affordable day-care options geared to people with a range of daily needs.

Older adults can also share their home with someone younger or healthier, in return for assistance and companionship. By temperament and habit, however, my parents were not good candidates for alterations in their daily lives. And there was my father's dementia. Always the dominant family member, what my brother and I used to describe— to our father's great satisfaction—as a benign dictator, he remained central and in a different way the dominant force in their lives as an older couple. For quite a stretch of time, his impairments left him aware enough to declare, sounding helpless, "I am losing my mind, I can tell." And he could tell much of the time. "We have a big problem here," he might state, waking up in a seemingly strange building that was identical to but was not his house; or wondering how he would get to his office on Monday, the office in Los Angeles he last entered twenty-five years before; or thinking he was in San Francisco searching for a mysterious property he owned, yet determined for some pressing reason to get home. A bemused smile might lighten his face while he grasped, however fleetingly, that he was at home when he had just felt for certain he was not. Or he might turn angry when I assured him this was his house, with his car in his garage, ready for me to drive him where he needed to go, angry enough then to protest, however halting his words, "I have absolutely no confidence in you whatsoever."

I heard that anger in a who-does-*she*-think-she-is resentment, the she being me. I became a focus for parental outrage at a child taking over, for what he spit out loudly were my "machinations," my "delusions of grandeur" in hiring people who bothered him, followed after him to see that he didn't fall, provided care that he didn't always comprehend and never wanted. I was naive to think being at home means independence. Certainly, we would not be free of bureaucracy and paperwork, of care that felt fragmented and uncoordinated, even with the best of individual caregivers in their various capacities, the several women and eventually one Ukrainian man who each arrived at my parents' door intending to do a good job.

More important, however, was my father's own person and autonomy, his right to choose how he wanted to live for however long it would be. I did not foresee ways we would all be subject to institutional pressures even at home. Perhaps it should be obvious that financial incentives might influence a private agency to identify need for a greater amount of care and government-funded Medicare to identify less. Nor did I think of an agency's liability until my father's doctor mentioned the word: by declaring that my father required constant assistance at literally every step, the private agency aimed to ensure he did not fall on its watch. Defined as a matter of safety, of preventing the potential falls, the requirement only made my anxiety soar. To my father, the alternatives were clear. The required surveillance and intrusion, the denial of autonomy and privacy, were far worse than falling. Who did I think I was to decide a bruise, perhaps a broken bone with complications, represented too great a risk? He would fall and presumably get up, as always before. I had to pull back, accept that he would fall, and assure his formal caregivers that they should do the same; the risk was mine.

My mother had learned well her generation's role, a dependence reinforced throughout a more than sixty-year marriage. Added to an engrained passivity were her own physical problems, limited energy and endurance, her failing memory, and then—classic characteristics of being a caregiver—her weariness and at times bewilderment, if not depression. Often she tuned out, whether as a function of neurology, a faulty or turned-off hearing aid, self-protection—intentional or not—or all of the above.

For a stretch of time, my father's bad days would come and go. Only the ratio changed steadily, with fewer days, and sometimes only hours, when he seemed to be here with us. At times he turned uncharacteristically passive, offering to do "whatever you tell me," or lying back silently on his bed, as if removing himself, as if he could disappear, while an aide and I pulled on his shirt and pants. And then again came anger, darkening over the months toward rage, not only at me but sometimes at my mother, or whatever unfortunate aide happened onto the scene. And then one morning I overheard my father crying, a sound I had never heard before in my life. Still in bed one morning, he was sobbing, telling my mother he was going to die. When she asked him why he was saying that, I expected to overhear his fear, but he answered, "Because I want to."

Gone were the days when I could savor a different relationship with my father, enjoy conversations we would never have had were he not so old, unable to read his magazines or his mail, pay his bills, or manage his bank accounts, forced but finally willing to concede certain authority. At his request I might help shave a straight sideburn to the same electric buzz of so many childhood mornings when I watched him glide the shaver through its daily pattern, pushing skin up and down, then splash from a long-necked greenish glass bottle that men's potion, aftershave, onto his face and, every once in a while as a surprise, onto mine. Sometimes he talked to me about his father, a man I never met, whose self-educated taste in books and music and art my father so admired. A temporarily prosperous businessman, my grandfather's loss of everything, including his life, during the Depression haunted my father still. He even spoke to me as never before about his own years as a lawyer, dredging from his mind the memories he could, as at other times he sat at his desk—a fine carved mahogany desk salvaged from his father's possessions—dragging from its drawers old files, crumbled brown accordion folders, to search out some document, real or imagined, or merely to feel that everything was still there.

Trying to keep my parents safe and content felt like trying to hold water in my outspread hands. The biggest problem was that one of my parents was too often just not mentally home. Although my father and one agency health aide finally tolerated each other well and even grew fond of each other, her time was but a fraction of the time, her shift one portion of the day, the week, the months. In a strange reversal I found myself fleeing to Lillian's, to a dull and quiet calm. Though I never feel that all is well in any such care facilities, as I signed the visitors' register and looked past the wheelchairs for Lillian, I could anticipate her pleasure at simply seeing me, a friend she recognized from visit to visit, even if she could never tell from where or when. With nothing for me to do but enjoy my time there with her, I could relax and even feel in some way a help by merely showing up.

MAKING CHOICES TODAY

This chapter's discussion of independent living has led inescapably through escalating degrees to its opposite. Indeed, immediate decisions for today's old most commonly require them to give up some measure of living on their own. For people considering what care an individual needs among current options, a few general truths prevail:

- Most people want to live out their lives at home.
- No one wants to end up in a skilled nursing facility, commonly known as a nursing home; one study of seriously ill patients found that more than a fourth would be very unwilling to live permanently in a nursing home, and nearly a third would rather die.[19] And in fact approximately 95 percent of people will not live in a nursing facility at the end of their lives.
- Most older Americans do not receive the type of health and social services that could best support living at home with chronic illness and loss of abilities during the latest years of life.
- Many aged people resist formal help they see as infringing on their independence, including within their home.
- The daughters and daughters-in-law who used to provide informal care are no longer as available; they have jobs, live far away, have their own children to care for.

The help traditionally provided by daughters and wives is increasingly provided by home health aides or the staff of assisted living facilities. As the stories of Lillian and my parents illustrate, decisions about the amount and type of help individuals need, and whether it can occur at home, depend on the following factors:

- Their ability, physical and cognitive, to perform the activities and chores required to maintain an acceptably safe daily life, and the nature and severity of physical and mental impairments that require assistance;
- Their support network of family, friends, organizations, and social and health-care services;
- The health and abilities of their primary informal caregiver, especially if an aged spouse;
- Their ability to pay for help at home or at a care facility;
- Their willingness (and their family's) to accept risk—for instance, of a fall, of a missed meal or medication (each of which can occur within a care facility as well);
- Their preferences regarding social activities and physical surroundings, as well as geographic locale.

For many people, a health crisis—a stroke, a broken hip—precipitates an immediate decision about care. An individual who requires skilled nursing and twenty-four-hour assistance will need deep financial pockets or extensive informal care, or most likely both, to remain at home. Absent a crisis, pressure to change the status quo builds gradually, with greater play of pros and cons. An enlarging physical and/or cognitive impairment may eventually trump desires for privacy and independence, necessitating a companion or health aide at home, or a move to assisted living. For some individuals, the ongoing effort and anxiety of trying to manage at home may sap enjoyment and threaten the safety of their daily lives; family caregivers run parallel risks. Certain dementias—with nighttime wandering, increasing physical needs, hallucinations, agitation, and combative behavior—may not only become extremely difficult to handle at home; home may not provide the environment best suited to advanced dementia care.[20] In fact, the vast majority of people with severe dementia (as high as 90 percent, according to some estimates) eventually move to institutional care.[21]

Families are generally on their own not only in reaching decisions but also in coordinating formal care at home, or monitoring the quality of an individual's life and care within a residential facility. Very few physicians will make a house call, and few physicians' practices include nurses or social workers who regularly visit patients at home, assess the need for and help to arrange support services, and help coordinate and maintain appropriate overall care. Yet geriatric specialists identify case coordination and a multidisciplinary team approach as most desirable for the oldest of patients.[22] In some parts of the country, as the advertisements cited above indicate, private elder-care managers offer case-management services to those who can afford them. (In Canada, national health insurance includes this service as part of long-term care within provinces.)

Many studies have demonstrated home care to be cost-effective when utilized appropriately. Results include reduced acute-care costs for specified conditions, shortened hospital stays and less frequent readmission, less decline in abilities needed to function at home, improved patient satisfaction and clinical outcome, more appropriate medication use, and reduced medication errors.[23] Although cost-cutting efforts throughout the 1990s aimed at lowering hospitalization rates, Medicare covers only minimal assessment and nurse visits at home following a hospitalization and, on a more extended basis, to manage medical conditions requiring intermittent skilled nursing for homebound patients. Medicare spending for home health care fell 45 percent between 1997, when Congress passed the Balanced Budget Act, and 2000.[24] The sharpest decrease was in visits by home health aides.[25] Medicare legislation passed in 2003 further lowered reimbursements paid for home health care (a reduction barely noticed in the glare of a new prescription drug benefit). Under Medicare's definition of homebound, moreover, patients who leave their home more than a few times per month for social rather than medical reasons, regardless of how difficult the effort, are not eligible for Medicare-covered skilled nursing at home, a policy that can only contribute to social isolation, or to placement in a residential institution.

As to private health insurance companies, approximately 1 percent of their budget covers home care (excluding long-term-care insurance, a commercial product only recently gaining sellers and buyers). All in all, one geriatrician describes the homebound as "a medically underserved population, [who] are usually invisible to physicians and would benefit from more regular physician contact."[26] In fact, they are more generally invisible and need additional social contact far more broadly. Finally, neither government nor private insurance covers comprehensive in-home programs aimed at preserving an old person's abilities to live there or at recovering functional abilities after acute illness, beyond the minimal therapy Medicare covers after hospitalization. Yet even minimal restriction of activity (defined as staying in bed at least half a day or cutting down usual activities) caused by illness, injury, or other problem can contribute to more general, ongoing physical decline and disability, and to a pattern of recurrent acute episodes.[27] Needed programs would center, for example, on extended physical therapy and daily exercise regimens and coordinated multidisciplinary services that support patients, as well as their home caregivers.[28]

This chapter has focused, so far, on the needs of today's old, needs that are a problem not only for the old but also, in many cases, for their adult daughters and sons and for society. Always lurking in the background for the larger society and for these younger individuals is the prospect of their future old age. The next chapter will examine more closely vulnerabilities of the old that can undermine independent living. However, first I will address how today's middle-aged women and men can begin to consider parallel themes that relate to their own later years.

DOING OUR OWN THING

For the population bulge whose young adulthood became identified with America's 1960s and 1970s, "do your own thing" became a popular mantra, a generational characterization applied by some people with pride, some with envy, by others with disdain. At middle age, few of the baby boomers maintain such trademark alternative lifestyles as living in a commune or rejecting material acquisitions. Yet all has not been lost from those heady years of seemingly boundless possibilities. The very idea of alternatives, at least, became engrained, the notion of choice highly visible. A shaping of society by this generation's demands, now largely commercial, remains an ongoing dynamic reinforced by their sheer numbers. Sandwiched between aging parents and their own children, this huge cohort entering and passing through their fifties can benefit from their past, but with a view toward their future. Seeing how parents or any of the old live today, now is the time to ask: How do people want to live as they age, and what baby boom steps, or what demands, will lead to the desired lifestyle? What can people presently at midlife be doing in order to live as they want—do their own thing—as they become America's old?

NETWORKING REVISITED

During the last several decades *to network* became an action verb for young entrepreneurs within the business world and, to a lesser extent, among professionals and academics as well. Meeting and staying in touch with people, whether through rolodex or e-mail, was a way to profit, to advance professionally, to feel well connected. The idea appears now worth retooling as a crucial factor in the way these same people and others are aging. Remaining enmeshed within a social network may contribute not only to general feelings of well-being, but more directly to physical and cognitive health. Put another way, maintaining connections with others can help people avoid potential risks of independent living as they age—the feeling of loneliness, and the drain social isolation may have on their health.[29]

Observers commonly note the loss within modern societies of the intergenerational support once available from the extended family, support consisting of such daily activities as childcare by grandparents, marketing for a sick elder, or less tangible support through ongoing social contact and traditions. Though such observations often ignore less desirable aspects of the good old days in small communities (when everyone knew everyone else's business, for instance), it is clear that most families are now separated geographically, and that everyday contact across generations is more the exception than the rule. As people age, moreover, additional characteristics of contemporary life can render isolation the path of least resistance. For instance, when people retire from work, they generally withdraw from social contacts at their place of employment. Older people commonly lose the mobility needed to reach other people; what's more, they simply lose the people most important in their lives when a spouse, siblings, or friends die first.

Evidence is now accumulating of a two-way relation between poor health status and degrees of social isolation. Social engagement, it turns out, may actually be better for our health.[30] Most directly, family and friends may provide more frequent and intensive help with daily tasks, lowering physical wear and tear on an older individual, and compensating for his early stages of decline. Someone is likely to check on the older person more often, catching a health problem sooner, assuring enough heat in winter, fans or air conditioning and fluids to drink in summer, even lessening the likelihood she will lie on the floor unnoticed after a fall. More intriguing, though less certain, neuroscientists speculate that ongoing contact and communication with other people may require more complex and frequent cognitive stimulation that prevents or delays dementia. And stimulation may also be immunologic. The body's disease-fighting abilities may gain in some way a physiological boost from satisfying and supportive connection to others. Conversely, social isolation may not only be a consequence of declines in physical or cognitive health but may contribute to such loss; feeling lonely and depressed, researchers hypothesize, may dampen an individual's immune response.

Though surveys report consistently that the old do not want to burden their adult children, they may gain from living near family or friends. Frequent visits, phone calls, and electronic mail all help maintain social connection. People's differing temperament and preferences will also go into the mix, defining the amount and type of social contact needed.[31] Isolation for one person may feel like a crowd to another. A woman cheered by group activities, enjoying the company and conversation, may prefer an assisted living residence if her only alternative is to live alone, with no easy way to get out and about.

In today's communities, getting out and about can be difficult, especially for people who no longer drive. Cities and suburbs sprawl, walking even short distances may be impossible, and public transportation may be negligible. Even if buses stoop to curb level for the old and disabled, there may be no place to go, no center for social gathering. Zoning ordinances may discourage creative alternatives to the single family home, such as shared dwellings or co-housing units clustered around communal buildings and spaces. Especially in less affluent neighborhoods, the physical surroundings just beyond the front door—excessive noise, inadequate lighting, heavy traffic, the absence of a stop sign at marked crosswalks—can be hazards in themselves.[32] And, as Lillian knew, moving into an institutional residence often removes the old from long established social networks, increasing their isolation in the company of strangers.

As baby boomers age, then, they will need to attempt once again to create alternative lifestyles, with emphasis on the plural. An immediate need, for their parents and later themselves, is to greatly enlarge affordable care services at home. In recent years, however, government support for home health care has moved in the opposite direction, with reduced Medicare coverage forcing many elders into institutional long-term care. The type of home individuals choose for late life—an apartment, single-family home, or shared housing—will vary. The goal is to generate a variety of forms that provide both social support and needed care (e.g., meals, personal assistance, nursing care, whether at home or in a residential-care facility), then let people find their right place. The idea is not revolutionary, not so different from parents seeking the right school for their child. Why expect old people, forced by finances and/or health, to fit into and feel content within even the best of inadequate choices? Just as I would not have long tolerated rural commune life even in my youthful twenties, I doubt that my preference in old age, should I live so long, will be group living. I will likely not want an amount of social activity that infringes on times for solitude, those capacious hours or days of quiet, when I enjoy feeling no obligation to talk. In this I am like my father, frighteningly so, we used to joke.

I looked at my father and asked myself so many what-ifs. What if my mother were not with him, and my family did not live so near? What if they could not afford the hired help, the insanely rising cost of their medicines and of keeping their home comfortably warm? What would this man do—his health failing, barely able to see, shuffling and unsteady when he walks, then far enough into dementia that he sometimes thinks it's all happening to someone else?

Old men alone can be a sorry lot, the rooming house men, the faces in windows of single-room occupancy hotels, my uncle in a San Fernando Valley nursing home where he might live to be a hundred. The numbers, however, are with the women, the wives or daughters or daughters-in-law who will take care of the men, who will outlive the men, suffer their own illnesses and disabilities, and then be alone.

AGING AS A WOMEN'S ISSUE

Throughout their adult lives, women interact with the medical world far more than do men, not only as patients themselves but as organizers and overseers of medical care for a spouse and children. For older women this role takes on added complexities as health care and aging concerns entwine. The baby boom generations know well the feminist and women's health movements, whether as participants or observers. Whatever the more recent disagreements over who is a feminist and what feminism has gained or wreaked, these women are living proof that, regarding aging and health care, the more things change, the more they remain the same. Overall, women today are more liberated than were their mothers in educational, occupational, and reproductive choices, in the nature of their personal relationships and in family configurations. Yet decades after American women began organizing to challenge their traditional roles and unequal status, they continue to bear the greatest responsibility for safeguarding the old in this country. Beyond the overwhelmingly female pool of hired aides and nurses within institutional residences and private homes, women provide most of the unpaid informal care (75 percent according to the Older Women's League);[33] and as the sandwich moniker denotes, midlife women are likely at the same time to be caring for their own children.

In one family out of four at the close of the twentieth century, at least one adult cared for an elderly relative or friend; the average length of time was eight years, according to a survey conducted for the Metropolitan Life Insurance Company.[34] With more than six million people already providing long-term, unpaid care for a physically or mentally impaired elderly family member,[35] one gerontologist predicted, "Elder care is to the 21st century what childcare has been for the last few decades." It is something of an irony: for a generation that came into maturity along with the women's movement, much of the sandwich filling—determined to hold together both child and elder care—is female. Indeed, a previous forecast may now be all the more telling. In the early 1990s, researchers assessed the legacy for elder care of this country's Reagan (and G. H. W. Bush) era, with its commitment to smaller government, its reliance on privatized care and free market forces. Their prediction: American women could expect to accumulate eighteen years helping aging parents and other relatives, along with seventeen years caring for their own children.[36]

Women can also expect to continue outliving men and to remain alone, with chronic disabilities greater in number and severity than men experience. In 2000, according to the Older Women's League, women constituted 80 percent of the over 9 million older Americans living alone. They faced inadequacies of American health care magnified by encountering them on their own, especially the difficulties of emergency room and hospital care, and of obtaining good follow-up care at home. Like today's older women, many who are now middle-aged will find themselves on their own during later decades of life. The impact of aging on women will expand, moreover, owing not only to the sheer size of the population passing now through their fifties, but also to altered characteristics of that population. More than a third of baby boom women will likely be single when they retire.[37] As the number of women who are divorced, never married, or without children rises, more women face the prospect of aging alone with less informal care and fewer economic resources than are now available to wives and widows, who may receive a husband's pension, life insurance, or Social Security benefits.

Individual stories of aging unfold to a considerable degree, then, as women's tales. A central, ongoing theme is financial. Not only do women generally earn less than men throughout their lifetime (including for the same work), but women's informal caregiving—for children and/or parents—often requires sacrificing full-time work, as well as the promotions, salary, benefits, and retirement plans attached to a more traditional male career ladder. The formal caregiver—again, for children and the old—earns a low, if not minimum, wage with few if any benefits. By the time women enter their own old age their financial health may be precarious, especially women who are alone, with no pension or retirement savings, and with a smaller Social Security contribution than men. At the end of the twentieth century, 60 percent of women eighty-five years or older were poor or near-poor.[38] For married women, the late chapter of their caregiving role jeopardizes their physical and psychological health as well. In this role, my mother becomes the demographic statistic. Currently, when a married man grows increasingly disabled with age, his wife provides most of his informal care. For many of these women, the caregiving job is full time, essentially requiring her to be on call twenty-four hours of every day.[39] This pattern holds even if she too suffers physical or cognitive difficulties. One study found, for instance, that among married women with at least two of the standard measurable impairments in the activities of daily life—including the ability to wash oneself, use the toilet, dress, eat, and get up from a chair or out of bed—20 percent are caregivers for their husband, while only 8 percent of similarly impaired married men provide informal care for their wife. Her care will most likely come, if at all, from a daughter, daughter-in-law, or granddaughter.[40]

As I observed when visiting Lillian, today's longer-living women fill most of the country's nursing-home beds, dining rooms, and hallways. In the late 1990s, estimates suggested that as many as one of every two women over the age of sixty-five would need some manner of long-term care for at least a year, compared to one of seven men.[41] At the same time, if the number of people moved to skilled nursing facilities continues to decline overall, as some social scientists predict, more severely disabled women and men will be living at home in the community. Yet Medicare cutbacks, most prominently the 1997 Balanced Budget Act and the 2003 Medicare legislation, reduced reimbursements for even short-term home care following hospitalization.

Older women generally rely more than do men on government programs to pay for health care and to ensure, through Social Security, a basic monthly income. One commentary in the *New England Journal of Medicine,* describing old age as "a territory populated largely by women," adds that beyond the age of eighty years, Medicare and Medicaid could be considered "women's programs."[42] Yet Medicare's focus on hospital stays and doctors' office visits is poorly designed to meet a substantial portion of health-care needs for the people it serves. These women, as well as men, tend "to have multiple complex, interacting, acute and chronic physical and psychosocial problems and to need long-term care and outpatient drug therapy, neither of which [has been] covered by Medicare. Medicaid provides for these major exclusions from Medicare, but Medicaid comes to the rescue only after impoverishment"—that is, spending down an individual's assets.[43] The new Medicare prescription drug benefit, slated to begin in 2006, does not appear to be likely to adequately meet the aging population's medication needs. (See chapter 3.)

In sum, concerns about independent living concentrate in women as both caregivers and survivors. My parents, at least, could afford to hire help, buttressing family caregivers living across the street. They could also afford to remain with their same primary care doctor, not needing to switch to an HMO, with its limited list of participating providers, in order to save money on prescription drugs and other services Medicare does not cover. They knew and trusted their doctor of twenty-five years; they found him reassuring, no small contribution to their ongoing care. He observed their individual ups and downs, the frail wife and strong husband replaced quite precipitously by a frailer, more disabled husband and a wife who managed to hold her own, until she too began losing ground. And to some extent, he was able to evaluate them "as a unit," as one study of older married couples put it, "in terms of their health status as well as the caregiving demands that exist in the home environment."[44] As is the case with many doctors, however, his attempt to focus simultaneously on the needs of both individuals remained limited and relied increasingly on reports from family members or other caregivers, delivered by phone calls or during fleeting office visits squeezed by Medicare cutbacks. Perhaps doctors feel their own sense of helplessness when they can do nothing to arrest a debilitating chronic illness or inexorable cognitive decline; patients with severe dementia especially become shells of the individuals doctors have cared for, often grown fond of over the last decades, so that finally doctors can help most, perhaps, by attending to a spouse.[45]

THE LUCK OF THE DRAW

"I never thought I'd be here, but I'm seeing from the other side now. I am disabled and old." Gerda Miller sits at the front of a meeting room on the ground floor of a large assisted living residence to which she recently moved. "I didn't age until the day when I fell with a stroke." This assertion raises a chuckle from her audience, a baker's dozen of silver-haired women and men. Some are her new neighbors, others longstanding Berkeley Gray Panthers answering Gerda's call for a meeting here in Oakland. She wants to begin organizing a new local chapter to address current political issues, especially the needs of children and immigrants, and everyone's right to health care supported by the government.

Gerda is a friend of Lillian's and like her a longtime activist. As she learns now to use a motorized wheelchair as well as a computer, Gerda's cognitive abilities, political views, and humor appear gloriously intact. She tells the group she is very content in her new home. In fact, this facility was the only assisted living residence that would take her after the stroke, on a trial basis only, to see whether she could care for herself without help from nurses. A widow for many years, she is managing largely with help from friends, a cross-generational network of social-activist colleagues. It's hard to weigh one against the other—the physical disability of a stroke, a broken hip, loss of eyesight, or my father's self-described loss of his mind. But maintaining good cognitive abilities predicts long-term independence better than does an individual's physical condition.[46]

My parents weathered removal of malignant tumors, beating impressive negative odds, although my mother's osteoporosis and chronic pain over many years did limit her activities and quality of life. My father's heart pacemaker and, at the age of ninety-two, new batteries certainly extended his life, but it became one trapped in a barely recognizable world of dementia. Driving to visit him during his week in the hospital my mother asked anxiously, and not for the first time, what we were going to do about what she called "his confusion"—as if a right solution

existed. After a silence, in a calm tone and with frankness on a topic unusual between us, she said, "I'm very lucky." She then listed friends who
either died young or were living with more severe health problems. She
mentioned my uncle living in a skilled nursing facility, unable to afford
any extras, his life savings spent long ago on a similar facility for my
aunt before she died. My mother knew she would not want for the extras that would help her live comfortably at home.

Lillian too is lucky, given the twists of her life circumstances. She has
knowledgeable friends connected to the world of long-term care, who
shepherd her to the better places.

I can't help wondering about my own years to come, already noticing
a bit nervously, along with friends my age, when we forget a name or
number, or a movie plot. With a husband ten years older, what caregiving will be my part? Will enlarged, improved resources exist to lessen
the strain when we and so many baby boom couples enter our decline?
And will my future include someday living on my own, alone? With one
child, a son, must I think now about this teenager someday married? Do
I need to hope he lives nearby and hope for a daughter-in-law who not
only tolerates—maybe even likes?—me but is willing and able to give
the informal care many women never receive?

My own doctor has joked, "We know what will get you," hearing
the family history of my parents' cancers and then my brother's rare malignant tumor diagnosed at a younger age than I am now. But of course,
my doctor and I can't know what or when. So far, my brother is luckier
than he was unlucky. After a year of highly aggressive and expensive
treatment, his periodic scans reveal no sign of cancer. Riding the first
wave of baby boom generations, my brother and I may be among the
first of this cohort to contend personally with the various dread diseases
of body and mind that become more likely with age.

Already the insurance industry peddles its baby boom solution: buy
long-term-care insurance now, the sooner the better for lowest rates, to
pay for the daily care you might need later in an assisted living or skilled
nursing facility or, with higher premiums, at home. This private market
answer, which surely has the Bush administration's blessing, plays on
common, well-founded fears about old age. The American Council of
Life Insurance asserts (no surprise) that "purchasing long-term-care insurance now when it's most affordable is *the most important thing baby
boomers can do to safeguard their financial future*" (emphasis added).[47]
Yet even if decades of premiums are preferable, say, to buying into a life-
care community later, buyers cannot rest assured of needed care; rather,

they must beware of loopholes—perhaps eligibility requirements for actually receiving benefits, exceptions not covered—ways insurers might avoid paying. Before rushing out to buy long-term-care insurance, this huge population of potential customers might well ask what kind of daily life the purchased "product," that bland term of commerce for all manner of health-care insurance, will actually buy them. Before plunking down the steep insurance premiums, people might ask what could be alternative visions of living and care for their long-term future?

The new century did not progress far before demonstrating just how uncertain the future can be. Even before September 11, 2001, Americans could see how inextricably tied to the country's economic health and political fortune are individuals' health and wealth. The haloed version of coming decades predicted increased numbers of people retiring early to enjoy extra independent years of leisure, travel, pursuit of unfulfilled dreams. Certainly, women and men well into their eighties now float on barges down the Seine, tour China's Great Wall, even trek up mountains in Nepal. However, a 1999 report on retirees in California found goodly numbers (46 percent under the age of fifty; nearly 30 percent up to seventy years) retiring from their jobs early because of poor health, including chronic back problems, arthritis, high blood pressure.[48] By that year's end, additional workers ages fifty to sixty-four were losing their job and health insurance to the country's recession, with layoffs accelerated after the terrorist attack.

For those who have not reached sixty-five, the current age for Medicare, loss of employment for whatever reason, or an employer's elimination of health insurance coverage, or death of a spouse whose employment brings insurance often means paying medical bills with reduced or no income, and with no health insurance at all. Moreover, they enter a vicious cycle: uninsured adults in their fifties face greater likelihood of chronic disease and declining overall health, jeopardizing future ability to live independently, than do those who are insured.[49] Adding insult to injury, if individuals attempt to purchase their own insurance policy, at considerable cost, they may be turned down due to a preexisting condition. (See chapter 4.) Lacking insurance, these individuals are less likely than insured age-mates to seek needed physicians' services or preventive care until they turn sixty-five, when the disparity disappears.[50]

The rapidly expanding U.S. population ages fifty to sixty-five will peak around the year 2010. By then, approximately 4.6 million can expect to be uninsured, up from 2.8 million in the mid-1990s. Almost 20 percent of the total population (nearly one of every five Americans) will be between the age of fifty-five and sixty-four by 2015, up from 8.7 percent in 2000. As of 1999, 16.1 percent of this age group were uninsured, up from 12.9 percent the year before.[51] As demographers, social scientists, and health professionals ponder the future, the good news is that baby boomers can expect a longer life than their parents' generation; the bad news is that they could be gaining quantity without quality, without adequate health care. Whether the added years will be free enough of illness and disability that they can live independently remains anyone's guess. Indeed, as the next chapter suggests, a major concern in the study of aging and longevity is just how healthy the longer years of living will be.

2

Patterns of Decline
Mind and Matter

Amoment in time: my mother-in-law phones from New York, there
is a pause, and then I hear, "Who am I talking to? Who did I call?"
When the voice I hear is my mother's from across the street, the
greeting is, "I can't remember why I called." On some calls, she then remembers, "Dad wants to talk to you." As he forces out words or parts
of words tied to his thought, I wait, trying to balance patience with
helping him finish what he means to say. I gave up talking with Lillian
on the phone months before hers was disconnected.

Of these four probably none would have lived to see the twenty-first
century without medical treatments developed during the last decades
of the twentieth. All have taken antibiotics, which as new wonder drugs
probably saved my mother's life in the 1940s. Their medications control
blood pressure to ward off strokes and stabilize a chronic heart condition. Two have pacemakers with tiny computer chips programmed to
keep their particular age-weakened heart beating. Three have undergone surgery to remove a malignant tumor. The most recent cancer surgery occurred more than fifteen years ago; as my mother prepared herself, she told the doctor, "I just want to live long enough to see my new
grandchild," the teenager who has provided a major portion of her informal care.

Yet at the time captured above, none could live on her or his own, owing primarily to a progressive loss of cognitive abilities, the particular impairments of varying types and severity. By the following year, moreover, the configuration of abilities and daily lives would be substantially rearranged. This chapter looks more closely at the vulnerabilities of age that threaten an individual's ability to live independently, especially the loss of mental abilities, ranging from modest memory loss to the dementias that can so devastate our later years. First, an overview of rapidly expanding knowledge about age-related cognitive decline may help people evaluate problems and support, to whatever extent possible, the way older individuals want to live. The chapter next considers depression, a psychological and physiological condition that often confounds the evaluation of cognitive, as well as physical, abilities, but one that for many older adults can improve with treatment. As in the previous chapter, the focus then shifts to implications for women and men currently at midlife, to ways these younger generations, my contemporaries and those who follow, might avert some of the major pitfalls ahead. In this context, the discussion highlights one risk already evident for these baby boom women and men: the commercial exploitation of a health and fitness culture that includes unprecedented amounts of medical information on age-related ailments of mind and body as they anticipate (or not) what will come next.

In light of what may seem an epidemic of chronic illness in an aging population, and of cognitive impairment—within a society that measures an individual's success in terms of work and mental tasks—this chapter raises important questions about aging and health care: have gains in quantity of life outpaced quality in people's added years? And what can younger people do to better maintain their cognitive as well as physical abilities so that whatever the length of their individual life, they need not feel it is too long?

MEMORY AND THE AGING BRAIN

"Did you ever see a brain going dead?" my father asked me now and then. At times he sounded at a loss, on better days merely amazed at what was happening to him. I did in fact view my mother's brain, in a magnetic resonance image (MRI) during one of our emergency room visits. I sat staring at the screen's glare beside a technician, an impassive white-coated woman deciphering whether the scan's squiggles or shadows were signs of a stroke. During that same time, my father's brain was revealing itself differently: his confusions about where he was and what he needed to do; his lost understanding of extended family relations, of bills and bank accounts; his unpredictable flares of memory arising from some experience somewhere between childhood and now; his inability to distinguish events in a dream from his life awake.

The pattern of his thoughts did not seem arbitrary and was in fact intriguing, though it feels a bit unseemly to react so with my own father. I couldn't help wondering what neurons were misfiring or depleted or lost, what taken-for-granted mental tasks had gone awry. Certain episodes resembled what neurologists see in younger patients suffering seizures or brain damage caused by an accident.[1] For instance, when my only brother visited, my father thought of him as three people: a dinner guest, a visitor who would sleep upstairs, and his son. They were all from the same town, working at the same job, which my father viewed as quite a coincidence. When we told him they were all the same person my father nodded in agreement, for a moment, until the strands of thought pulled apart, like a broken zipper. At times he lost the differing perspectives of himself and others: when handing me a dollar he thought I was giving money to him. What he would soon do—take a shower, stay home, go to a doctor's office—he thought was instead happening to me, or my mother, my son.

My mother-in-law's mental decline was more memory-focused. She didn't so much forget what she had heard a few minutes before or what she had done that day; it seemed that words, information, and experiences never registered at all. Each visit to New York revealed significant jumps and new problems—getting lost on her way to the beauty parlor; asking what street we had just passed at every block, though they were numbered and we were riding on her usual Broadway bus; worrying about us at night because she did not remember we went to a play; then not worrying because when we went out at night she forgot we were visiting, staying there in her apartment. My own mother, about five years younger, now sounded like my mother-in-law had about five years earlier.

Captured in generations past by the label *senility*, the loss of cognitive abilities and memory appeared to some people as an unavoidable reality of being old. Others fought back. In her classic study of old women and men at a Jewish seniors' center, the anthropologist Barbara

Myerhoff describes the efforts people took, "directed at convincing others, and then themselves, that they were in charge of their life . . . Underlying this was the unspoken, enormous fear of senility. Clear-mindedness and self-possession were signs of being intact. They regarded any indicators of senility, decay, and dependence as more alarming than an illness that might terminate in death. A forgotten word, an outburst of temper, a non sequitur, a misplaced object, a lapse of judgment or reasoning were all scrutinized as ominous portents that the process of decay was beginning."[2]

For most people, either observing others or noticing themselves, problems start with memory. As with the label of senility, however, memory loss is far too global a term, obscuring crucial distinctions. So too is Alzheimer's, used too loosely as a catch-all encompassing various dementias. Diagnostic categories for cognitive impairment are rough, even controversial, among researchers and physicians; the defining criteria are fluid, particularly at early stages. Methods most commonly used to assess cognitive changes as people age—for instance, the questions a doctor asks when trying to determine if a patient is showing early signs of Alzheimer's disease—have been quite primitive.

What is certain, as the population ages, is that the numbers of people experiencing memory loss and other cognitive problems are rising, as are the numbers of people wondering if they or a parent or friend are still mentally with-it. Also certain is that the effort to refine the meaning of "with-it" is moving apace. The aging brain is a hot topic of research, with new findings announced continually from a range of scientific and medical disciplines, using ever-more sophisticated study techniques. As with cancer, further research will doubtless identify more clearly several disorders sharing some common symptoms and biological processes but also differing in severity as well as in the way the condition typically progresses. Differing treatment and, perhaps, preventive measures may develop as well.[3]

While the science and technology grow increasingly complex, basic information of more immediate benefit to anyone concerned about an aging mind, their own or someone else's, is now emerging as well. A key question is what conditions reflect abnormal processes or diseases of aging rather than the norm. Some consensus is now jelling within the medical community around several categories of memory and other cognitive problems that become more common as people pass through their fifties.

AGE-ASSOCIATED MEMORY IMPAIRMENT

Sometimes called "benign forgetfulness," because it does not generally interfere with daily life, AAMI is a fancy name for greater difficulty remembering names, phone numbers, the plot of a movie or novel, where you put the car keys. Some estimates put this mild-to-moderate memory decline at 50 percent in people over the age of fifty. Whether this type of forgetting falls within a range considered normal for older people, or when and why it spills over into an abnormal process, is not yet clear.

MILD COGNITIVE IMPAIRMENT

In concert with lowered efficiency of other mental abilities, MCI indicates more severe and consistent memory lapses that begin to impinge on an individual's regular activities. A crucial characteristic distinguishing this broader cognitive loss from simpler memory problems is the individual's inability to function as before. For example, what you forget more frequently is how to balance a checkbook or get to the beauty parlor or post office. You may begin forgetting to pull together daily meals, or how to turn off the car's ignition and remove the key. This category seems the most amorphous, the criteria uncertain and too inclusive. Assessing initial declines from an individual's previous abilities is bound to be imprecise. As one *Lancet* review article put it, MCI "is a term in evolution," with research "suffocated by too many heterogeneous definitions."[4] Researchers are attempting to distinguish patients for whom MCI reflects a transitional stage into dementia—for instance, individuals whose memory impairment is initially out of proportion with their loss of other cognitive abilities and more severe, on average, than memory lapses in age-mates.[5] In years to come, greater knowledge about various types of normal and pathological age-related cognitive declines will likely break down MCI into subgroups, particularly describing conditions that cannot be called mild and that more likely presage dementia if the individual lives several additional years.[6]

DEMENTIA

Characterized by still broader cognitive loss, dementia describes a constellation of symptoms that worsen over time in somewhat predictable patterns, though at varying rates. Not only do individuals forget information or where common objects belong and lose the ability to perform certain daily tasks, they also lose the ability to solve problems (say, how to find missing car keys or the car). Unable to maintain emotional control in such circumstances, they may experience great upset. More generally, recent study of dementia has identified a strong component of psychiatric and behavior disorders along with cognitive loss. As many as 90 percent of people with dementia develop some combination of depression, anxiety, euphoria, personality change, agitation, apathy, irritability, hallucinations, delusions, and eating disorders.[7] Symptoms attached to these facets of dementia become major contributors to caregivers' stress and the admission of dementia patients to residential institutions. Substantial, progressive, and global decline affects abstract thought and at least two of the following areas of mental function essential to living independently—language, memory, visual and spatial ability, judgment, mood, and personality. An estimated 3 to 10 percent of people over the age of sixty-five suffer some degree of dementia, which increases to 25 percent of those over seventy-five years, and 40 percent over eighty.[8] Beyond the earliest stages, an individual with dementia cannot live alone and requires escalating levels of care.

TYPES OF DEMENTIA   *Alzheimer's disease* is the most common of several diseases and other physical conditions that can result in dementia. Although accurate numbers and rates of Alzheimer's, other dementias, and other types of age-related cognitive decline are not yet available, given diagnostic uncertainties, estimates at the start of this century for Alzheimer's disease in the United States hover between 2 million and 4.5 million, with most favoring the higher number.[9] The second most common disease that can cause dementia is *Parkinson's*, an illness characterized by worsening tremors, stiffness and rigidity. Among an estimated 1.5 million Americans with Parkinson's, between 40 and 70 percent will develop dementia over the course of their illness. Parkinson's dementia is diagnosed at least two years after initial motor symptoms appear, though often after a ten- to fifteen-year lag.[10] (Complicating matters for physicians and patients, medications commonly used to treat Parkinson's frequently cause dementia-like side effects over time.) Parkinson's and the closely related *Lewy body disease* account for approximately 10 to 15 percent of dementias. The latter illness appears to mix Alzheimer's symptoms with the stiffness or slowness of Parkinson's disease. Memory loss may not appear in early stages, though day-to-day fluctuations in attention and alertness are common. Early in the progression of this dementia, individuals often experience hallucinations, paranoia, or other psychiatric symptoms, as well as temporary losses of consciousness and falls.[11]

Research is also identifying other brain disorders that may account for dementia and are distinguished by certain distinctive symptoms. One such syndrome, named for its apparent brain locale, is *frontotemporal lobe dementia.* In contrast to Alzheimer's disease, early symptoms appear in personality and social skills, affecting memory later. Individuals with this dementia often experience unusual cravings (as for sugar), and many express noticeable creativity in art or music. *Pick's disease* shares symptoms of Alzheimer's, though symptoms generally appear between forty and sixty years of age. Rare diseases that can result in dementia include *Huntington's* (an inherited degenerative disease) and *Cruzfeldt-Jacob* (a neurological prion disease).

Multiple small strokes that do not initially result in observable symptoms, sometimes labeled mini- or silent strokes, may contribute to dementia by damaging tissue in crucial areas of the brain (called *multiinfarct* or *vascular dementia,* describing clots or hemorrhaging of blood vessels in the brain). The particular area injured may account for the type of behavior, thoughts, and mental deficits an individual experiences. One recent study found more than twice the risk of global cognitive loss and dementia among individuals whose MRI scans show such strokes.[12] Estimates that vary widely indicate from 10 percent up to 50 percent of dementias are of this vascular type. While some specialists describe vascular dementia as second in frequency to Alzheimer's, research is only beginning to unveil its relation to Alzheimer's disease and other dementias.[13] In fact, current studies suggest the prominence of mixed types of dementia, including subgroups of Alzheimer's disease, rather than pure, clearly distinguishable conditions.[14] Research is also identifying less common types of dementia. For example, *primary progressive aphasia* is an atypical dementia characterized by relentless loss of language abilities (word finding, speech patterns, spelling) even as memory remains relatively intact.[15]

It is important to recognize that memory decline, confusion, and other symptoms of dementia may also appear in cases of psychological depression, head injury, adult hydrocephalus (fluid accumulation in the brain, difficult to diagnose and treat, with symptoms that often include gait and balance problems, loss of bladder control), brain tumors, thyroid abnormality, adverse reaction to medications, severe and prolonged alcohol abuse, dehydration (as during hot weather), nutritional deficiencies (especially vitamin B_{12} and, perhaps, folic acid), or infections (AIDS, meningitis, urinary tract infection). Recent studies suggest that about 50 percent of patients recovering from heart bypass surgery experience cognitive decline, most reversing during ensuing months, but some deficits persisting.[16]

DIAGNOSING DEMENTIA   As the most common and commonly feared dementia, Alzheimer's disease receives the lion's share of attention. A major concern among the public and health-care professionals is whether an individual's initial, relatively mild problems are early signs of Alzheimer's. Preliminary study does suggest that people previously diagnosed with mild cognitive impairment are more likely than others to be among the approximately 360,000 new Alzheimer cases diagnosed in this country each year. Again, estimates vary widely; a few studies suggest about 10–25 percent of older people with MCI progress within a year to Alzheimer's, compared to 1–2 percent of non-MCI elders. Close to 50 percent are diagnosed with Alzheimer's after four years.[17] With diagnostic criteria and tools very much works-in-progress, boundaries separating loss of memory from cognition, or mild loss from moderate, are neither clear nor definitive. The significance of onset age—say, of developing MCI at seventy-eight years or ninety-two—remains unclear as well.[18]

Typically, an individual's physician performs an initial assessment, prompted by concerns the patient or a family member expresses about memory loss or episodes of confusion. The doctor needs to talk with family or a close friend to help assess recent changes in a patient's abilities (see figures 2 and 3). Unlike many individuals who complain to their doctor about memory loss, patients who are in fact developing dementia may be unaware of their own cognitive problems or decline.[19] The evaluation includes questions that test basic mental abilities and orientation to the present world—who is the president, what is the month and year. A Seven-Minute Screen developed in 1998 (its title particularly apt during the managed-care era) assesses verbal ability, recall, and understanding of time, the latter through clock-drawing tasks. A longer, standardized Mini-Mental State Examination asks patients to complete additional mental exercises—to count backward from one hundred by sevens, spell certain words backward, or draw geometric figures. Additional cognitive assessment includes a verbal fifteen-word learning test.[20] To rule out other conditions, the doctor checks basic neurological function, such as reflexes, sensitivity of hands and feet, and the ability to walk a straight line, balance on one foot, and coordinate

2. WARNING SIGNS AND CHARACTERISTICS OF DEMENTIA

Characteristics and their prominence vary by dementia type; categories listed below overlap and interrelate. Most significant are characteristics and behaviors that occur *repeatedly* and reflect *changes* in that individual.

MEMORY LAPSES

Recall of new information: misplaces objects; repeats words, phrases, and questions in same conversation; misses appointments; forgets what happened earlier in day (e.g., Did I have lunch? Where was I? Whom did I see?)

Routine tasks: forgets to pay bills, turn off stove, make morning coffee; forgets family occasions (e.g., birthdays, anniversary, holidays)

Complex tasks (especially ones requiring a series of mental steps and actions): forgets how to pay bills, balance checkbook, use basic math; unable to perform usual job activities, hobbies, to shop for and cook a meal

DECLINE IN REASONING ABILITIES

Experiences difficulty and anxiety over making choices

Shows inappropriate simple daily judgments (e.g., choice of heavy winter coat on hot summer day)

Makes poor financial decisions

Has trouble problem solving (e.g., what to do if car gets flat tire)

LOSS OF LANGUAGE

Forgets simple words, often using longer, circuitous, descriptions

Substitutes wrong or made-up words

Has trouble following and participating in conversation

DIFFICULTIES WITH ORIENTATION IN SPACE AND TIME

Gets lost on familiar route, unable to find way to destination

Does not recognize familiar surroundings and landmarks

Loses track of time (e.g., spend hours in market), of day and night, month and year

Wanders away from familiar places and people

UNUSUAL MOODS AND BEHAVIORS

Is irritable, agitated, suspicious, angry, passive and unresponsive, or anxious

Exhibits extreme mood swings (e.g., euphoria/depression)

Has disturbances in sleep

Places objects in odd, inappropriate places (e.g., umbrella under bed, keys in oven)

Loses interest in previously enjoyed activities

Exhibits inappropriate eating and sexual behavior; undresses inappropriately (disinhibition)

Displays unusual physical and/or verbal aggression

PSYCHOTIC-LIKE CHARACTERISTICS (MOSTLY LATER STAGES)

Has delusions, hallucinations, paranoia

3. WHEN TO SEEK EVALUATION

PROBABLY NO NEED FOR CONCERN	TALK WITH DOCTOR (ESPECIALLY IF PROBLEM RECURS)
Forgets street address for appointment but is able to find building	Gets lost in familiar neighborhood, unable to find way home
Forgets where car is parked in a lot	Unable to track car down or devise ways to remember next time
Leaves stove on but checks before going out of the house	Leaves stove on until someone else checks, does not recall using it
Forgets name of new acquaintance or blanks on familiar name/word	Can't recall name of good friend, relative, even when reminded
Asks same question as yesterday but remembers when told	Asks same questions several times in single conversation, does not remember when told
Complains and jokes about own memory problems (including to own doctor)	Unaware of and denies memory (or related) problems when others express concern

hand-eye movements. Blood tests can detect vitamin B_{12} deficiency, high or low thyroid hormone levels, diabetes, and other metabolic abnormalities. Further evaluation may include a geriatric specialist or a neurologist. A psychological consultation can help identify a more exclusive depression, although dementia and depression commonly coexist, with complex interactions, in the old.

Misdiagnosis of the various dementias does often occur, in part because research is only beginning to reveal interrelations—for instance between Alzheimer's, Parkinson's, and multi-infarct—and distinctive characteristics. In fact, a diagnostic catch is that greatest certainty must await death, when laboratory analysis of brain tissue can reveal abnormalities not otherwise observable. Protein deposits called plaques and tangles are hallmarks of Alzheimer's, while different forms and patterns of nerve cell pathologies characterize Parkinson's, Lewy body, and Pick's dementias. Autopsy of the brain can also reveal damage caused by mini-strokes.

Short of autopsy, a thorough diagnostic process of elimination—ruling out other ailments of the live but aging brain—can identify, with over 90 percent accuracy, probable Alzheimer's disease, according to the

Alzheimer's Association. Increasingly sophisticated imaging technologies now providing new windows on the brain are not yet recommended generally as part of a routine diagnostic evaluation, although some specialists recommend obtaining a baseline scan for suspected dementias.[21] Certainly, MRI and CT (computed tomography) scans are allowing more comprehensive and detailed views than simple X-rays of the size and shape of brain structures, as well as evidence of fluid buildup, damage from stroke or physical trauma. PET (positron-emission tomography) scans now visualize the brain at work, colorizing like in an old movie the metabolism of glucose, the circulation of blood, the areas activated when an individual thinks, talks, remembers. Currently used primarily for research, these technologies are further delineating and identifying the various dementias.

SEARCHING FOR CAUSES OF COGNITIVE DECLINE

A data trove on cognitive decline comes from an ongoing study focused on Alzheimer's disease that includes brain imaging and then autopsies of the participants, aged nuns living their last years within convents dotting this country's midwestern and mid-Atlantic regions.[22] Since the project began during the early 1990s the nearly seven hundred nuns have undergone periodic brain imaging, as well as blood tests, and tests of physical and cognitive abilities. Of crucial importance, all agreed to donate their brain for study when they die. The research also includes genetic analyses (a bonus: some of the nuns are biological sisters as well) and draws on a wealth of information about participants' lives and family background. Included within convent archives are especially rich and unusual documents: autobiographical statements that each woman wrote, as much as seventy years earlier, when initiated into the School Sisters of Notre Dame. The nuns' study essentially recreates its subjects' young adulthood, catching up and following them as old women. All have experienced similar stable lifestyles within similar stable communities throughout their adult lives, minimizing differences resulting from their environment during those years. By the age of seventy-five or eighty, some begin a progression through advancing stages of Alzheimer's, while others remain cognitively sharp, in several instances beyond a hundred years of age.

Among the most surprising findings, once deaths began to accumulate: the extent of Alzheimer's plaques and tangles did not always correspond to an individual's diagnosis before she died. Brain pathology appeared in some of the nuns who never showed symptoms of dementia, performing well on cognitive tests until their dying days. That is, while autopsy could confirm observed Alzheimer's symptoms, researchers also discovered a similar type and degree of brain pathology for certain women who had remained symptom-free at the same age. Furthermore, the stage of disease diagnosed in nuns who did show Alzheimer's symptoms was not always reflected in the plaques and tangles. Individuals who died at an early clinical stage might show more severe Alzheimer's pathology at autopsy than others diagnosed with more advanced dementia, and vice versa. The autopsy findings suggest one key factor underlying this disconnect: whether the brain also shows evidence of past small strokes. Nearly all (93 percent) individuals with Alzheimer's pathology and signs of strokes had been diagnosed with Alzheimer's disease before they died; the rate of diagnosis dropped to 57 percent for those with Alzheimer's pathology but no strokes. Among individuals with evidence of strokes but no plaques and tangles, only 2.5 percent had demonstrated signs of dementia; the mini-stroke link held only in coexistence with Alzheimer's pathology.

During these initial phases of data analysis, researchers are hypothesizing that damage from small strokes, arteriosclerosis (thickened, hardened artery walls), and cardiovascular disease more broadly can lower the threshold or act as a trip-switch for developing Alzheimer's disease. While cardiovascular and neurological disease may develop independently over several decades, the combined effect disrupts communication within the brain such that observable Alzheimer's symptoms emerge.[23] Moreover, as the 43 percent of stroke-free nuns with Alzheimer's autopsy pathology attest, the human brain appears able to tolerate and compensate for some degree of age-related damage without apparent cognitive decline. If individual thresholds depend in part on what other damage a brain has also sustained, another part of the equation may be what the researchers call brain reserve. Individuals may be born with and/or develop early in life varying brain capacity to compensate for similar levels of damage. The nuns' study investigators cite participants' early writing samples, which exhibit striking differences in richness of vocabulary, complexity of sentences, and density of ideas. After scoring the autobiographical statements along several dimensions, the researchers found that low scores on overall idea density predicted with 80 percent accuracy who would be diagnosed with Alzheimer's disease decades later. Perhaps the compositions by those women in their twenties indicate a brain already compromised in some way and, therefore, susceptible to developing more plaques and tangles characteristic of Alzheimer's disease without an ability to compensate. Conversely, the most idea-dense statements may reflect a brain already better equipped to limit, circumvent, or work around plaques and tangles and other injury throughout life—for example, by establishing alternate paths of communication connecting nerve cells—a brain exhibiting greater plasticity, flexibility, a greater reserve.[24]

As of 2001, 295 nuns were still alive. Data collection will likely continue another twenty years, with researchers poring through the findings much longer. Already the nuns' study offers intriguing preliminary clues that, along with research from many scientific disciplines, will help answer questions about

· the relation between development of dementias, depression, cardiovascular disease, and stroke;

· the role more generally of such intangibles as personality and temperament, emotion, social support, faith, and outlook on life;

· the genetic contribution that may predispose an individual to, or protect against, Alzheimer's disease and other dementias.

Finally, the lead investigator of the nuns' study, Dr. David Snowden, poses questions familiar to me and to others who have observed dementia close at hand and have repeatedly wondered just what our parents and friends could comprehend of the world as they once knew it. Were individuals suffering from dementia attempting to communicate more than they were able, trapped behind a loss of language more severe than their loss of perception or thought? Did some web of memory survive longer than anyone could know, some manner of relating their present circumstances to their past? Did they maintain preferences and desires for their daily lives, their loss of autonomy suffered more keenly than even the most empathic caregivers might imagine?

The particular world of these nuns—a secure, accepting, and intentional lifelong community—raises also a rather different point: dementias and other mental impairment entail social definitions as well. Within the religious sisterhood, aged individuals who develop dementia not only receive loving care, they remain highly valued members of that small community, engaged to whatever degree their impairment allows in daily activities perceived as worthwhile. Beyond the convent, however, is a highly cognitive society that measures an individual's social position, as well as cognitive decline, largely in terms of work and education-related mental tasks and abilities. In addition to age-related biological changes that can result in serious impairment of mental processes, the ways society defines demented or senile as compared, say, to eccentric or slowing down shapes the ways families, other caregivers, physicians, and government policy makers react and provide care to impaired individuals. Not only can social definitions marginalize individuals, isolating them from a wider community, the reactions and type of care provided may, in turn, intensify or minimize behavioral symptoms, such as the agitation or emotional outbursts observed in residents of nursing facilities and even, I would eventually see, in individuals living at home.[25] That social definitions might create unhappy impacts seems all the more possible given our limited insight into the way individuals with dementia experience their surrounding world—their perceptions, understanding, and fears. The study of Alzheimer's among elderly nuns is emblematic, more generally, of the most consistent link between individuals who develop the disease: age and gender. Less than 2 percent of people sixty years old suffer Alzheimer's disease. For those older than eighty-five, reports on Alzheimer's rates range from nearly 30 percent to as much as 50 percent.[26] Among people diagnosed with Alzheimer's, 43 percent are between seventy-five and eighty-five years old; women outnumber men 2 to 1 owing largely to women's greater longevity.

Although scientists search the human genome for genetic messages underlying Alzheimer's and other dementias, genetic testing has so far provided only limited information. Like the breast cancer genes identified, with much fanfare, during the 1990s, suspect inheritable Alzheimer's gene mutations appear to cause a small proportion of diagnosed cases (probably less than 10 percent); these cases share a distinct pattern of symptoms appearing at an early age (often younger than sixty-five), among an unusually large number of family members over several generations. So far, only Huntington's disease shows an identifiable link between dementia and a single dominant gene mutation, with genetic testing able to confirm a diagnosis and accurately predict which family members will inherit this fatal dementing illness. In contrast, attempts to diagnose Alzheimer's in its early stages are invariably accompanied by such qualifiers as "questionable," "possible," and "probable."

Even among the 90–95 percent late-onset cases, Alzheimer's disease likely encompasses heterogeneous risks and processes.[27] Current evidence suggests that genetic variability within the human population—normal but differing alleles of a gene, especially the gene labeled

ApoE—may interact with environmental factors (such as diet, exercise, stress, head trauma) to confer increased susceptibility or resistance to cognitive decline, altering the risk for developing dementia, including Alzheimer's, and the age at which symptoms appear. Reduced efficiency and repair of genes involving learning, memory, neuron survival, and brain plasticity may become significant by the age of forty.[28] The critical mechanism may involve not genes that cause aging or dementia but rather the absence of genetic contributions that increase an individual's disease risks, along with protective genetic contributions that promote durability of the human organism—that is, longevity—as reflected in extremely old women and men who remain cognitively intact. People who now live to one hundred years of age are often in relatively good health. Some protective mechanisms, likely a combination of genetic and environmental factors, have allowed them to survive rather than succumb to illnesses fatal to most people in their eighties and nineties. Researchers note, moreover, that extreme old age (over ninety-seven) runs in families; compared to the general population, these related individuals age slowly and greatly delay or escape age-related disease and disability.[29]

For most of today's middle-aged, however, evidence suggests a rather chilling thought: cognitive impairment evident among the oldest old may reflect late phases of a continuous process beginning, in many cases, when they were in their twenties or thirties, if not before.[30] Research on how the brain normally functions throughout life, orchestrating the intricate and highly complex mental processes of human living, may contribute to developing preventive measures. Neurochemists are analyzing, for instance, how billions of nerve cells communicate their chemical messages to move our every muscle and thought. Using new imaging techniques, scientists are mapping various types of mental processes carried out in different areas of the apparently normal brain and identifying the structural and neurological changes that do come with age. Cognitive scientists are defining a range of mental processes necessary for planning, initiating, and completing a sequence of behaviors.[31]

One such process, *working memory,* is in constant demand and appears especially vulnerable to weakening with age. Working memory entails temporarily storing new information from the external world, as well as completing mental operations (called executive functions) to analyze that information, focus attention on some aspects but not others, and reach decisions based on additional recalled information. That is, the mind must be able to process information from outside and retrieve information from internal memory banks. These mental tasks are essential to the decision making, judgment, and planning required to live with some independence in the community. Without working memory, new information essentially evaporates. The brain cannot work on new mental input even as long-term memories remain settled elsewhere in the brain's network, at least for a while longer. Thus, for quite some time my mother-in-law could retell stories from her childhood in Turkey and her young married life on the Greek island of Rhodes, including fleeing Nazi occupation with other Jewish families. For the life of her, however, she could not remember what you told her five minutes ago.

My mother-in-law's loss of recent memory, my father's and Lillian's dementias broadened and grew more severe as each moved past ninety years of age. Some individuals show little decline in memory retrieval or ability to perform very familiar mental tasks, particularly if they do not live to such an advanced age. Most common is a slowing of mental abilities (say, in memorizing new information or recalling a familiar name). Paying attention to several simultaneous activities or information sources may take greater effort (talking on the phone while cooking or driving, remembering what you were saying if interrupted, or why you entered a room if the television is on). Often, a slowed rate of receiving, processing, and retrieving information is not generally apparent, as most activities do not require rapid and complex mental processes. Moreover, as the nuns' study and other research suggest, the healthy brain compensates for many age-related changes, substituting new pathways and areas of heightened mental activity when previous systems begin to fail. Although some brain cells die and certain areas shrink in size after middle age, current evidence suggests that lessened efficiency of memory processes—considered benign and even expected—results primarily from alterations in biochemical communication across synapses separating cell from cell. These age-related changes differ from pathological types of synapse interruption and damage with eventually more substantial loss of brain cells or deterioration of structures characteristic of Alzheimer's disease, other dementias, and, probably, a subset of what is presently labeled mild cognitive impairment.

WHY BOTHER KNOWING?

In frustration, at times I wondered what difference it made if an individual, like my father, my mother-in-law, or Lillian received a diagnosis of Alzheimer's or some other cognitive impairment. Why find out whether my mother's increasing forgetfulness was labeled as still benign? No small reason for most people is reassurance: faulty memory or slowed mental abilities will not look like Alzheimer's, as they may have feared. They can then concentrate on better concentrating, supporting day-to-day memory not only with such simple aids as lists and calendars, but also with mental tricks that focus their attention on new information, so that it registers and can later be more easily recalled. Additional efforts that may bolster attention and memory include getting adequate sleep, correcting vision or hearing problems, avoiding excessive alcohol and unnecessary drug use, and improving circulation and alertness through regular exercise.

TREATMENT

A possible dementia gives all the more reason to find out, and sooner rather than later. For one thing, some dementias or dementia-like symptoms can be reversed or their severity modulated, their progression delayed. Given the uncertainties enveloping diagnoses of memory loss and early dementia, evaluation of any apparent cognitive impairment should consider conditions that are reversible:

- · by stopping, changing, or reducing dosage of medications that commonly exacerbate, if not cause, memory loss, disorientation, and confusion (see figure 4);
- · by initiating vitamin B12 injections to counter lowered absorption of this nutrient as people age (20 percent of people at sixty years and 40 percent at eighty years lose the ability to absorb vitamin B12), in addition to a basic vitamin and mineral supplement;
- · by ruling out or treating a thyroid problem, dehydration, alcohol abuse, an infection, or the less clear-cut diagnosis of depression (which I discuss below).

Conditions reversible through surgery (such as some brain tumors and hydrocephalus) require detection before it is too late. Otherwise, damage to the brain may become irreversible, or potential complications of the surgery itself, which increase with age, may eliminate the surgical option.

4. DRUGS THAT CAN FOG THE MIND

antibiotics
anticholinergics (for motion sickness, Parkinson's disease)
antihistamines and decongestants
antiemetics (for nausea)
pain control medications
blood pressure drugs
corticosteroids
muscle relaxants
heartburn and ulcer drugs
antidepressants
antipsychotics
sedatives, sleep aids, anti-anxiety medications
alcohol and recreational drugs

Based on *Consumer Reports on Health,* vol. 12 (April 2000).

"Before it is too late" may also apply to the drugs doctors prescribe in an attempt to slow or delay symptoms of Alzheimer's and other dementias. Although data on efficacy remain scanty, one type of medication increases the amount and activity of a neurotransmitter, acetylcholine, thought to be deficient in Alzheimer's patients; if treatment begins during early stages, these cholinesterase inhibitors (Aricept, Exelon, Reminyl brands) appear to provide some modest beneficial effect on cognitive and neuropsychiatric symptoms related to memory and thought processes, anxiety, or agitation.[32] Though they won't provide a cure, easing symptoms and slowing the disease could not only improve the quality of people's immediate daily lives but also mean some individuals never experience the most harsh and devastating later stages. Perhaps they can maintain more remnants of independence for the rest of their lives. Yet now that prescribing such drugs is standard practice, knowing their true effect is virtually impossible. Neither doctors nor family members know whether the medication is holding off something worse. Despite medical journal advertisements claiming that persistent use of Aricept can delay nursing-home placement for nearly two years, no good evidence substantiates the manufacturer's (Pfizer) claim.[33] And, although some studies suggest that inflammation affecting the brain may contribute to developing dementia, anti-inflammatory drugs have not proven effective so far in averting or slowing cognitive decline.[34] However, for people already in later stages of Alzheimer's disease (moderate to severe), clinical trials of a different type of medication, memantine, indicate some slowing of further cognitive deterioration, especially among patients already taking a cholinesterase inhibitor.[35] In addition, identifying the type of dementia may be important in selecting treatments. For instance, while early psychiatric symptoms are common in Lewy body disease, this illness can also bring severe adverse reactions to the antipsychotic medications prescribed increasingly to dementia patients experiencing such symptoms.[36]

With researchers actively pursuing newer medications, including a vaccine to halt development of Alzheimer's disease and drugs that target pre-dementia cognitive decline, enough delay in the onset of symptoms could allow many people to live out their lives, dying of other causes with neither doctor nor patients aware that the latter were, in fact, on a track toward dementia. Slowing disease progression could allow people experiencing early phases of cognitive loss today to benefit from improved treatment still a few years away. By then, greater understanding of the origins and processes of Alzheimer's and other dementias will enable doctors to differentiate among dementias and other cognitive loss and better distinguish which medications are effective for which patients.[37] There are, however, several caveats. First, if such developments currently represent the potential good news, the bad news is that for many people the cost of these drugs will be prohibitive. With hundreds of dollars needed to fill prescriptions each month, patients cannot always follow their doctor's orders. Second, there are risks and trade-offs even in identifying problems early. An individual may live longer under the cloud of Alzheimer's. That cloud will surely affect the individual psychologically; it may also affect prospects for maintaining or obtaining employment, not to mention health insurance. Finally, diagnosis will be less certain and more subject to error. These early but misdiagnosed patients may be prescribed medications that they do not need, and thus take on the risks of medications without any counterbalancing benefits.

Whether or how much current dementia medications improve an individual's condition remains uncertain. Would my father's progression have been worse had he never taken Aricept? Would his late life have been better had he started sooner? Or was the drug's effect primarily on us, his family caregivers—a placebo effect that made us feel better because we thought the medication might be helping him?

MENTAL ABILITIES AND DAILY CARE

The prospect of treatment—to reverse, slow, or modulate cognitive loss and to buy time until improved medical treatment develops—is but one crucial reason to evaluate the type and degree of impairment an individual is experiencing. As scientists better distinguish differing types of dementia, they may also identify useful nonpharmacological interventions, as well as conditions unlikely to respond. Such interventions may relate to an individual's mental abilities and daily care: Does an evaluation indicate the need for changes in the logistics of daily life, now or in the months and years to come? Cognitive impairments do require planning for what can be many years, extending far beyond the time when independent living becomes too difficult and dangerous. Although onset of any type of dementia is difficult to pinpoint, most people with Alzheimer's disease, for instance, live between three and eight years after diagnosis; they may live twenty years, especially as diagnoses come earlier.[38]

As with such physical ailments as arthritis, poor eyesight, and hearing loss, adaptations in daily habits and physical surroundings can help compensate for common memory gaps and slowed mental skills. Certain characteristics of more profound cognitive impairments and dementias may also improve with alterations in an individual's environment, and with far less risk than medications.[39] For example, a study of Alzheimer's patients living at home demonstrated physical and mental health benefits following a three-month home exercise program combined with training for their caregivers. Caregivers learned to continue an individual's exercises, find other pleasurable activities, and increase the patient's social stimulation; they also learned techniques for better handling specific behavior problems.[40] More generally, simplifying an individual's surroundings and routines, reducing noise and other distractions, creating visually calming indoor spaces and a simple and secure outdoor garden path may ease behavior problems as well (see figure 5).

Efforts to maintain, as much as possible, a person's safety and autonomy depend not only on the most obvious considerations—the who and where and what of daily care, and how to pay for it. Family and friends interacting with the individual day after day and night also will need to change their own behavior, attitudes and routines, adaptations best informed by knowing how the impairment will likely progress and by taking part in training and ongoing support as caregivers. In some com-

5. ADAPTING TO DAILY LIFE WITH DEMENTIA: RECOMMENDATIONS FOR CAREGIVERS OF IMPAIRED INDIVIDUALS

Reduce clutter and noise; try quiet music

Keep conversations calm, choices or questions easy

Don't argue with or try to convince individual; try to perceive individual's reality

Simplify and allow extra time for daily routines

Facilitate simple, enjoyable, and diverting activities—arts and crafts, watching videos, looking through photo albums

Monitor and treat other health problems—including pain, constipation

Monitor and treat other psychological problems, including with nondrug interventions

Hide or lock away medications

Camouflage doors to outside; if available, sign up with "Safe Return" (through local Alzheimer's Association) in case individual gets lost

Take walks with individual

Enroll individual in well run dementia-focused day care

munities, day-care programs provide social and recreational activities geared to people with dementia. Such programs can benefit not only the individual suffering dementia. They provide crucial respite for family caregivers.

Dementia does create a particular set of demands for caregiving. One study followed 1,200 Alzheimer's patients and their family caregivers over four years, including the last year of the patients' lives. The caregivers—half of them spouses, others primarily adult children (84.3 percent were women)—felt they were on-duty day and night needing to provide or coordinate full-time supervision and care. Over time the daily physical care (bathing, toileting, dressing and undressing, preparing and serving meals, taking the person in a car, etc.) became additionally burdened by loss of communication with a loved one who no longer recognized them, by that individual's angry outbursts, and by their need to prevent him from wandering away (54 percent of the patients were men). Moreover, caregivers were eventually handling end-of-life care, including increased physical problems (such as incontinence, loss of mobility, trouble eating and drinking), and the patient's need for pain control and comfort care. Beyond the sheer physical difficulty of care, the most immediate danger is the toll from accumulated

6. TEN WARNING SIGNS OF STRESS IN CAREGIVERS

denial
anger
social withdrawal
anxiety
depression
exhaustion
sleeplessness
irritability
lack of concentration
health problems

Based on Alzheimer's Association materials, www.alz.org 2003.

stress, which may take different forms in different caregivers: see figure 6 on the warning signs of harmful stress in caregivers. Nearly 60 percent of family caregivers become clinically depressed, according to the Family Caregivers Alliance. (Other types of serious ongoing illness can cause similar stress.) The impact is all the more worrisome when a caregiver is herself aged. Evidence now suggests that chronic stress of such caregiving is "a risk factor for mortality," particularly for a spouse, whose intense, unique support relationship does persist through better and worse (that is, stress may shorten an aged caregiver's life).[41] The long duration of most dementias and the nature of cognitive decline mean that family caregivers also experience a long span of grief and bereavement for loss of the person who is still requiring increasingly difficult and ever-vigilant care. If that person moves to a residential institution, depression and anxiety remain high (especially in a spouse).[42]

Fairly early in dementia's progression, the need for care will extend to financial and legal matters as well. Someone close to the individual, often an adult daughter or son, will need to pay the bills and manage bank accounts, do the taxes, determine the end-point for credit card use, banking, and driving. Determining more broadly whether an individual maintains the capacity to live independently, assessing the risk to himself and others, will loom as a complex but inevitable quandary.[43] (A doctor can help determine when a patient should no longer drive and, if necessary, initiate revocation of a license.) Awkward questions about a will, a trust, end-of-life wishes, about designating a power-of-attorney for legal, financial, and health-care decisions must be addressed while the individual can understand and decide. Aside from an acute and obvious change such as a stroke or heart attack, no obvious moment will announce the time when someone else needs to take over, a determination that may also become the impaired individual's accusation. More likely, taking over will happen gradually and reluctantly, after second and third notices of unpaid bills arrive, when the refrigerator and cupboards are too often empty, the untended stove left on—until the gray area and fuzzy borders of competence, legal and real, are clearly left behind. In my parents' case, an earthquake fault forms the divide. My father had failed to renew earthquake insurance, complaining of the cost (which they could afford), although their house sits astride California's Hayward fault, a geologic rift due to convulse any time now with the big one. In a brief telephone query to their lawyer asking when my power-of-attorney would be activated and such decisions would become mine, he mentioned their best interest and advised, "Just do it" (see figure 7).

It is a difficult balance between providing too little help too late, on the one hand, or too much too soon, on the other, since the latter can contribute to a learned and exaggerated helplessness in someone experiencing cognitive loss and in the person (probably a spouse) providing daily care.[44] How can the timing and type of help not feel like taking over, as my father and Lillian put it? How can daughters and sons avoid failing to provide assistance that will ease a parent's anxiety about managing on her or his own?

Such judgments are especially difficult when older people lose words and language that might convey what they truly understand and how competent they do remain, as well as what they see and hear and want. And, whether assistance is too much or too little, or relatively appropriate, those individuals are in fact losing control over their own lives. Perhaps the hardest question of all, then, is: Do people maintain some ultimate right to reject offers of help and live, or not, with the consequences?

For many of today's oldest old, taped phone menus and answering machines alone, not to mention e-mail, Web sites, or online transactions can make daily life impossible to manage. The way individuals compensate for their own loss of abilities may mask initial signs of decline, making early detection of impairment more difficult. Extensive use of memory aids may delay the time when their condition becomes obviously worse than benign, affecting daily activities. Only in retrospect do

7. ASSEMBLING AN INDIVIDUAL'S LEGAL AND FINANCIAL RECORDS

PERSONAL INFORMATION

Full legal name, Social Security number, date and place of birth, legal address
Names and addresses of spouse and children
Location of an up-to-date will and/or trust
Location of birth, marriage, divorce certificates, citizenship papers
List of employers and dates of employment
Records of education, military service, religious affiliation, other organizations
Names and addresses of close friends, other relatives, doctors, lawyers, financial
advisors

FINANCIAL INFORMATION

Income and assets (pensions, interest, property, stocks, other investments, etc.)
Social Security, Medicare/Medicaid and supplemental health insurance, life insurance (and policy numbers)
Location of bank accounts (checking, savings, credit union) and safe deposit boxes, with all account and box numbers; location of all valuable personal items (jewelry, family keepsakes)
Copy of recent income tax returns, property taxes
Documentation on mortgages and debts—how and when paid
Credit card and charge account names and numbers

I realize why my father became so irritated when someone altered his arrangement of papers and pens on top of his desk or put the stamps or scissors in the wrong drawer. Not only was his eyesight failing more dangerously than I knew, he also must have been trying to overcome a faltering ability to stay organized, to hang on to the facility with which he had always managed the family's financial affairs.

As I began to learn about care for aged parents, the most immediately helpful understanding was that my father's thoughts and behavior were not idiosyncratic. He was not being stubborn or willful. He was not being domineering in his fatherly way. His confusions were par for the course, a course that moved along the same general phases of dementia tracked by countless others. There were ways to better communicate with him. Tracing his thought to recent or past experience, or identifying the words he was trying to say—and most importantly, learning not to argue with his reality—could decrease both his frustration and ours.

And there seemed, at times, a tenuous logic still present in my father's dementia, as if his diminished brain struggled to make sense of a disturbingly unfamiliar world. For instance, his questions about the army bivouac arose when he slept away from his own bed and his wife, sharing his nighttime space with another man, as had last occurred while he served in the army (albeit nearly sixty years earlier). The imagined search for San Francisco property could, perhaps, reconstrue his hardfought effort, as a newly minted lawyer during the Depression, to salvage a single piece of real estate for his widowed mother's income out of his father's otherwise total loss. His persistent questions—"Who is running this place? When are we going home?"—reflected, perhaps, some awareness that he was no longer in charge; he and my mother must, therefore, be trapped on some unwanted, enforced vacation away from home. Talking to him, attempting to uncover his train of thought suggested responses that reassured and calmed him, at least temporarily, until the focus of his puzzlement shifted. Or perhaps I searched unrealistically for links in his mind, clinging still to my father's former self.

With time, I better recognized my mother's ways of coping as his spouse of six decades plus and, in recent years, his main daily support even as she herself was slipping. That the two of them resisted help, especially from a hired stranger, was to be expected, I learned. Not only were they maintaining a claim to independence, a refusal to give up control over their own lives; their perception of their own limits was itself limited. She would do what he asked even as the requests became unreasonable. That was, after all, her longstanding role, exaggerated now by a more organic inability to question or contradict, to grasp my father's condition and exert sound judgment. No wonder, then, my mother saw no reason not to take my father on errands, just the two of them, even after the time he fell on the sidewalk, able to get up thanks only to the nearest passerby. Why not take him to the bank, though his concept of amounts allowed for any expanse of zeros at a number's end? And later, as my father's condition and her abilities deteriorated, it was no wonder that she inexorably disengaged and withdrew.

DEPRESSION, WITH DEMENTIA OR NOT

My uncle in Los Angeles, living in a nursing home, did not reach the age of one hundred. My father, unable to travel for one last visit with his brother or to attend the funeral with their few family and friends, grieved at a distance in his own way. It was during the weeks after my uncle died that my father said, "I feel depressed," an unusual declaration from a man who had always been stoic, not given to sharing emotions. My first thought: antidepressant brand names—Prozac, Zoloft, Paxil—are common vocabulary, so what took us so long to consider this possibility? Although his sadness had surely been heightened with his brother's death, perhaps his ongoing anger and frustration, volatility, and spells of agitation were something more than dementia and his reaction to it. And that something, depression, might respond to medical treatment.

In fact, some geriatricians and psychiatrists argue that too often physicians fail to identify depression in older adults, and so they fail to provide helpful treatments, including medications and individual or group psychotherapy. Doctors and their older patients may interpret symptoms of depression as a more acute grief over the death of a spouse or sibling or dear friend, an experience common in this population. Doctors may not take the time needed to recognize depression by talking with a patient, especially with only an allotted fifteen-minute appointment. If an antidepressant seems warranted, a primary care doctor may not have experience with the various types or may not monitor the medication's effects on that individual, adjusting the treatment if necessary. Furthermore, definitions are imprecise, subject to varying perceptions and interpretations, especially by family members and doctors. Individuals may experience symptoms that are not severe or numerous enough to constitute the standard psychiatric diagnosis of major clinical depression; characteristics of depression in the old may differ from depression in younger people. And symptoms may wax and wane.[45]

A doctor may attribute depressive symptoms to other health conditions that accumulate as people age. Although depression may coexist with other health problems, whether heart failure, cancer, a chronic illness, or dementia, doctors do need to rule out or treat such conditions as thyroid abnormalities, diabetes, cardiovascular disease, sleep problems, chronic pain, hearing and vision loss, alcohol abuse, and misuse of prescription or over-the-counter drugs.[46] Doctors should also rule out the well-known syndrome of overmedication by doctors—Is a medication causing depressive symptoms?—before prescribing yet another medication to treat what looks like depression.

Depression is not an inevitable or normal condition of aging; most old people do not become depressed. Estimates of the numbers vary, as current understanding of depression and other psychological dimensions of aging does not allow diagnostic accuracy. The National Institute of Mental Health puts the rate of major depression at 3 percent of people over sixty-five living at home; looking more narrowly at doctors' visits, the estimate rises to between 5 and 10 percent. The rate is higher among nursing-home residents. "Significant symptoms" of depression appear in 15 to 20 percent of the old.[47]

Distinguishing depression from dementia presents an especially perplexing diagnostic puzzle. Symptoms can be similar: confusion, memory loss, sleeping too much or too little, inability to concentrate, withdrawal from social interactions. More broadly, however, the relation between late-life depression, cognitive decline, and dementia, as well as physical disease, creates many newly recognized avenues for research. Among older adults, studies suggest that those with Alzheimer's disease are more likely to experience depression than are their healthy counterparts. Specialists now think as many as 50 percent of people with dementia may also suffer depression. Although depression can reflect a psychological reaction to the experience of early dementia, evidence also suggests that the reaction and symptoms may change in later stages, reflecting more directly the dementia's systemic deterioration.[48] Individuals suffering depression at a younger age are nearly twice as likely to be diagnosed years later with Alzheimer's. That is, chronic depression may be a biological risk factor, predisposing them to more global cognitive deterioration. Or the conditions may both be outcomes of a shared origin and pathway. For example, mini-strokes and other cardiovascular or neurological pathology could affect brain structures and processes involving cognition and emotional feelings or expression. Untangling cause and effect, the confounding dynamics of neurological, endocrine, immunologic, vascular, psychological, and social factors, is difficult in research, as it is in any individual person.

While scientists attempt to pinpoint the origin, physiological processes, and neurological locale involved in depression and dementia, the pressing concern for affected individuals and their families revolves around potential treatments, as well as daily interactions and care. Knowing the substantial risks and overuse of medications for the old, I initially favored nonpharmacological efforts for my parents as a safer strategy to ease depression and other psychological and behavioral symptoms.[49] Such efforts include adjusting the physical environment or other aspects of an individual's living arrangements, eliminating sources of pain or discomfort, and correcting hearing and vision loss. In some instances, individuals may respond to psychotherapy, peer counseling, senior center social activities, increased physical activity, a rediscovered hobby or musical instrument, companionship of a pet. My parents did not seem likely candidates for any of these approaches, however, particularly my father. And he was the more immediate problem.

Identifying the point at which the benefits of medical treatment outweigh the risks is a difficult call. I found myself following a common medical approach: rely on the best diagnostic information available and then proceed with a trial-and-error process. In other words, use it if it seems to help, as long as the side effects remain tolerable.

For my father, antidepressant medication did appear to help, for at least some stretch of time. Not only did his emotional condition improve—with fewer episodes of crying or anger or saying we would all be better off if he were dead—so too did his speech and cognitive focus. He could follow more lines of thought, seeming more often to rejoin us. We could sit at the dinner table and engage in some level of conversation once again. He could comprehend, sound amused, and laugh at something funny. Whether the apparent cognitive improvement resulted from lifting depression itself or from the medication's more direct physiological effects—a neurochemical bonus that parallels antidepressant effects—was not clear. Nor was medication a cure. He did not regain his former mental abilities or personality, and with time the improvement dissipated into the continued decline of dementia.

My own medical philosophy required greatest scrutiny when the next question became: Should my mother also begin taking an antidepressant? I knew that depression is a risk among family caregivers, especially a spouse. Overall, more women experience depression than do men. I knew too that as a younger adult, my mother had experienced a depressive bout, as did other women on her branch of our family tree. Yet the thought of both parents on antidepressants created for me a conceptual barrier. In principle, I feared using a blanket approach to meeting the psychological needs of the old with drugs. Aside from concerns about side effects, I worried: Should everyone saddened by circumstances of their old age be medicated, to dull the grief and mourning that come with loss of people and perhaps also of their own former existence? For many doctors, the answer is a quick yes, a tendency strongly encouraged by drug company promotions. As one doctor joked, he'd like to put Prozac in the water supply. If depression is an individual's response to some manner of life review toward its end or anticipation of death, is that less reason to ease psychological pain than if its basis is a physiological deficit or imbalance, say, of serotonin or other neurotransmitters? (Said another doctor, "If your mother weren't depressed she'd be crazy.") And why my hesitation over an image of everyone on Prozac, while liberal use of medications to ease physical pain gives me no such pause?

Propelled by the common and urgent desire among patients, their family, their doctor, to do something that might help, and by the irresistible possibility that we might be missing an answer that was out there, I adjusted my concerns in principle to the reality at hand. Not everyone would be taking Prozac, just everyone in that household: two very old individuals living a personally difficult day-to-day existence. They were not experiencing acute grief from which they could expect to rally. Rather, along with more global cognitive decline, they were showing symptoms of depression that, in my father's case, had improved with medication. My mother, even more than he, had gradually withdrawn and become disengaged from conversation and activity. The goal was not to create a sunny disposition, a uniformly happy though numbed demeanor. But their days and nights should at least be bearable, not spent in psychological pain.

And so my mother too began taking a low dose of Prozac, then slightly more. There seemed, perhaps, some improvement, some return of the animation that had drained out of my mother's face, from her entire being. But her response was shallow and short-lived, perhaps again an observer's placebo effect, so strong was my desire to see it work. Several months passed, with both parents on Prozac. For my father, depression became the least of it; we added medications aimed to soften his agitation and combativeness and to moderate the depth of his delusions. My mother was the quiet one. She was not difficult or disruptive; she hewed to the daily routine. Her daily naps grew longer, however, her words fewer and farther between. There was no denying the obvious: if depression was the problem, Prozac was not the answer. Perhaps a different antidepressant, I repeated to their doctor, knowing that several other brands compete avidly for Prozac's market. Yet that *if* nagged at me. She didn't cry or express feeling hopeless. She never said she was unhappy, when asked. But then, she didn't say or do much of anything. The only way I could describe it, to friends or family, to the doctor: she just seems to be not there.

"I had a patient like that once," their doctor recalled, his clinical memory jarred by my description over the phone. What had helped her was not an antidepressant but a stimulant, an amphetamine. As he put it, that old person needed "a kick-start." We would wean my mother off Prozac and try her on speed.

It took a good two weeks, longer than the doctor expected, and then the change was abrupt, as if she awoke one morning and was suddenly awake. The first hint: a full sentence I overheard her say to her daytime caregiver, the mere fact that she said it as telling as what she said ("It's a long day"). And then, she made a phone call on her own; later looking out her bedroom window she told me, "That tree needs trimming," which it did.

An explanation, possibly, came by chance soon after, in a medical journal article shared with members of a biweekly eldercare group at the university. A retired psychology professor, whose wife's uncharacteristic behavior probably reflected early Alzheimer's disease, had discovered a review of studies describing a little-recognized and poorly understood syndrome captured by the label *apathy*. Behavioral symptoms, looking much like depression, reveal a distinct pathology that captured almost perfectly my mother's demeanor. The core characteristic, loss of motivation, appears in an individual as diminished initiative, poor persistence, reduced physical activities and speech, lack of interest in activities, indifference, fatigue, social withdrawal and low social engagement, blunted emotional response and expression, lack of insight.[50] For that individual, such behaviors and emotion mark a change rather than a lifelong pattern or temperament, a change that may be gradual enough that even close family fail to appreciate its full extent.

Fortunately, I was able to obtain more solid confirmation of the nature of my mother's impairment. I realized, belatedly, that she could be assessed by a highly experienced psychologist who participates in the team approach at the Over 60 Health Center. So I arranged a consultation with Dr. Laura Carstensen, of Stanford University, to gain a firmer basis for sorting out depression and dementia and deciding about appropriate medications. Indeed, after talking with my mother and administering tests of memory and other mental abilities, Dr. Carstensen observed no evidence of depression. For instance, my mother responded to her and to other people socially and even with some humor, seeming to enjoy the interaction. She did, however, exhibit significant short-term memory loss and a deficit often seen in dementia—an inability to initiate and pursue, on her own, cognitive activities. In fact, at her level of dementia, the signs of which had probably first appeared four to five years earlier, she likely no longer retained enough memory to be depressed.

As is the case in much research on dementia, the most studied patients are people diagnosed with Alzheimer's disease, in whom apathy may be the most common behavioral aspect, occurring in as much as

90 percent of cases.[51] Evidence also suggests that people (like my mother) with other types of dementia experience this syndrome. Measured by the most widely used screening tests, the crucial impairment underlying the behaviors and emotional characteristics reflects most prominently a loss of mental processes that select, plan, and implement cognitive and behavioral tasks, a deficit in organization and direction termed *executive cognitive dysfunction*. For my mother, I came to realize, the effort to initiate and formulate her own thoughts, to order events and intentions and meanings, then express them in full sentences and in actions had become, in a sense, overwhelming and exhausting.

This concept of apathy represents more than a change of descriptive terminology. Key questions focus not on what cognitive abilities an individual has lost, but on what she can still do, given a motivational push, the kick-start. And what type of push is best, pharmacological or not? Such questions, in turn, are central to the way family members, friends, and caregivers perceive and interact with that individual. First they must recognize that the problem is not primarily that an individual has given up or doesn't care; then they can introduce activities, social stimulation, and daily routines that bring out his existing abilities through engagement with the world.

Clearly, attention to an apathy syndrome adds to the complexity of identifying and treating dementia and depression, as well as to determining rates of these conditions among the old. Furthermore, the research suggests that any bandwagon approach toward diagnosing depression and prescribing antidepressants may bypass a more helpful tactic for many individuals. I gained some reassurance from reported pharmacological evidence supporting use of stimulant medications, amphetamines. To my consternation, however, certain antidepressants, Prozac for one, may actually cause symptoms of apathy. For all I know, then, my mother's improvement resulted not from taking an amphetamine but from no longer taking Prozac, though I like to think both of these simultaneous changes helped.[52]

Apathy and depression may coexist within an individual, and studies suggest they do so at varying rates for people with differing types of dementia, findings consistent with considering apathy a distinct syndrome (see figure 8). So too, individuals with minimal cognitive deficit, whose behavior does not display apathy, may suffer depression. In these individuals, the most prominent characteristics of depression are easier to tease apart. Although symptoms of low interest, energy, and activity may be common to both conditions, depression is marked by a strong

8. COMPARING SYMPTOMS OF APATHY AND DEPRESSION IN PEOPLE WITH DEMENTIA

APATHY	COMMON TO BOTH	DEPRESSION
Blunted or absent emotional response	Diminished interest	Dysphoria or sadness
Indifference	Slowed psychological and motor abilities	Suicidal thoughts
Low social engagement	Fatigue, excessive sleep	Self-criticism
Diminished initiation of activities, speech	Lack of insight	Pessimism or feeling of hopelessness

Based on Landes et al. 2001, table 3.

emotional dimension that psychologists call dysphoria: sadness, guilt, self-criticism, hopelessness, and helplessness. In contrast, apathy is notable for the lack of emotional response. As explained in the research review: "The loss of interest seen in depression may be related to feelings of despair, pessimism, and hopelessness, and it is this cognitive perspective, as well as the dysphoria of depression, that distinguishes it from apathy. Self-criticism and negative thoughts about the future that are common in depression are also absent in the apathetic individual, who instead shows a lack of concern."[53] In this scheme, regardless of my parents' psychological history as younger adults, in old age it was my father, not my mother, who was more clearly depressed, and far from apathetic.

As with their health care more generally, the most effective depression treatment for older adults may employ a team approach, which might include medication and/or psychotherapy, rather than relying on a primary care doctor, who may or may not prescribe an antidepressant.[54] In the team approach, a nurse or psychologist would coordinate care with the patient's primary care doctor, a psychiatrist, and family members. Very importantly, this care coordinator would maintain ongoing contact and follow-up with the depressed individual. Agencies already serving a community's older adults may be able to incorporate such home-based mental health care.[55]

As research continues to piece together the mental puzzle comprised, at the least, of dementia, depression, and apathy, several concerns are already clear:

- Caregivers and family can easily overlook apathy and other signs of cognitive impairment and dementia, particularly when the affected individual lives in the shadow of others who are agitated and disruptive, whether a spouse at home or residents of a care facility. As in a school classroom, the quiet ones may not receive their fair share of needed attention and stimulation, the routines and interactions that support cognitive abilities and social engagement. Independent of my father, my mother could enjoy seeing people and hearing music at a nearby senior center; after her medication change, she could again choose to sit in the garden on sunny days after lunch. And we could recognize and attend to her experience of dementia.

- Older adults may be subject to undertreatment of depression overall, but also in many cases to inappropriate treatment for those individuals not clearly or exclusively depressed. That is, doctors may prescribe an antidepressant, then never look back to reassess a patient's condition and monitor responses to the drug. (My own theory, based on a sample of two: any neurochemical jolt may produce an initial but transient improvement.) Furthermore, if an antidepressant is ineffective, perhaps the individual is not depressed; simply trying other antidepressants may not help. Indeed, stopping the antidepressant may provide greater benefit and lower risks.

- Pharmaceutical manufacturers market heavily their costly brand-name antidepressant and antipsychotic drugs as the modern medical approach. No drug company promotes an older, cheaper, generic medication—such as long-available stimulants—that may be the more appropriate choice. Nor do drug manufacturers inform doctors of effective nonpharmaceutical methods of handling various behavioral problems of patients experiencing dementia, depression, and/or apathy. (In addition, doctors may hesitate over the more tightly regulated and monitored prescribing process for amphetamines.)

- Older adults metabolize drugs differently than do younger patients or the subjects in drug tests, a physiological process affecting how quickly a medication clears out of the body, whether it accumulates, how soon effects on the central nervous system will be observable, and how long effects will last.[56] Older patients' responses may differ, therefore, from what a doctor expects, requiring particular care in monitoring beneficial and adverse effects.

· Just as drug manufacturers drum into doctors' and consumers' heads a medication's name and patients' need for it, doctors and the public need to drum into their heads that cutting back or eliminating a drug may be the appropriate choice. Most important, finding the right drug and dose for any individual requires time and attention and patience. For my mother-in-law, a new antipsychotic medication eased her nightly anxiety at feeling she was not in her apartment; but with time she grew lethargic, and slept most of the day in her chair, barely able to talk with family or caregivers. Taken off the medication, she regained energy and alertness. However, anxiety did creep back in, requiring a finer tuning of her particular drug regimen.

As with other mental disorders, research is revealing underpinnings in brain chemistry and structure that may contribute to depression and apathy, as well as to dementia. Biological explanations are appealing for reasons beyond greater understanding and potential for developing remedies. Most prominently, as in cases of bipolar disorder or schizophrenia, whatever onus was placed previously on individuals who experience depression, apathy, dementia, or other cognitive loss—some personal weakness or fault, failure to try hard enough—can rightfully be dismissed. Yet the danger is that biological explanations, and hope for a medical fix, can remove onus and responsibility from society, minimizing social resources committed to nonpharmacological treatment approaches and care that extends beyond custodial. Mental health care has long received scant reimbursement support from Medicare and other insurers.[57]

Limits of bioneurology may be most evident with regard to depression. To whatever extent depression reflects an individual's perception of his life and surroundings, and however such perceptions interact with physiological processes, there is a question of why many old people feel unhappy, hopeless, and helpless in their living situations. What is it about how the old live, how society defines their role and their behaviors, how they interact with other people, and how other people—including family members, doctors, other caregivers—perceive and relate to them? Especially important, what choices do individuals perceive for themselves, what resources, what alternatives to institutional living or isolation at home, what activities and relationships that seem worth pursuing? Must a patient feel she has "nothing left to live for," telling her doctor she is "so very, very tired of living . . . [she] just wants to die?"[58] Indeed, turning the biological explanation around a bit, the question should perhaps become: Does life as an old person in this country result, for some individuals, in psychological as well as physical disease?

GRASPING AGE

I could have done some things differently as my parents aged. Encouraging greater mental stimulation and social interactions would surely not have hurt. I can imagine repeatedly insisting that my father try the magnifying devices he rejected, on the chance he might ultimately agree. His near blindness from macular degeneration, loss of reading, of seeing faces and other sights likely exacerbated his cognitive decline. I can imagine reading to him daily and encouraging my mother to do the same, an activity good for her as well. Though I couldn't help viewing my parents as a couple blended by long marriage, I could also have better recognized two individuals and paid equal attention to the passive, quiet one. I could have pushed my mother to maintain and join new social activities in the community, to continue sewing or quilting classes, in a greater effort to prevent her withdrawal from other people into stultifying isolation. Such imaginings, as if grown children are able to shape the way aged parents live their lives, spring from two concepts, reflecting current though incomplete knowledge about aging.

> *The usual need not be considered normal.* Though everyone experiences age-related changes in health and in physical and mental abilities, nothing delineates normal aging as an immutable, inevitable sequence of physical and cognitive loss. Unlike child development, with its sequence of milestones describing normal cognitive and physical growth, older aging varies considerably among individuals of the same chronological age and within individuals over time. Many physical and mental declines now attributed to old age are symptoms of disease or disability, not part of healthy aging. While greater age can diminish elders' physiological reserve, many remain quite resilient. Along with appropriate treatment of disease, exercise and dietary changes can at least slow the decline. Researchers note the brain's plasticity, which allows for relearning or remembering in different ways. Cognitive

training can improve memory and reasoning skills in people sixty-five and older, although overall effects on performing daily living tasks are not yet known.[59]

Mind and matter intertwine. Most people beyond seventy years experience simultaneous chronic conditions that can impinge on daily life in complex ways. Mild chronic illness or depression, for example, can slow response time, an intricate mental and physical action essential for such daily activities as driving. Depression may also exacerbate arthritis pain and stiffness.[60] Incontinence has a neurological component more complex than an aged bladder; moreover, a sudden urge during the night can lead to falls. My father's difficulty climbing up or down steps, a physical therapist explained, resulted not from a lack of strength but from a neurological lack, an inability to coordinate his brain and muscles through motor planning or follow verbal instructions— where to put his feet on the steps and hands on the rail. Later, he would essentially have to remember, prompted by verbal cues, how to walk each morning, to bend his knees and deliberately move each foot forward, one after the other, in order to get out of bed and move across the room. Eventually, the intertwined nature of physical, cognitive, and psychological conditions can create a spiral of susceptibilities and deterioration. Among the clearest examples: hospitalization of the old, especially with surgery and anesthesia, can result in delirium, mental declines, and a cascade of complications requiring additional intervention.

The dichotomy between body and mind that characterizes Western medicine and its specialized, fragmented approach does not serve people well as they age. With health concerns involving pain, depression, sleep, the loss of physical and mental abilities and of social contacts, attempts to untangle the physiological and psychological dynamics can be particularly difficult, and often nonproductive. The impact of stress reduction on an individual's health and longevity remains poorly understood and understudied (see figure 9).

The role of satisfying and stimulating social interactions in maintaining physical and psychological health remains an enigma as well. Among older adults, the brain's capacity for relearning or rerouting mental messages in response to age-related cognitive decline, the underpinning of memory and other mental abilities, may depend at a basic physiological level on maintaining adequate communication between

9. SYMPTOMS NOT NECESSARILY CAUSED BY AGING

confusion
memory and other cognitive decline
anxiety
depression
mania
insomnia
sexual problems
shortness of breath
weakness
urinary incontinence
balance and mobility problems

Based on *Consumer Reports on Health,* vol. 16 (April 2004).

nerve cells. Yet scientists' speculation regarding these neurological pathways broadens immediately to questions about the source for such cellular communications; for instance, mental stimulation of interaction within a complex social environment involves not only specific cognitive tasks but also activities, thoughts, language use, interpersonal relationships that come with social engagement and feelings of "useful connectedness." Interestingly, one recent study of social networks and dementia found that quality of social contacts was more important than quantity.[61] For example, individuals who had unsatisfactory contacts with their children were more likely to develop dementia than those with no children. Purposeful and satisfying interactions tended to be two-way, in contrast to only receiving assistance or social visits. Being single or living alone was not so much a problem as living alone *and* having no friends, relatives, or other close and satisfying social ties.

Threats to health and well-being for older adults can be surprisingly simple and common. Falls, for instance, become a significant source of fractures, head injury, skin wounds and subsequent infection. Among people over sixty-five years, more than a third fall each year, and half of these are recurrent fallers, including "abnormally frequent fallers."[62] Of those who break a hip, 50 percent never regain their pre-fall mobility or independence, and 25 percent die within a year.[63] The list of reasons for falls is long and can be quite involved. Poor eyesight, of course, makes tripping more likely. Dizziness and poor balance are obvious though overlooked culprits that may in turn relate to problems with sleep or blood pressure or nutrition and weight (over- or underweight, diabetes or low blood sugar). Some medications commonly used to treat health problems themselves contribute to dizziness, sudden drops in blood pressure, imbalance, and falls, especially sedatives and other sleep medications, antidepressants, or combinations of several medications whatever their type, a frequent practice among the old. In addition to prescribed and over-the-counter drugs, excessive alcohol consumption, often a form of self-medication, leads to falls. Or the inability to bend over to tie or even to see shoelaces may mean an individual, like my father, falls. Moreover, an older individual's fear of falling causes more serious health consequences than most people realize. The fear itself can lead to lost mobility and strength, perhaps to depression and then antidepressants (or excessive alcohol)—any of which in turn increases the risk of actual falls (which can precipitate nursing-home placement, a realistic element of many people's fear). This fear is serious and frequent enough to merit a front-page *New York Times* report, as well as attention from gerontologists.[64]

Prevention can include simple measures: removing slippery throw rugs and low objects that invite a fall, adding grab bars and a shower chair in bathrooms. With bone fracture a major concern, particularly for postmenopausal women with osteoporosis, a physician may prescribe medication intended to strengthen bone. While appropriate for many older women with dangerously low bone-density measures, and while underprescribed for some high-risk women, medication for osteoporosis presents a classic prescribing dilemma. Thus, a doctor laments that her own eighty-plus-year-old mother currently takes Fosomax although any benefit is marginal, given her age and already long-existing osteoporosis. The prescribing physician had never taken time to discuss risks and benefits. He is not a bad doctor, the daughter comments, merely a participant, along with everyone else, within "a badly broken health care system. . . . Meanwhile, my mother continues to fork out $66.47 for [four Fosomax pills], while the scatter rugs still litter her hallway floor."[65]

Additional measures, less profitable for drug manufacturers, may help prevent falls. For example, recent studies suggest vitamin D supplements reduce fall risk by increasing muscle strength as well as increasing bone density.[66] Doctors can play a more central role in preventing older women's and men's falls and fractures.[67] When patients reach their seventies, doctors can ask yearly about the occurrence and circumstances of falls. Along with regular evaluation of vision, blood pressure, muscle strength, and other health conditions affecting balance, doctors can assess a patient's balance and steadiness when walking. They can recommend bone-strengthening exercise and advise wearing shoes with slip-resistant soles (and avoid walking barefoot altogether). They can alter an individual's medications, minimize use of sedatives, and reduce the total number of drugs, as well as employ methods to avert prescription errors and monitor medication's effects. Nonmedical alternatives for pain control, such as acupuncture and biofeedback, are effective for some people and avoid drugs' dangerous side effects. Psychotherapy or peer support groups are helpful in treating some depressions.

For older adults who are already frail, doctors can enlist a physical therapist to work on strength and balance exercises, on the use of a cane or walker. An occupational therapist can focus on the ability to navigate safely at home, including identifying and eliminating physical hazards (loose rugs and cords, stairs without railings, poor lighting) and risky behaviors (carrying laundry or packages down stairways, standing on an unsteady chair to reach high objects). Exercise programs at home can help maintain abilities and recover them after acute illness or hospitalization.[68] In fact, a recent study indicates that a combination of exercise, home safety measures, and vision correctives most effectively reduces falls (16 percent over eighteen months). Among these interventions, exercise to improve leg strength, flexibility, and balance, by itself or with the other measures, provided the greatest benefit in preventing falls.[69]

Walking four hours or more per week, even standing rather than sitting, can lower bone fracture risk.[70] More broadly, recent studies of longevity, and especially of aging with minimal disease and disability, find that moderate but regular physical exercise—including walking, tai chi, light aerobics, and strength training—helps older people maintain not only better physical condition, with improved balance and flexibility (reducing likelihood of falls), but also better cognitive function and mental outlook.[71] Research focused on aerobic exercise and cardiovascular fitness in older adults indicates improved brain efficiency, plasticity, and adaptability, and improved performance of cognitive tasks; as in animal models, these results may reflect more adequate blood supply and nerve cell communication, as well as new nerve cell development.[72]

Unfortunately, the measures cited here do not commonly receive the push that medications and technology do. Doctors are not trained to encourage these other interventions, nor do such measures profit corporations involved in medical care. Medicare reimbursements do not encourage preventive and health-supporting care. And at some point certain measures bump hard against individual borders of personal autonomy and will. For my father in his nineties, despite recurrent falls, attempts to supervise his walking or showering or climbing stairs (carpeted) were infringements with which he simply refused to live.

Falls, of course, are a single slice through an older person's daily existence. As memory becomes less trustworthy or signs of dementia appear, added safeguards become essential for people living at home—for example, coffeemakers, irons, heaters, and gas appliances should be equipped with automatic turn-off switches. Homes of the future will undoubtedly feature other inventions designed to accommodate aging in mind and body, a positive dimension of commercial marketing to baby boomers.[73] Future generations may also benefit from their greater familiarity and comfort with nonmedical alternatives for pain or depression, with goals more generally of preventive health care and wellness promotion. Even so, they cannot dodge worry about acquiring physical ailments and, even more, about losing their mind. And now the latter worry starts much earlier, I can attest, by about the age of fifty. It arises from observing the oldest old and repeated commercial messages, but also from knowing that mental abilities are so fundamental to defining ourselves and to living independently, and that ideas about prevention, about ways to protect ourselves, are currently so tentative at best.

SEARCHING FOR HEALTH AND LONGEVITY

"When you break a bone . . . and you will," my doctor said, conveying my risk given a precocious development of osteoporosis. An overly pessimistic, alarmist view? Or a realistic assessment shared with a well-informed patient deciding whether to take medication that brings risks of its own? For many people, the search for health and longevity takes sharpest focus within the doctor's office, the scatter of information and anecdote concentrating into personal do's and don'ts. How today's midlife women and men pursue their personal health quest, what they can draw from their parents' generation, and from ongoing research on aging, is the focus of concern here.

I try to remember when our kitchen counter was not so cluttered with pill bottles. The collection started small: basic daily multivitamins, then extra vitamin C to fight colds, then calcium. By the time middle age was no longer a novelty, the collection included vitamin E, said to help prevent cancer and possibly Alzheimer's disease; estrogen (later eliminated) and a nonhormonal drug to prevent bone fractures by slowing the osteoporosis I was too late to prevent; a progesterone to avert the uterine cancer risk from the estrogen; my husband's daily aspirin to prevent heart disease and the most frequent type of stroke, caused by blood clots (though it may contribute to brain hemorrhage, the less frequent type). My latest added bottle is lutein, which my eye doctor said he would take, even on the meager preventive evidence, if he had a parent blinded by macular degeneration. I do try also to eat leafy greens. When I take ibuprofen for aches and pains, which seems often, I remind myself of preliminary suggestions that long-term use of such drugs may help ward off Alzheimer's disease by fighting an inflammatory process in the brain, even though early studies of anti-inflammatory medications have not supported this hypothesis.[74] My husband and I line up behind older people for flu shots each year (absent a vaccine shortage). We have passed through our oat-bran phase but remain aware that monounsaturated fats are far preferable to saturated or to trans fats, the newest and most threatening demon. The diets followed by friends and relations range from macrobiotic and vegan to the protein-larded Atkins', their exercise regimens from walking to running, from stationary bicycles to the full-blown twenty-four-hour health club with personal trainer included. Yoga proceeds in rooms that are comfortable or hot. No one smokes.

American medicine has long aimed most of its resources at curing disease, often through heroic surgical or aggressive chemical treatments. Now the hunt is on, within the medical world and the alternative domain, for ways to prevent, or at least postpone and minimize, age-related illnesses and disabilities, including such formidable targets as cancer, heart disease, stroke, dementia, and arthritis. The list of preventive measures—medications, herbs, diets, and nutrients—changes in the specifics, as promising possibilities appear, receive their moment of fame (and, for some promoters, fortune), then fade for lack of evidence that they prevent anything. For the baby boom generations who coined the term "proactive," taking health-promoting and -protective steps is natural (as much of the material used supposedly is).

As with medical treatments, however, many preventive measures require individuals to weigh the desired benefits—less chance of developing a disease or disability—against known and potential risks of the measure itself. Widely used examples include postmenopausal estrogen replacement, cholesterol-lowering drugs, and anti-inflammatories. Often information for such a decision is incomplete and changing, as well as clouded by unsupported promotional claims.

Beyond the continuous appearance of uncertain, controversial, and frequently failed preventatives, the list has retained several mainstays, as well as a few apparently little-harm-in-trying protective measures. Among the mainstays that may preserve mental health, including cognitive abilities, are several recommendations that also benefit cardiovascular health by controlling blood pressure (hypertension) and cholesterol, lowering the risk of heart disease and stroke, and possibly protecting against some cancers as well. These measures include not smoking (the clearest way to prevent lung cancer as well as an ever-broadening range of other health problems); controlling weight; exercising regularly; eating nutritious foods that are low in saturated and trans-fat but high in monounsaturated fats (olive oil and nuts) and in beta-carotene, calcium, B-vitamins and folic acid, antioxidant vitamins E and C (see figures 10 and 11).[75] Frequent but not excessive alcohol consumption may also be good for cardiovascular health. And, although following such measures into older age benefits overall health, some research suggests that individuals who reach their late eighties without significant cardiovascular disease were probably at low risk for cholesterol-related problems in the first place. For others, early detection of hypertension or heart disease may suggest more aggressive intervention with medications.[76] A rather different type of preventive measure stems from evidence that head trauma at any age may predispose an individual to later dementia, suggesting the need, at any age, to use vehicle seat belts, wear helmets when bicycling, take precautions when playing sports, and forgo boxing.[77] Identifying and treating depression is important, as well as following recommendations that can bring mental health benefits, more generally, including stress-reduction measures, adequate sleep, stimulating and satisfying life activities.

Especially noteworthy is the accumulating evidence that an essential proactive health measure may be activity itself, physical and mental. A study following white middle-class women through middle age, for example, found that those who remained active (taking walks each day,

10. FACTORS THAT MAY INCREASE RISK FOR COGNITIVE DECLINE

GENETIC FACTORS

Female gender

Apoe4 genotype

MEDICAL CONDITIONS (ESPECIALLY COEXISTING CONDITIONS)

Hypertension (high blood pressure)

Heart disease

Diabetes

Elevated low-density lipoprotein cholesterol (LDL)

High homocysteine levels (an amino acid)

Transitory ischemic attacks (TIAs, "mini-strokes")

Head trauma

Environmental toxic exposure (especially to lead)

LIFESTYLE CONTRIBUTIONS

Smoking

Substance abuse, including alcohol and drugs

Lack of physical activity

PSYCHOLOGICAL AND SOCIAL FACTORS

Low educational attainment

Isolation or lack of social interaction

Lack of stimulating leisure activities

High stress and excessive response to stress (elevated cortisol levels)

Based on Institute for the Study of Aging 2001.

---

gardening, swimming, playing tennis or golf) were more able to perform daily activities on their own into their seventies than were sedentary age-mates.[78] Among even sedentary women and men over the age of sixty-five, increased physical activity results in lowered mortality rates; for people over seventy, just one day of restricted activity, due to illness or injury, contributes to more general functional decline.[79] Regular physical activity (including walking) throughout adult life helps maintain mental abilities as well.[80] In addition, mental exercise (participating in classes or discussion groups, learning to speak a new language or use a computer, working on crossword puzzles, engaging in regular social interactions) can contribute to mental acuity and emotional satis-

11. MEASURES THAT MAY PROTECT AGAINST COGNITIVE DECLINE

Challenging mental activities

Physical activity

Social activities and interactions

Sensory aids if needed—hearing aids, eye glasses, magnifying equipment

Daily stress-reduction techniques—e.g., leisure activities, meditation, yoga

Informal and professional help for depression, grief, loneliness

Adequate restful sleep at night

High-nutrition, moderate-calorie diet, including antioxidant fruits and vegetables

Daily multivitamin/mineral supplement, but not excessive doses

Safety measures to avoid head trauma—seat belts, bike helmet, no boxing

Not smoking

Moderate alcohol consumption at most

Appropriate treatment to control high blood pressure, high levels of undesirable
  cholesterol, diabetes, and heart and other cardiovascular disease

Based on Institute for the Study of Aging 2001.

---

faction. Particularly important, according to some psychologists, is novelty, challenging the mind with new, stimulating, nonroutine tasks.[81]

The importance of a stimulating environment for the cognitive development of babies and children has long been demonstrated. Recent neurological research, however, is contradicting long-accepted views that the brain's physiological development halts after childhood. Significant and initially controversial studies of primates show that the adult brain can generate new brain cells, a process previously considered impossible.[82] New brain cells or not, mental activity throughout early and middle adulthood may help establish a crucial reserve of nerve cell connections. Performing new and challenging mental tasks, researchers suggest, activates and thereby maintains nerve cell receptors that transmit chemical messages between cells. One case-control study of people diagnosed with Alzheimer's disease found that they had engaged in fewer nonoccupational activities between the ages of twenty and sixty than similar people without Alzheimer's. The diversity of activities and their intellectual challenge were two characteristics of "environmental complexity" that most distinguished the latter group.[83] These results are consistent with a prospective study of 469 women and men over seventy-five years old to identify those who developed various types of dementia during an approximately five-year follow-up.[84] As with the nuns' early writing samples, a simple association cannot determine cause and effect; that is, fewer challenging mental activities could be an outcome of early, subclinical cognitive impairment rather than a cause contributing to the later Alzheimer's loss. The findings, and possible underlying relations, are intriguing nonetheless.

In sum, current knowledge on extended development and then decline of the brain indicates that all of us, including laypeople and their physicians (even pediatricians), need to pay greater attention to the way various health problems (e.g., hypertension, cardiovascular disease, obesity, depression), treatments (medications, surgeries), activities (reading, aerobic exercise, soccer, or boxing), habits (diet, using seatbelts and helmets) might affect mental capacities. Moreover, rather than a medication or other substance to ingest, "use it or lose it"—and especially "try it" in novel ways—may be a nostrum that applies to an increasing number of characteristics defining good mental and physical health at any age.

AVOIDING HYPE

Long before my doctor's prediction of broken bones I could conjure up an alarmist view, if not from personal acquaintance then surely from the frail, bent women featured in advertisements for calcium supplements or new bone-enhancing drugs. Or, in place of scare tactics, a commercial counterimage might inspire me: the active, vigorous, gray-haired tennis player, the arthritis-free gardener. The positive image more closely matches an emphasis shaping many current studies in epidemiology and public health, the pursuit of "successful aging." The goal is to identify characteristics, behaviors, and interventions that allow people to avoid disease and disability, maintain good physical and cognitive functioning, remain engaged in productive activities and in satisfying social relationships.[85] This goal marks a shift in the study of aging from a focus on curing specific diseases and extending the length of life, still the emphasis of much medical practice, to concern with identifying factors that support a good quality of life in later years.

Those now or soon to be middle-aged already enjoy some prospect of preventing certain of the health problems seen in their parents and of benefiting from emerging treatments for chronic, degenerative, and life-threatening disease. Yet this same population also faces the daunting challenge of sorting the helpful from the hype. While the media, popular writing, and commercial interests portray successful agers as fit, healthy, and wealthy, there seems little hesitation to take advantage of common middle-age fears about old age. Among the most blatant of sales pitches: a full-page advertisement announcing a new, advanced, memory-enhancing dietary supplement, indeed touting it as "the *next generation* in memory enhancement" (emphasis added). In the largest print above a very middle-class, middle-aged woman (as well as on the product's box): "You don't have to be a senior to need Senior Moment." (On the company's Web page I also saw information on lawn and garden, pet and agricultural products.) That message aims, of course, at what a recent report on longevity and "cognitive vitality" describes as "perhaps the greatest fear of old age . . . losing one's mind."[86]

Any number of commercial products now lay claim to all manner of cure—herbal memory concoctions compete with Senior Moment in the twenty-first-century battle against what our parents' generation called senility. Major-brand beverages boast additives that combat arthritis, alleviate anxiety and depression, stimulate the immune system, and relieve everyday stress. Another full page of newsprint advertises a specific combination of amino acids and nutrients that, sprayed into the nose, speeds and increases the body's release of human growth hormone, claimed essential to staving off the aging process, satisfaction guaranteed (no mention of already known risks, let alone the unknown). Asks this ad, "Do you suffer ANY of these signs of aging?" Of course, anyone over the age of thirty-five skimming this list of twenty signs would have to answer yes. A pamphlet arrives in the mail: "Pinpoint the true cause of aging and memory loss." Such promotions are a long way from earlier Clairol hair coloring or Grecian Formula to cover the gray. Like so many patent medicines of a previous century, the unregulated potions and pills flood the market with little regard for safety or side effects and no valid data on efficacy. One scientifically controlled study of a widely used ginkgo biloba product found no improvement in memory or other related cognitive tasks, contrary to the manufacturer's claims, among healthy older adults.[87] Whether such products benefit more seriously impaired individuals remains unknown. Most herbal remedies have never been studied to determine benefits or risks. Though often assumed benign by virtue of being natural, herbs and other added substances can provoke harmful side effects or dangerous interactions with prescription and over-the-counter medications.

The lines are not always so clear between commercial exploitation of fears about old age, on the one hand, and information pertinent to lifestyle or medical decisions, on the other. Today the public has ready access to numerous health newsletters written for laypeople (published by the *New England Journal of Medicine*, the Mayo Clinic, Harvard Medical School, UC Berkeley School of Public Health, and Consumers' Union, to name a few), some with a focus on aging. Print media, radio, and television pour out medical information, while the Internet—that most recent and least tamed mix of help, hype, and sheer fiction—now reigns as a major medical resource for a public searching day and night the innumerable medical Web sites. Drug manufacturers have long blurred boundaries between prohibited promotional claims and allowable educational communication. The process is already gathering steam regarding unproven though potentially lucrative preventive medications for unproven though possibly pre-dementia symptoms of memory loss and mild cognitive impairment. As with the assisted living facilities discussed in the previous chapter, commercial promotions for memory medications, antidepressant drugs and vitality drinks target today's middle-aged, who may be thinking first about their parents, but then, before long, before it is too late, about themselves.

LIMITS OF LONGEVITY

When I was a child, my unlucky friends were those whose parent died young, usually a father who dropped dead from a heart attack. Notable progress in preventing and treating heart disease means today's children need not dwell on that particular fear. During the intervening forty-five or so years, many of the men and women who parented the baby boom have avoided heart attacks, as well as influenza, pre-vaccine polio, pneumonia, and other causes of early death. These survivors represent the first cohort living long enough to display in significant numbers the memory loss and dementia age can bring, loss of sight from macular degeneration, Parkinson's disease, osteoporosis, various cancers, and a range of chronic illnesses and disabilities.

Seeing among today's oldest old both the hardy and frail, the cognitively sharp and severely impaired, the middle-aged are wondering: Will I live that long? Will I be physically strong and mentally with-it? These personal questions have their more scientific versions. While biologists investigate how the human organism works, how and when it breaks down, epidemiologists are studying rates and patterns of mortality (death) and morbidity (illness, disabilities) in human populations, and attempting to project changes over the next decades. Today's middle-aged should be aware that epidemiologists disagree about health prospects as this cohort grows old; the argument arises over two potential futures, one sounding distinctly more morbid than the other.

The optimistic prognosis envisions fewer adult years of illness and disability, resembling the notion, cited above, of successful aging.[88] As people live longer, according to this assessment, they will gain more healthy and vigorous years, pushing illness and disability into a shorter time span, closer to the age of death, which will occur on the average at eighty-five years. Improvements in health quality and a delay in developing chronic and terminal disease will outpace increases in length of life.[89] This forecast, known as the *compression of morbidity* and proposed initially twenty-five years ago, gained preliminary support from a recent study sponsored by the National Institute on Aging.[90] Among Americans older than sixty-five, the proportion with chronic disabilities (including effects of stroke and dementia) declined significantly throughout the study period (1982–99), particularly during the late 1990s. The investigators cite greater attention to diet and exercise, fewer people smoking, and increasingly effective medical treatments as reasons for the improvement. Similarly, another research group, noting that Americans who reach the age of sixty-five presently average an additional eighteen years of life, found that the individuals with fewest cardiovascular risks at middle age (nonsmokers with healthy blood pressure and cholesterol levels, no heart abnormalities) scored higher than others in their cohort on quality of life and disease measures twenty-six years later (at an average age of 73.2 years).[91] With baby boomers even more attuned than their parents to preventive measures and healthful living, coming decades could see this trend accelerate.

Yet a population over the age of sixty-five encompasses a broad age span and a number of subgroups. Already, trends toward improvement appear most robust among better educated, more affluent Americans.[92] Beyond persistent socioeconomic and racial disparities, the health of Americans sixty-five to seventy-five or even up to eighty-five may be quite different from that of those approaching ninety and beyond. As a species, humans may be genetically endowed to live until about eighty-five; favorable environmental conditions, including diet, exercise, and other preventive health measures, may help individuals reach this genetic potential. As mentioned earlier, a small proportion of the population may carry genetic combinations that lower their susceptibility to illness and/or increase their biological sturdiness, protecting them against cancers, heart disease, dementias. Research on how these favorable genetic variations work may contribute to future interventions that improve health over a longer life span. Eventually, so too might the experiments of biological scientists focused on genetic information within cells; researchers are attempting, for instance, to manipulate critical chromosome regions in order to lengthen the life span of the total being (telomeres, or end regions, are recent candidates, at least in worms).

The complexity of human beings and of their development, however, anchors such eventualities within the very hypothetical domain. Efforts to apply knowledge about genes to people's illness and health are proving more difficult than some scientists predicted.[93] Moreover, aging affects a wide spectrum of abilities that decline at varying rates and result in varying consequences for daily life. Some age-related declines profoundly impact a person's daily functioning, others remain quite manageable. For now, the rising numbers of women and men moving through their eighties could also mean the epidemiological data will take a turn for the worse, a prospect suggested in projections that yearly diagnosis of new Alzheimer's disease cases could double by 2050, as the last of the baby boomers become the oldest old.[94] Such a turn would create a decidedly different pattern, known as the *expansion of morbidity.* The nearly thirty-year increase in human life expectancy during the twentieth century, this model notes, resulted primarily from improved public health measures: sewage treatment and sanitation, cleaner drinking water, better nutrition, vaccination against major childhood diseases.[95] The time people are now gaining by living longer will amount to more years of chronic disease and disability, conditions avoided in earlier times by earlier death. The great reduction in mortality in youth or middle age leaves more people reaching old age, accumulating a number of health problems for a longer amount of time. They have not prevailed over environmental threats faced by previous generations. Unlike today's hardy survivors, essentially the fittest of their generation, more people will be living past eighty-five on "manufactured survival time," the time produced by improved public health, nutrition, and medicine.[96]

Today medical treatments and technologies do allow individuals to live longer with seriously debilitating, eventually fatal diseases. Heart attack survivors live with chronic heart disease, cancer patients with recurrences, stroke victims with severe incapacitation. Women and men with Parkinson's and Alzheimer's survive into advanced stages of the disease. As one gerontologist puts it, overall "the surviving population, which is already frail, lives longer with a disability that tends to worsen as a function of age."[97] From an evolutionary perspective, explains another, it's not that the human species is "programmed to die, [but] merely insufficiently programmed to survive" so long after the reproductive years.[98] Thus, Dr. Sherwin Nuland, an eminent Yale surgeon and medical historian writing about the process of dying, notes that around 85 percent of the aged population dies from complications resulting from at least one, and usually several, of seven major conditions: atherosclerosis, hypertension, adult diabetes, obesity, Alzheimer's and other dementias, cancer, and lowered resistance to infection. Although he also notes that attributing deaths simply to old age is not politically correct, that diagnosis is basically Nuland's view, one he considers consistent with an ancient Chinese physician's explanation: a man dies when he "can no longer overcome his diseases."[99]

In fact, some characteristics beneficial for early development and reproduction may become liabilities in old age (the process of cell division, essential to early growth, may lose control mechanisms in later life, resulting in cancers). Even granting some delay in onset of morbidity (many of our parents are generally doing well into their eighties), those last years feel stretched unbearably by each individual's deterioration. In other words, the legacy of twentieth-century health-care advances may, in a sense, mean that some people do presently live too long, their bodies holding out beyond what their minds can endure, let alone enjoy.

Unfortunately, this pessimistic projection does sound like my parents, Lillian, my uncle, though they qualify only as anecdotes, not verification. Determining how the next generations will fare late in life awaits population data from years to come. Whichever epidemiological prediction wins, with or without further gains in human life span, the urgent question is not how long people live, but how they feel while still living.

IMAGINING AGE

Toward the end of Gabriel García Marquez's novel *Love in the Time of Cholera,* one of the lovers finally acknowledges his aging. As a younger man, after his mother's death, "the rust of routine . . . had protected him from an awareness of his age. . . . He had behaved as if time would not pass for him but only for others. . . . And he continued in the same way even after his body began sending him the first warning signals. . . . When he had just turned forty, he had gone to the doctor because of vague pains in various parts of his body. After many tests, the doctor had said: 'It's age.' He had returned home without even wondering if any of that had anything to do with him." Now, during a weekly cemetery visit, taming rosebushes that crept over his mother's tomb, he was reviewing his life, "and only then did he realize that his life was passing. He was shaken by a visceral shudder that left his mind blank, and he had to drop the garden tools and lean against the cemetery wall so that the first blow of old age would not knock him down. 'Damn it,' he said, appalled, 'that all happened thirty years ago!'" (218–19).

It is one thing to observe health problems and needs for care in the old, even to acknowledge you are no longer in the bloom of youth yourself. It is quite another to grasp ahead of time the vulnerabilities of aging discussed in the previous pages, or to know just how you want to live when old. Imagining ourselves old may be a key to thinking about our future health and health care. Yet this effort runs against an opposing human tendency—a disconnect between chronological age, especially an aging body, and how an individual feels inside. The anthropologist Sharon Kaufman finds this "ageless self" during interviews with people over the age of seventy. As one eighty-four-year-old woman claims, looking at a photograph of herself at twenty-nine years, "I feel the same now as I did then . . . The only way I know I'm getting old is to look in the mirror. But I've only *felt* old a few times—when I'm really sick."[100] My mother uttered nearly the same words, viewing her shorter, thinner, wrinkled self in a mirror and adding, "How did I get this way?" And in the words of a poet, A. R. Ammons, "Old people don't see much age in old people's faces: they see a young woman in a wreck."

Perhaps it is impossible, then, to really know before getting there how it feels to be old; and the old seem to be the only ones who don't see themselves that way. Something about the way we perceive ourselves and others does strange things as we age, bestowing some neurological gift that helps individuals maintain continuity throughout a long life of many changes. All around me, in lines outside a movie, at restaurants and stores, people grow younger looking. By now, students crowding the university walkways could be fresh out of junior high, the assistant professors barely adult. On television, reporters and spokespeople, the expert consultants look to me like young kids. And yet, aside from a few physical complaints, I would say I am basically me about thirty years ago. Adaptive as this phenomenon may be personally, it does not spur a person to plan for living old, to take needed, or at least prudent, steps while there is still time.

This chapter has considered the vulnerabilities that can undermine an aged individual's ability to live independently. Indeed, watching from close quarters as old age weakens people, both mentally and physically, leads to one dominant conclusion: no wonder the old are vulnerable. They are prey to outright con artists with financial scams that exploit poor memory, confusion, inattention, as well as poor vision or hearing, physical frailty, and immobility. Businesspeople making propositions that are considered more legitimate confuse and take advantage as well: the aggressive young banker bearing new investment opportunities; the phone company caller, phoning to switch service, long-distance or local, whereas most elderly residents don't know which service they already have, let alone knowing one from the other. Until my mother-in-law gained her full-time companion, the family worried about the people she befriended sitting outdoors on the Broadway bench. We worried about phone calls my father answered, or the doorbell, with solicitations imagined and real.

The chapter also suggests potential for the not-yet-old to modify and eventually manage their later years. But today's middle-aged need to bear in mind that the pursuit of successful aging and longer life brings for them its own particular risks. One risk is creation of the worried well—basically healthy individuals overly concerned with every ache or pain or memory slip, potential health hazard, and possibility for preventing disease, never allowing the reasonable indulgences. Certainly, a fine line separates wise concern from hypervigilance. However, the latter surely fuels, even as it is fueled by, commercial development of CT and MRI scans of heart, lung, colon, full body. This latest method is now advertised widely for consumers to monitor their own health (though they are not to worry about the procedure's radiation risks), targeting especially the middle-aged and older, the middle class and above. ("My body scan was the best gift my family ever gave me," declares a happy middle-aged recipient surrounded by that family in December advertisements for gift certificates, covering a choice of scans, appearing in local newspapers directly above a competing advertisement for the $50,000 Jaguar S-Type.) Or an individual can purchase at-home hormone tests detecting age-related declines, with treatment to attain more desirable hormone levels, presumably to slow aging or at least feel younger, merely a toll-free phone call or Web site click away.

The goal of successful aging brings also the related risk of blaming individuals and their chosen lifestyle for inevitable failures. How else to react when magazine articles-cum-advertising supplements declare,

"You're only as old as you feel," or "How quickly you age is largely a choice"; when a publication by the modernized, redefined American Association of Retired People (AARP) claims "Age is just a number, and life is what you make it"; when media and merchants blame too much of what ails us on choices reflecting less-than-wholesome habits. Yet statistics suggest that individual lifestyle behaviors account for less than 25 percent of risks to living a long life. Far more powerful are our socioeconomic circumstances, reflected especially by large disparities in income and the healthfulness of neighborhoods and work environments.[101] And, although white middle-class American women and men can generally count on living into their eighties, there can be no guarantees. Even the wealthy cannot rest assured of filling out the image of fit and healthy. No one can be certain of attaining a personal compression of morbidity, a quick and easy death at a comfortable old age. For the less advantaged in this country—people with less income to spend on prescription drugs, eyeglasses, hearing aids, on health clubs or therapists or fresh fruits and vegetables; people living in unsafe neighborhoods and locked into stressful life circumstances more generally; the uninsured patients spilling into emergency room hallways—the aging process is that much more difficult. Few people will have a genetic forecast or fix, the Human Genome Project notwithstanding. Everyone risks a less than successful effort, with no way to know if and when health problems will arise, how severe or disabling they might be, how gradual or rapid the age-related declines, how much care she or he will need, of what type and at what cost. Described in chapter 1 as the luck of the draw, this certain uncertainty forms the backdrop for the next chapters, which look more closely at aspects of health care that have major impact as people pass through middle age, focusing first on the booming business of prescription drugs.

3

The Pharmaceutical Age
Taking Our Medicine

Three physicians' groups share the waiting area for my parents' doctor; the space is large and open. Without fail, the pharmaceutical representatives stand out from the typical Berkeley assortment of patients middle-aged and older. Known in the past as detailmen, these young men and women are well dressed and coifed. They tote large black carry cases and talk frequently on small cell phones. They talk also with each other about their territory and wares, as might any traveling salespersons whose paths tend to cross. Their pitch to the doctors inside may highlight a new drug their company is pushing; in fact, much of the information doctors obtain about current medications comes from drug manufacturers. These representatives leave free samples, sometimes packaged as "starter-kits," aiming not only to start doctors prescribing and patients taking that product but also to establish brand loyalty for the longer run. They leave logo-embossed pens, Post-its, and prescription pads with drug names conveniently listed. Depending on the season, they may leave free basketball, baseball, or football tickets as well.

This inner-office routine, replicated daily throughout the country, is but one interchange within the much broader and problematic relationship linking patients, doctors, and drug makers. This chapter examines two basic questions about that relationship, highlighting concerns no detailer or marketing tactic will publicize. One is a medical question of appropriate and timely use of prescription drugs, the mainstay in treating health problems that become increasingly common as people leave their fiftieth birthday behind. The other is the question of cost, rising steadily beyond the means of many middle-aged and older adults. The discussion then turns to strategies the pharmaceutical industry employs to influence both prescribing and cost: the constant but generally unseen marketing to doctors and, more recently, very visible advertising directly to consumers; persistent stretching of drug patent protection to maintain high prices and shut out less expensive competitors; selective compliance with or maneuvers around Food and Drug Administration (FDA) regulations intended to safeguard the public; and finally, political lobbying, generously financed, especially during legislative and electoral battles that give shape to American health care—for instance, over Medicare coverage for prescription drugs.

Although prescription drugs play a role in people's lives at any age, the 13 percent of Americans old enough for Medicare account for more than 35 percent of prescription expenditures. Nearly 3 percent of their total household spending goes to medications. Among older Americans, nearly 90 percent fill at least one prescription a year; more than 80 percent take at least one prescription drug each day and average a stunning 18.5 prescriptions in one year.[1] As the baby boom generations move through middle age, they already experience some increase in health-care needs (beyond care for their parents) and will doubtless see medications become even more central to lowering health risks and managing chronic conditions, including many cancers. For such development to proceed with the public's best interest as the ultimate goal, people need to understand something of the medical and political context that surrounds current prescription drug-related policies, how they have evolved, and where they may be heading. Toward that end, the following discussion includes brief sketches of selected aspects of that context. By better appreciating the likely impact of pharmaceutical industry and government actions and inactions on their own health in years to come, people may also recognize needed alterations in policy directions, before it is too late.

THE MEDICAL QUESTION

A troubling paradox imbues the prescription drug enterprise: something so necessary, good, even lifesaving can bring such potential for harm and even death. For older Americans, much of the harm arises when a doctor misprescribes a medication—the patient should not be taking that drug, or that amount of it. Studies of what the medical world calls inappropriate prescribing reveal rates approaching 25 percent among patients over the age of sixty-five.[2] Consumer advocates (one is Public Citizen's Health Research Group) suggest the rate is higher. In addition, as patients age and take greater numbers of medications, they increasingly misuse in various ways what may be a medically sound prescription drug.

TOO MUCH AND TOO LITTLE

Evidence of serious problems with the prescribing of medications to older women and men centered initially on their excessive use for nursing-home residents. Not only was this captive audience easiest for researchers to study, nursing facilities far too often employed heavily sedating tranquilizers and antipsychotic drugs to keep residents quiet and manageable day and night. This approach surely required less cost and less expertise than assurance of a calming environment, adequate numbers of well-trained staff, daytime activities, and regular exercise for people who might be agitated and disruptive and have difficulty sleeping at night, owing to their physical or mental health condition and to their surroundings.

By the 1970s, such overuse of psychoactive drugs was emerging from institutional shadows. Concern broadened to prescribing practices, more generally, for elders living in the community. In some ways more hidden, or at least harder to detect within doctors' offices and private homes, the use of too many medications and dosages too high commonly characterized health care for the old. Such *polypharmacy,* a term describing this particular health condition, contributes to symptoms commonly attributed to old age itself: dizziness, falls, incontinence, lethargy and sleepiness, confusion, agitation, poor appetite, memory loss, and other cognitive impairment. Not only can such symptoms lead a doctor to prescribe yet another drug, they can result in life-threatening complications. For example, infection may develop after surgery for a broken hip resulting from a fall.

The twentieth century ended with greater recognition of complexities in medicating the generations of people who had benefited from the post–World War II arrival of lifesaving wonder drugs, most prominently antibiotics. Research was demonstrating that standard dosages appropriate for younger adults, the age group that participates in most drug testing, are often too high for older individuals. With age, the body metabolizes drugs differently. Kidneys function less efficiently, slowing the body's elimination of medications, resulting in greater accumulation over time and increased risk of harmful side effects. Age reduces the safety margin-of-error for medications, increasing susceptibility to direct kidney damage. Drugs may cause sudden drops in blood pressure and fainting; they may affect central nervous system functions for a longer stretch of time in older individuals, enlarging risks, for instance, of falls and their array of harmful consequences.[3] If people take several medications, as is common in the older population, dangerous interactions between various prescription and over-the-counter drugs, as well as herbal remedies, are more likely to occur (see figure 12). A full gamut of substances can cause problems: common painkillers known as nonsteroidal anti-inflammatory drugs (NSAIDs, including aspirin, ibuprofen, and prescription anti-inflammatories); opoid-type painkillers (morphine-based); various cholesterol-lowering drugs; medications for high blood pressure and heart disease; antibiotics; antidepressants; blood thinners; diuretics.

The need to rein in and modify common prescribing practices persists. An analysis of ten-year trends, through 1996, estimated that 2.6 percent of people sixty-five and older took at least one of eleven medications an expert panel determined should "never be used."[4] An additional 9.1 percent used drugs categorized as rarely appropriate for this age group, most commonly propoxyphene (brands: Darvon; Cotanal 65), a sedating and potentially addictive painkiller with efficacy similar to aspirin or acetaminophen. Doctors prescribed drugs in the final category—minimal benefit, generally to be avoided—to 13.3 percent of patients over sixty-five; most common was amitriptyline, an antidepressant used also to treat chronic pain, for which newer, safer alternatives exist. Recent reassessment showed no substantial improvement, especially regarding pain killers, sedatives, and antianxiety and antidepressant drugs, especially for women.[5]

Clearly, inappropriate medicating of older patients involves more than doctors' overeagerness to prescribe too many new drugs, whether starting with free samples or responding to patients convinced by now-ubiquitous direct-to-consumer advertisements. Physicians' habit may keep patients on long-used but outmoded drugs. Doctors may not reevaluate an individual's need to continue taking specific medications or monitor for harmful side effects requiring lowered dosages, shortened

12. POPULAR HERBAL SUPPLEMENTS THAT MAY MIX POORLY WITH PRESCRIPTION DRUGS

Types of known interactions (which vary from drug to drug)

1 = reduction in drug's efficacy
2 = potentially dangerous increase in drug's accumulation, effects
3 = increased likelihood of drug's side effects

Echinacea: 1, 2
Garlic: 1, 2, 3
Ginko biloboa: 1, 2, 3
Ginseng: 1, 2, 3
Grape-seed extract: 2
Milk thistle: 1, 2, 3
Saw palmetto: 1, 2
St. John's wort: 1, 3
Valerian: 2, 3

These and other supplements (e.g., DHEA, Ephedra, glucosamine and chondroitin, kava, iron, vitamin A from retinol) can themselves occasionally cause or worsen various health and psychological problems in some individuals, as can most types of prescription drugs.

Based on *Consumer Reports on Health*, vol. 14 (November 2002).

duration, or immediate cessation of a medication. The problem is even more complicated, however. While older adults are notoriously over-medicated overall, current patterns reflect that doctors often fail to prescribe beneficial medications for pain, depression, osteoporosis, hypertension, and cardiovascular disease.[6] Beyond what one pharmacologist describes as a "perverse mix of overtreatment and undertreatment," yet another source of harmful, even lethal, medicating has enlarged in recent years: human error.[7] Greater numbers of drugs on the market and greater numbers of older people taking several of them, combined with cost-control staffing cutbacks in hospitals, pharmacies, and doctors' offices mean that mistakes happen more frequently.[8] A staff person mislabels a medication or misreads a label. A doctor or pharmacist confuses similarly named drugs (see figure 13).[9] A doctor prescribes new medication, for instance a blood thinner, but does not instruct the patient to

13. CONFUSING DRUG NAMES—BRAND AND/OR GENERIC

Accupril (hypertension)	Aciphex (heartburn, ulcers)	
Ambien (insomnia)	Amen (menstrual cycle regulation)	
Celebrex (arthritis)	Celexa (depression)	Cerebyx (seizures)
Fosomax (osteoporosis)	Flomax (enlarged prostate)	Volmax (asthma)
Lamictal (seizures, bipolar disease)	Lamisil (fungal infections)	
Oxycontin (pain)	Oxybutynin (urinary incontinence)	
Rimantadine (flu)	Ranitoidine (heartburn, ulcers)	
Paxil (depression)	Plavix (heart attack and stroke prevention)	
Pravachol (high cholesterol)	Propranolol (high blood pressure)	
Serzone (antidepressant)	Seroquel (antipsychotic)	
Singulair (asthma)	Sinequan (depression, anxiety)	
Xanax (anxiety)	Zantac (heartburn, ulcers)	Zyrtec (allergies, asthma)

Approximately 15 percent of reported medication errors involve name mix-ups, which may result from a doctor's poor handwriting on the prescription or a mispronounced or wrongly remembered name.

Based on *Consumer Reports on Health,* vol. 15 (March 2003).

stop using the old, resulting in a potentially deadly overdose. A nurse injects the correct medication into the wrong patient. Whatever the immediate error, an individual faces the risks from a wrong medication, wrong dosage, or dangerous drug interaction.

Such errors can occur, of course, with patients of any age. Still, people passing through middle age, who gradually take more medications to treat more ailments, often seeing several physicians who don't know what the others prescribed, are subject to probabilities—a greater likelihood of mistakes. Moreover, older patients become a more likely source of error themselves. I have witnessed many of the ways: my mother sharing her prescription painkiller when my father's backache flares; my father dropping his pill, unable to see to find it; each confusing one bottle for another or forgetting to open their respective pillboxes, divided by days of the week to help them remember their various pills. And that does not include stopping an antibiotic before completing its full course.

Medical information systems and other procedures now exist that could, with judicious use, help avert prescription errors.[10] Hospital, pharmacy, HMO computers store data recording which doctors prescribe what drugs to individual patients; they can store and cross-check drug side effects, interactions, and individual histories of health conditions, previous drug allergies, or toxic reactions as well. Already some hospital computers provide physicians immediate feedback on drugs considered for an inpatient's condition. In fact, many older individuals are hospitalized because of toxic interactions from drugs known to carry this risk, interactions that could have been avoided.[11] Pharmacists could more actively join patients' health-care teams, alerting doctors at the office and customers about excessive amounts and risky combinations for certain medications taken at home. Implementing such monitoring, however, adds expense to be borne by individuals or institutions somewhere along a line already burdened by cost.

THE COST QUESTION

While human error explains why some older adults fail to take their prescribed medications, too frequently the reason is cost. As the public learned during the 2000 presidential election campaign, if not before, Medicare generally has not covered prescription drugs outside hospitals or skilled nursing facilities. Medicare recipients who can afford private supplemental insurance have been able in part to fill this major gap; the higher a yearly limit on amount covered, the greater a policy's expense. My father's Medicare supplement, for instance, was always less generous but also considerably less expensive than my mother's, as he took no prescription drugs regularly until later years, and she took several. Dementia medication and the addition of an antidepressant, prescribed not with clear evidence but just in case they might help, demonstrated to me how easily Medicare recipients can accumulate hundreds of dollars in monthly prescription sums. By midsummer I was startled by a jump in what my father had to pay for his prescriptions. A pharmacy computer printout explained the sudden increase: he had "exceeded plan benefit cap limitation." For the remaining four months of that year, it said, his "co-payment is 100 percent."

Though 100 percent makes me wonder about the "co-," health-care insurers contend that requiring consumers to share costs through co-payments, deductibles, and yearly coverage limits helps deter unnecessary purchases. Cost-conscious shopping may dampen conspicuous consumption of other products, but prescription drugs and the health-care market generally follow more dangerous rules. Most consumers and many doctors lack the pharmacological knowledge to separate necessary medications from the superfluous. Moreover, current knowledge about many medications is tentative, pending further study. Complicating matters further, drug manufacturers do not always provide full and accurate information about what is known. Neither I nor my father's doctor could know whether expensive dementia drugs improved his late life. With clear-cut knowledge often lacking, how are consumers to choose which purchase to forgo in the interest of economizing?[12] Consumers cannot comparison-shop when drug manufacturers set prices, especially for a brand-name medication that may be the only available version. That is, the drug's manufacturer has a monopoly on the market, and buyers become the captive audience, with inadequate information to determine whether they truly need the product—a circumstance ripe for egregious abuse. Medication should not be a product that requires bargain hunting in the first place.

Prescribing a drug in case it might help, though with little scientific evidence that it will, is an exceedingly common practice. Doctors, patients, and patient family members want to do something for an ailing individual, an inclination encouraged strongly by drug manufacturers. This practice is costly and often brings risks in the absence of countervailing benefit. The tendency of doctors and patients to rely on drugs, to the neglect of less expensive, less risk-laden measures, is reflected in a scientifically controlled study reported in *Lancet,* focusing on an unusually low-tech intervention for chronic back pain of no specific detectable origin.[13] Challenging many doctors' long-held recommendation that patients suffering this condition should sleep on a firm mattress (advice often supplemented, on the one hand, by wooden boards and, on the other, by escalating pain medications), this clinical trial determined that a mattress of medium firmness more effectively lessens back pain. This finding, the authors suggest, could reduce the use of drugs and save their concomitant cost. In fact, some researchers assert that most back pain will improve without drugs (or surgery), while about 10 percent of people suffer intractable pain that prescribed drugs (and surgeries) will never relieve.[14] With more than 70 percent of adults experiencing back pain at some time (about one-third within any given month), the implications are striking. And there are other aches and pains that develop with age, annoying though not serious, that may better be treated as part of life, like the skinned knees in childhood, soothed by nonpharmacological means.

To some extent, then, in a rather perverse twist, a drug's high cost may confer an inadvertent benefit: an older patient fails to purchase an ineffective and possibly dangerous medication that she should not be taking anyway. Yet evidence is mounting that rather than eliminate only unnecessary medical treatment, the high cost of drugs impairs older consumers' health, in that they fail to obtain needed medications. Medicare patients with heart disease but no supplemental drug insurance less often receive newer, more expensive medications demonstrated to be more beneficial than previous treatments.[15] HMO formularies (the medications covered) select cheaper alternatives that are less effective and/or bring greater adverse side effects—for example, older, now generic antipsychotic drugs that can cause difficult side effects when prescribed to agitated patients with dementia.[16] Patients who pay increased shares of the cost or exceed yearly caps on the amount covered cut back on essential medications for chronic and acute conditions, resulting in higher rates of emergency room visits, hospital and nursing-home admissions, and mortality, clearly undesirable outcomes that, moreover, cost far more than the drugs. Patients cut pills in half to stretch the dosage. Some do without, paying instead for food, for rent, for heat in winter months.[17]

Among members of Medicare HMOs, an additional strategy is to switch plans midyear on reaching their prescription cost limit, but this move risks significant disruptions in their health care, often requiring a change of doctors and medical treatment.[18] Indeed, a major lure of Medicare HMOs (an option through which members sign over their government-insured benefits to a commercial managed-care plan) during the 1990s was prescription drug coverage. However, the track record is not reassuring: not only do most of these managed-care plans require co-payments and set annual prescription caps, many HMOs cut back or eliminated the drug benefit (complete coverage down from 80 percent in 1999 to 40 percent in 2000, according to the Henry J. Kaiser

Family Foundation) or precipitously dropped their Medicare patients altogether, finding this population unprofitable after all, owing in large measure to the expense of their medications.

Unlike my parents or HMO members, at least a fourth to as many as half of Medicare recipients (at least 10 million people) had no prescription drug insurance at all in 2003, when Congress legislated a new prescription benefit set to begin in 2006.[19] These individuals paid out of pocket double the price charged to "favored" customers—for instance, large HMOs, government employees, the Department of Veterans Affairs (in total less than 15 percent of nonnursing-home Medicare recipients in 1995). One source of lower prices still beckons those unfavored customers living within range of Canadian or Mexican pharmacies: for them, international travel by car, bus, or train can prove cost-effective. These neighboring countries, like all other developed nations, impose some manner of price regulation. Although bringing home their prescribed purchases violates a federal ban on drug reimports (with a few specific exceptions), these personal expeditions generally proceeded unhindered—until the travel, especially to Canada, became virtual. Over six months ending in early 2003, individuals' boundary-crossing Internet purchases from Canada for gastrointestinal medications jumped 73 percent compared to the previous six months (total Canadian sales rose 9 percent). American Internet purchases of cardiovascular drugs rose 60 percent during that time, and Internet sales of cholesterol-lowering statins were up 55 percent (compared to 5 percent and 9 percent throughout Canada). Total prescription medication sales by Canadian pharmacies to Americans paying approximately half the American price, in person or via the Internet, amounted to over $1 billion in lost U.S. sales.[20]

By 2003 American pharmacists and their customers were arguing an obvious solution: make prescription drugs more affordable in the United States, for instance by negotiating prices with manufacturers, as Canada does. Meanwhile, one of the world's largest drug manufacturers, GlaxoSmithKline, was attempting to cut off this northern supply in a different manner. According to a coalition of organizations from both countries working to maintain affordable sources of prescription drugs, Glaxo was refusing to provide any of its products to Canadian pharmacies and wholesale distributors selling to Americans. A second manufacturer, AstraZeneca, soon threatened to do the same, with others likely to follow. In September of that year, pressured by pharmaceutical companies, the U.S. Department of Justice initiated steps to close down a more organized and fast-spreading commercial effort, a chain of drug storefronts opening throughout the United States to help consumers procure drugs over the Internet from Canada.[21] Interestingly, during the same time a number of city and state officials were considering, and a few were starting, programs to obtain less expensive drugs from Canada for employees, retirees, prisoners, and other enrollees of government health plans or in some states, for all residents.

In Congress, a proposed amendment to Medicare prescription drug legislation, seeking to legalize reimportation of American-made medications from Canada, went down to defeat in the face of stiff opposition from the pharmaceutical lobby. The only allowable exceptions—say, for cities and states—would require the secretary of Health and Human Services to guarantee the safety of imported Canadian drugs. Although Bush administration secretary Tommy Thompson declared initially that he could not provide such guarantees, mounting political support for imports (including from key congressional Republicans and state governors) combined with ever-worsening Iraqi war news during a presidential election campaign year weakened his resolve. New legislation allowing imports, he conceded, appeared inevitable. Pharmaceutical industry resolve, however, remained stalwart—for instance, lobbying for international trade agreements that would stymie drug imports.[22]

In Mexico, the personal version of free-trade cross-border shopping may well carry greater risks. The many medications available in Mexico without prescription are as easy to obtain as aspirin. This ease of purchase magnifies legitimate safety concerns. Dangers arise most prominently from counterfeit drugs (i.e., fakes with no active medical ingredient), expired or improperly stored drugs, differing inactive filler ingredients that cause adverse reactions, and drugstore substitutions for the medication or dosage prescribed by American doctors. Such dangers notwithstanding, an affordable Mexican medication seems better to many Americans than their only alternative—remaining unable to pay for any medication at all. Whether purchasing medications in Mexico, Canada, or over the Internet, many patients must now weigh the potential risks of obtaining prescription drugs from these sources against benefits the drug may provide, adding yet another consideration to what should be more purely medical-pharmacological decisions.

Although major drug manufacturers offer charitable programs to help low-income patients buy medications, the bureaucratic requirements of 175 differing programs with differing forms and eligibilities overwhelm the stretched staffing resources of community health clinics nationwide. Moreover, according to Health and Human Services investigators, drug companies have repeatedly overcharged community clinics and public hospitals (along with Medicaid), in defiance of legal limits.[23] Indeed, the various consumer strategies—eliminating or halving pills, switching health plans, crossing borders, relying on community clinic subsidies—are no match for the drug industry's repertoire of powerful tactics.

THE PHARMACEUTICAL INDUSTRY

As national health-care costs accelerated with the new century, following several years of a slowed pace, prescription medications made up the fastest-growing piece of the pie, hovering between a 15–19 percent yearly price increase.[24] By 2002, prescription drugs accounted for nearly 25 percent of Americans' out-of-pocket health-care expenses, and for over 50 percent of the yearly rise in the amount of health-care costs they face.[25] Whatever share consumers or insurers pay, drug manufacturers remain the country's most profitable industry, up 33 percent in 2001, about five times the average of the Fortune 500 companies, a profit pattern consistent over the previous decade.[26] Adults at midlife and beyond remain their most lucrative customers, especially those nonfavored individuals who pay retail pharmacy prices.

In 2004, two reports documented escalating costs specifically for older adults. A study sponsored by AARP tracked the rise in prices from 2000 through 2003 of nearly 200 brand-name drugs commonly used by Americans age fifty and above. Compared to a general inflation rate of 10.4 percent, cumulative drug price inflation averaged 27.6 percent, and the increase picked up speed through those years. On average, individuals were paying nearly double for the same medications purchased in 2000.[27] The second report, by the health consumer organization Families USA, focused on the thirty drugs most widely prescribed to Medicare recipients. These prices rose an average of 6.5 percent during 2003, 4.3 times general inflation (excluding energy). From 2001, drug prices were up nearly 22 percent, or 3.6 times general inflation. The increases were fast and frequent, with the five top sellers clocking in as follows:[28]

Lipitor, to lower cholesterol: 5.5 × inflation

Plavix, to prevent blood clots: 5.3 × inflation

Fosomax, to treat osteoporosis: 4.6 × inflation

Norvasc, to lower blood pressure: 6.6 × inflation

Celebrex, to control arthritis pain: 5.4 × inflation

Obviously, over the years the pharmaceutical industry has developed effective means of maintaining its extraordinary and sustained profitability, through marketing, legal and regulatory maneuvering, and politics.

MARKETING

To cite heavy advertising of pharmaceutical products cannot convey fully the extensive, expensive, and perpetual campaign to increase prescription drug sales. Drug manufacturers have long employed various approaches that persuade doctors to prescribe their products. Over $19 billion of persuasion in 2001 (up from $12 billion spent in 1999) included $4.8 billion for detailers (about 83,000 of them) and another $10.5 billion for the free samples they distribute, at a rate of approximately $8,000–13,000 per doctor per year.[29] This generous budget covers not only the detailers circulating with samples and gifts through doctors' offices and through medical convention exhibit halls, cocktail lounges, and dining rooms. Marketing money pays also for continuing medical education meetings (primarily to disseminate information about the company's products) held at winter ski resorts or summer beaches; pays for free lunches and dinners, with a brief sales pitch, to hospital physicians; pays for study notes and, perhaps, a first stethoscope given to medical students; and, of course, pays for the advertisements as well as supplements that thicken and subsidize medical journals. Especially flagrant are generous and direct payments to doctors who agree simply to prescribe a certain drug or participate, at least by attaching their name or enrolling patients, in manufacturer-designed and -funded clinical trials.[30]

More recent is the flood of direct-to-consumer advertising since the Food and Drug Administration lifted prohibitions in 1997: $2.7 billion-worth in 2001 and rising to $3.8 billion by 2004.[31] Although the advertised product is often merely a higher priced brand than equivalent medications (for example, medications for pain, hypertension, ulcers, and heartburn), the ad campaigns are highly effective in creating consumer demand that many doctors apparently can't refuse. Indeed, they agree to about three-fourths of all such patient requests, not only satisfying patients but also, in these days of managed care, keeping appointments short. According to a General Accounting Office (GAO) study, an estimated 8.5 million or more Americans (5 percent of the country's consumers) who follow an advertisement's advice each year to "ask their doctor" for the particular prescription get what they ask for.[32]

Furthermore, the FDA reprimands drug manufacturers about the content of their advertisements (more than seventy-five times between 1997 and 2001), often for several serious violations—including false statements about effectiveness and minimization of risks—as well as failure, at the outset, even to submit the advertisement for review as required. In some cases, the regulatory agency has warned a manufacturer repeatedly for one advertisement after the other. Among offenders, according to the GAO report, are medications used heavily by adults middle-aged and older—for example, Prilosec for ulcers and heartburn, Actonel for osteoporosis, Lescol and Lipitor to lower cholesterol. Since 2000, procedural changes introduced by the Bush administration have slowed this oversight process, allowing inaccurate and deceptive ads to continue running until their commercial lifespan ends (roughly 33 percent of advertisements run for only 1–2 months, 30 percent 3–6 months, almost 30 percent 7–12 months, the remainder longer). A new requirement for internal agency legal review before regulatory letters go to manufacturers, says the GAO report, "has sharply reduced FDA's effectiveness in issuing . . . warning letters in a timely manner" (2002, 22). For example, FDA regulators determined that advertisements for Prevacid, a medication for serious heartburn (gastric reflux), were misleading in suggesting their use for occasional indigestion. The regulatory letter, however, sat mired in the new review process for more than ten weeks, a turnover process that previously took several days. And, although the Bush administration claimed the new policy would promote the industry's voluntary compliance, the actual upshot was that people continued seeing the advertisements, asking their doctor, and taking the medication—often inappropriately—until time arrived for a new advertisement, one not yet reviewed and cited by the FDA. Nor is delay the full extent of the problem. The FDA is pursuing fewer misleading or false advertisements altogether. Although the number of complaints about false and misleading advertisements has remained steady, the number of FDA regulatory letters to manufacturers dropped from 158 in 1998 to 26 letters in 2002.[33]

The new century also brought more subtle and sophisticated methods for targeting a drug's potential market. For example, by developing profiles of doctors' prescribing and patients' purchasing, obtained when drug companies gain access to computer records of large national pharmacy chains, a manufacturer can design more effective promotional efforts, including direct mailings to patients. While surely beneficial for the drug company's bottom line, such methods violate the confidentiality of patients and doctors alike.[34] Whether recent privacy laws will successfully curtail such marketing tactics, and what new methods will emerge, remain to be seen.

Just how consequential the drug manufacturers' promotions to doctors and to consumers can be for a patient's health and finances received a rare public airing in late 2002. Widespread media coverage announced newly published findings from a study of drugs used to treat high blood pressure (hypertension), a chronic condition linked to a range of the most common and serious, often fatal, cardiovascular and neurological ailments as people grow older. Contrary to marketing claims by makers of popular and profitable brand-name medications introduced in recent years (two differing types known as calcium channel blockers and ACE inhibitors), a much cheaper, older type of hypertension drug—diuretics, sometimes called water pills—more effectively lowered blood pressure and the rate of strokes, heart failure, and heart attacks.[35] This large, well-designed, and federally sponsored study, its participants fifty-five years and older, demonstrated that for most patients with high blood pressure, doctors should first prescribe diuretics, as was standard care before drug manufacturers weaned doctors and their patients away, introducing them to the new products. Not only are these newer medications much more expensive, prescribing them provided less benefit compared to risk for the millions of patients better off on diuretics. The only problem for makers of the newer hypertension medications: diuretics are generic drugs, long off-patent and available at a small fraction of the brand cost to patients and insurers, a fraction that does not contribute to brand drug manufacturers' profits.

This study was striking for another reason. Pitifully few comparisons of competing drugs exist, as manufacturers are required to demonstrate safety and efficacy compared only to a placebo. Not until 2004, for instance, were results available comparing differing doses of two popular cholesterol-lowering medications, Lipitor and Pravachol.[36] Hypertension and high cholesterol are but two health conditions for which commonly prescribed medications need comparison studies, among competing brand-name drugs (including costly cancer medications), with older generics, and even with over-the-counter drugs for some ailments. For instance, as became evident during the 2004 Vioxx uproar, much uncertainty remains about the risks and benefits of new arthritis medications, called COX-2 inhibitors, in comparison or in combination with over-the-counter drugs (naproxen, ibuprofen, aspirin). A commentary in *Lancet* notes "intensive direct-to-consumer advertising in the USA" as well as abundant sales. Criticizing the FDA's role, and excessive prescribing, the authors continue: "It is hard to imagine the justification for this extraordinary adoption of [the new drugs] in light of marginal efficacy, heightened risk, and excessive cost. . . . If only a small fraction of the direct-to-consumer advertising costs or revenue were appropriately channeled for clinical trials, we might be able to have an enhanced perspective and make sound recommendations for our patients."[37] With comparative data, that is, prescribing doctors and patients could reach more fully informed decisions about available medications. Were the government to sponsor a full array of comparison studies or require drug manufacturers to subsidize the studies (both prospects unlikely), not only would consumers gain health benefits, they and their insurers could save considerably on prescription costs.

Congressional concern over potential Medicare spending for prescription drugs may eventually alter this status quo. Only through direct comparison of competing medications can Medicare (or any purchaser or prescriber) know whether a more costly drug is better for patients. Despite pharmaceutical industry opposition, an amendment to the 2003 Medicare prescription drug bill provided a small amount of funding for drug comparison trials. However, just months later President Bush eliminated this money from his 2004–05 budget, to the consternation of even his own party's Senate majority leader, Bill Frist (a physician), as well as the amendment's primary sponsor, Democrat Hillary Clinton.[38]

Current medications used to treat dementias have no direct comparison studies, nor do they have any generic competition yet. In fact, beyond questionable claims in medical journals regarding benefits for dementia patients, drug manufacturers are busy expanding this relatively new market of older women and men by stretching boundaries of a condition for which these medications are approved. Targeted symptoms would encompass what could be dementia's early signs, not only the newly coined but little understood mild cognitive impairment (discussed in chapter 2), but also forgetfulness or trouble finding words, as some advertisements put it. Safe and effective early treatment would surely be a boon for adults middle-aged and older; however, aggressive marketing proceeds despite scant evidence demonstrating whether and how much these medications (which bring significant side effects) actually ease dementia, despite inadequate knowledge more generally about dementias and treatments appropriate for the differing stages and types.

Expanding the definition of a disease needing medication may also be occurring with bone density and fractures. Doctors presently disagree about the range of bone density considered dangerously low (osteoporosis), for which benefits of available drugs to reduce chances of immobilizing, even life-threatening bone fractures outweigh medication risks. Scientists do not yet thoroughly understand the role of bone density in age-related fractures.[39] While drug makers may encourage treatment to prevent fractures when bone density is only slightly below the norm (known as osteopenia), there are no data on the relation of this condition to likelihood of breaks, and no evidence that medications will in fact provide protection.

Beyond exaggerating benefits, a drug manufacturer's highly selective information to physicians and the public commonly conceals negative results of clinical tests, and in some instances evidence of potential harm. For pharmaceutical companies marketing rival products to doctors and consumers (Aricept, Exelon, Reminyl brands of dementia drugs, rival osteoporosis medications, statins), or any manufacturer seeking the largest possible sales, time is of the essence, particularly during a new drug's first two decades, when manufacturers most profitably cash in.

PATENTS

For each newly developed FDA-approved drug, a manufacturer enjoys twenty years of patent protection for its brand-name product, shutting out from the market far less expensive, generic versions of the same chemical compound. The patent holder guards vigorously and often seeks to lengthen the span of years during which generic competition is eliminated. These exclusive sales rights, the industry argues, generate revenue essential to ongoing research and development of breakthrough medications. However, numerous analyses reveal a substantial proportion of "me too" drugs offering nothing new or improved over existing medications. In 1997, according to one such review, forty-two of the hundred top-selling prescription medications fell into this category. In 2002, only seven of the seventy-eight drugs newly approved by the FDA represented improvement over existing medications.[40] Even more troubling, a new drug may bring greater risks than the existing alternatives.

Moreover, taxpayers already subsidize a major portion of drug development through research that receives government funding. All the while drug companies pour huge sums, approximately double their research and development expenses, into the marketing that generates abundant sales. Industry profits soar beyond what many analysts consider fair return on the manufacturers' investment, ensuring high executive salaries and stockholder gains.[41]

Just as I was startled by the monthly cost of my father's Aricept, a dementia drug safely under patent, I was startled also by a sudden drop in price for Prozac. Transformed into the generic fluoxetine hydrochloride on the day Prozac's patent expired in late 2001, my parents' antidepressant seemed quite a bargain. Not that Prozac's manufacturer gave up completely: the Eli Lilly Company repackaged its fluoxetine under a new brand name, Sarafem, a drug for women, newly approved to treat a different set of symptoms—the irritability, breast tenderness, bloating, and other signs of a newly labeled condition, premenstrual dysphoric disorder.

For drug companies with a popular, widely prescribed medication, the patent's temporary extension can accrue several millions of dollars a day, and so they have developed well-orchestrated methods to gain the most such days. For example, AstraZeneca, having successfully drummed into the public head its purple pill Prilosec (though with misleading advertisements), sued a generic company to delay its entry into the heartburn and ulcer market. At the same time, the company introduced a barrage of new advertising urging people to switch to its next purple pill, even naming it Nexium, a product chemically jiggled enough to earn a new patent. The new advertisements aimed to establish brand loyalty before no further delaying tactics remained and the cheaper generics finally arrived in December 2002. Even the Bush administration, in the person of Medicare and Medicaid chief administrator Thomas Scully, balked at the expense of this new brand-name me-too drug. "The fact is, Nexium is Prilosec," he stated. "It is the same drug . . . a mirror compound."[42]

Among brand-name company tactics, filing with the FDA spurious claims of patent violation has automatically postponed by thirty months FDA decisions about particular drugs, thereby postponing the availability of a generic. Beyond such maneuvers, efforts to extend a patient's life at times cross legal bounds. For example, brand-name manufacturers have paid other companies to delay release of a generic version, an anticompetitive practice violating Federal Trade Commission regulations.[43]

THE FOOD AND DRUG ADMINISTRATION

Throughout development, approval, and marketing of prescription drugs, pharmaceutical companies have functioned in uneasy, at times incomplete, cooperation with the government agency overseeing and regulating their activities. Along with the deceptive ads and false patent claims, drug companies have at time skewed research and failed to report a product's harmful side effects. Shifts in power and authority have always marked their interactions with the FDA, but questions about undue industry influence have grown more pronounced since the late 1990s. With the Bush administration and a Republican Congress firmly in place, as noted above regarding FDA surveillance of drug advertisements, the cooperative relationship has shifted increasingly toward cozy.

Drug approval, based on studies demonstrating safety and efficacy, has always depended on manufacturers' data and documentation to supplement independent FDA-sponsored research. In 1997 Congress established speedier, but less stringent, approval requirements. The revised process placed even greater reliance on not always reliable data provided by a drug's manufacturer, and on internal FDA drug reviewers paid with pharmaceutical industry fees. Changes in the approval process for new medications pose particular dangers for older adults. While the goal of faster drug approval can benefit people with AIDS or cancer—diseases that may soon kill them—the outcome for sufferers of, say, arthritis or cardiovascular disease, even influenza, has not always been for the good. Most prominently, FDA officials have overruled reviewers' recommendations against approval, or health risks that did not appear during streamlined testing of new prescription drugs have surfaced after sales to the public began.

For example, the FDA issued a warning about Plavix, used commonly to prevent blood clots, two years after approval, and about Relenza and Tamiflu, two drugs for treating influenza, after only six months. Regarding the flu medications, the FDA's own expert panel recommended against approving Relenza (by a 13–4 vote) because its unimpressive benefits—perhaps shortening flu symptoms by at most one day—did not outweigh its several risks. According to the FDA scientist writing up the evaluation, agency superiors pressured him not to mention that the panel advised against approval but rather to state that the data are unclear. The manufacturer's petition for approval prevailed, repeating a common pattern of negative scientific evaluation trumped by too closely aligned agency/industry interests.[44] Later, even FDA officials expressed concern that the manufacturer's heavy advertising was prompting doctors to prescribe the new drugs inappropriately to patients with potentially lethal influenza complications requiring a different treatment, conditions such as pneumonia, seen frequently in elderly flu sufferers.[45] Only then did the FDA escalate the required warnings manufacturers must provide about these medications.

Similar problems shadow several of the most widely prescribed and heavily advertised medications for older adults' chronic health problems. In 2001, the manufacturer of Baycol withdrew this cholesterol-reducing drug from the market after thirty-one reported deaths were linked to the new medication, described in the *New York Times* as "wildly popular" and "highly profitable." The physician directing this FDA drug evaluation commented that Baycol offered no greater benefit than similar available drugs, only greater risks. However, this business section pharmaceutical report stated a clearly nonmedical outcome of major concern, patients' death notwithstanding: "Investors are shocked by the loss of a cholesterol medication."[46] More shocking are documents revealed later, in the course of lawsuits by injured consumers, that company executives knew of Baycol's excessive risk yet failed to report problems to the FDA up to two years before pulling their product off the market.[47] A few years later, Baycol served as a case study, in the *Journal of the American Medical Association*, demonstrating flawed FDA oversight of the safety of newly approved prescription medications—especially the unequal information available to patients and doctors compared to a drug's manufacturer, and an "almost insurmountable conflict-of-interest" for manufacturers who become aware of unfavorable data.[48]

Nor has Baycol been the only hazard within the class of cholesterol-lowering drugs known as statins. Indeed, these widely used medications capture the unhealthy dynamics in the FDA approval process, intense industry marketing, and high drug prices. In August 2003 the FDA approved the sixth statin, Crestor (rosuvastatin), following a delay over serious safety concerns. Not only did preapproval studies indicate toxic effects on patients' kidneys not seen with three similarly beneficial statins already available, Crestor appeared even more likely than Baycol to cause fatal muscle destruction. Even as Crestor's manufacturer, As-traZeneca, introduced its estimated $1 billion of first year promotional efforts (including repeated advice, in television commercials, to ask your doctor), a *Lancet* editorial, "Statin Wars," lambasted the corpora-tion for "unprincipled" marketing that "raises disturbing questions about how drugs enter clinical practice and what measures exist to pro-tect patients from inadequately investigated medicines."[49] Noting "con-trived" studies, "twists in the statistical wind," and "blatant marketing dressed up as research," as well as the availability of safer alternatives, the *Lancet* joined other critics in wondering, "What possible clinical justification can there be for licensing an unproven statin?" Not men-tioned in this debate was a major drawback that other available, safer statins share with any newly patented competitor: their excessive ex-pense. At a cost of $2 or $3 a day, many patients cannot afford the med-ications' benefit, or they end up postponing this purchase until their health has deteriorated all the more. Not mentioned as well: a study in-dicating that diets low in fat and high in fiber, nuts, plant sterols, and soy products equal statins in reducing cholesterol for otherwise healthy adults.[50]

Also in 2001, the *New York Times* reported in its business section that two arthritis drugs (also "wildly popular"),Vioxx and Celebrex, "may not be as safe as they were initially believed to be." Analysis of data available from the manufacturers of the new COX-2 inhibitors raised questions about a heightened risk of heart attack and stroke. Some heart specialists worried especially about older patients, prime targets for arthritis pain medication, with their already elevated rates of cardiovascular problems. The report noted that many users "request [the arthritis drugs] from doctors after seeing television advertisements paid for by the two companies [Merck and Pfizer], which are locked in a fierce marketing battle." A physician participating in an FDA review of the new evidence cited an "unbelievable" amount of marketing, re-sulting in "many people out there who are taking these drugs that should not be."[51]

Although the FDA failed to request additional safety studies (the agency currently has no legal authority to require such post-approval studies), the agency did warn Vioxx's manufacturer that its $100 mil-lion advertising campaign was misleading the public by minimizing such risks. The agency did not halt the ads, however, and not until 2004—over 80 million patients later (with $2.5 billion in 2003 sales alone)—did the manufacturer, Merck and Company, announce the largest ever withdrawal from the market of a prescription drug. Its own new studies, seeking a new FDA approved use and expanded market for Vioxx, demonstrated clearly the increased risk of heart attack and stroke compared to a placebo.[52] Even though Merck's research director claimed to be "stunned" by these new data, most analysts questioned the company's long delay in responding to the earlier evidence. In fact, a cumulative analysis of relevant studies determined that increased cardiovascular risks were evident by 2000, and that these effects are "substantial and unlikely to be a chance finding." Furthermore, Merck executives apparently knew of these troubling early findings and sought to disguise them (for instance, an e-mail memo labeled "Dodge Ball Vioxx" instructed detailers how to answer questions about these risks), leading *Lancet*'s editor to comment that the FDA "sees the pharmaceutical industry as its customer—a vital source of funding for its activities—and not as a sector of society in need of strong regulation." This relationship may help protect the agency from political pressure and protect the company's executives from stockholders' dissatisfaction, but it jeopardizes consumers' trust as well as their health.[53]

The main COX-2 competition, Celebrex, rushed new advertisements to fill the Vioxx void. These ads ran only briefly, however, as a cascade of year-end revelations about potential risks soon swamped all such drugs, even raising questions about over-the-counter alternatives. A month *after* Pfizer stopped running these Celebrex ads, the FDA issued a letter warning that they exaggerated benefits and minimized risks. As with Vioxx, evidence also surfaced of unpublished data as early as 1999 indicating the increased risks—information the company did not report to the FDA. With the agency considering stronger warning labels or withdrawal of Celebrex from the market (it ordered the labels in February 2005 but must negotiate content with the manufacturers), the public was at least seeing evidence of how flawed FDA oversight can be and how successfully drug manufacturers convince patients and doctors to use their new products. Such persuasion proceeds despite uncertainty, at best, and at times with data hidden about risks to be weighed against often questionable benefits. In the case of these pain medications, aggressive advertising to consumers greatly enlarged the number of Americans who faced the risks, who experienced a heart attack or stroke, and who died. (An estimated 88,000–140,000 extra cases of serious cardiovascular disease, many of them fatal, can be attributed to the use of Vioxx, since its approval, in place of other pain medications).[54]

Unfortunately, concerns that reach the media and general public about dangers of recently approved drugs are merely the tip of an iceberg. Although one FDA responsibility is to monitor new drugs for unforeseen problems after sales begin, no good mechanism to do so has ever existed. Doctors and patients rarely report adverse side effects to the agency, and the agency does not go looking. Drug manufacturers receive 90 percent of the reports on adverse drug reactions but do not always pass on this information to the FDA. Described in one analysis as a "passive system for voluntary reporting," another critique comments, "This system works well when there are no serious problems identified after marketing."[55] Even with thorough preapproval testing, less frequent but dangerous reactions may not become evident until larger numbers of people in the general population take a particular medication (the largest experimental phase). Their numbers grow beyond the population with the condition for which a drug is approved as safe and effective, as doctors commonly prescribe for additional off-label uses, a practice drug manufacturers encourage. Such prescriptions account for most of the sales of many drugs. While such doctors' prescribing is legal, manufacturers' promotion for unapproved uses is not. Drug companies frequently circumvent this prohibition by claiming their communications, packaged as scientific reports in company-subsidized meetings or journal supplements, are educational, an allowable purpose.[56] With an increasing number of drugs receiving speedier approval, the need is that much greater for efficient post-marketing surveillance. Failure to accomplish this task is especially perilous for people older and less healthy than typical drug testing subjects. Individuals who are more frail, who may have several chronic health problems and take several medications, are more likely to experience harmful drug reactions that the testing did not predict. Moreover, their doctor may then add yet another treatment in response, threatening a cascade of additional complications caused by a medical intervention itself.

In 2002, a study of drugs newly approved and available to the public found that 20 percent produced severe side effects not revealed during the approval process, adverse effects prompting the FDA to require either an additional label warning for physicians, called a black box (reserved for risks of serious injury or death), or the drug's withdrawal from the market.[57] Many such drugs offer no substantial benefit over long-used safer options. In the absence of known advantage—advertisements notwithstanding—the study's authors advised that doctors and patients wait several years before choosing new medications, allowing enough

14. OLDER DRUGS THAT MAY BE PREFERABLE

For most patients, older drugs (generics or brand name) may generally be preferable—at least for an initial trial—because of lower cost and greater knowledge of side effects, compared to newly approved medications.

DRUG TYPE	OLDER, GENERALLY PREFERRED	EXAMPLES OF NEWER MEDICATIONS
Statins to lower cholesterol	lovastatin (generic)	Lipitor, Crestor (brands of chemically altered statin)
Blood pressure lowering	diuretics (generics)	beta-blockers, ACE inhibitors ARBs (angiotensin-receptor blockers)
Nonsteroidal anti-inflammatories (NSAIDs)	aspirin, ibuprofen, naproxen (nonprescription)	COX-2 inhibitors (e.g., Celebrex, Vioxx, Bextra)
Chronic heartburn relief	H2 blockers (generics, Pepcid, Zantac)	Proton-pump inhibitors (Nexium, Prevacid, Prilosec)

SUGGESTIONS FOR PATIENTS

If the medication you are taking is effective, with acceptable side effects, don't change to a newer drug except for a compelling reason (such as much greater proven benefits)

Discuss thoroughly with your doctor the known side effects of a new medication and means to monitor its effectiveness and adverse effects (for example, changes in blood pressure, heart rate, blood chemistry)

If you switch to a new drug, ask for two prescriptions—one for a one-week trial, the other for a full-length prescription

Report any new symptoms or possible side effects to your doctor (such as changes in mood or appetite, problems with memory or other cognitive skills, or muscle discomfort, lack of coordination or balance, faintness, or falls)

Based on *Consumer Reports on Health,* vol. 15 (March 2003).

---

time for unknown dangers to emerge (see figure 14). Additionally, the editors of *JAMA,* among other medical researchers, propose establishing a new agency—independent of the FDA as well as the pharmaceutical industry—specifically empowered to actively monitor drugs for harmful effects after their FDA approval and public availability.[58]

In recent years consumers have seen dramatic evidence that, unfortunately, they cannot rest assured with every longstanding, widely prescribed medication either. The lengthy pro-and-con saga of hormone replacement therapy (HRT) for women during and after menopause reached a peak of upheaval in 2002: researchers announced they were halting early most of the studies comprising the Women's Health Initiative (WHI), the largest, most rigorously designed clinical research on combined hormones (estrogen and progestin) taken daily by millions of women. Data already gathered during this government-funded project clearly indicated greater overall health risks (increased breast cancer, heart attacks, strokes and blood clots) than benefits (reduced hip fractures, colorectal cancer, hot flashes, and vaginal dryness).[59] Consistent with findings of small but significant increase in these risks in other recent studies, the new report forced reassessment of a hormone regimen that drug manufacturers and some physicians recommended for essentially all women at midlife, for the rest of their lives.

Throughout the year following announcement of these early findings, a stream of additional research reports not only failed to substantiate once-hinted benefits of HRT, they confirmed added risks. Final results from the Women's Health Initiative revealed no cardiac protection but rather a possible increase in risk of coronary heart disease among healthy postmenopausal women, especially during the first year of using the combined estrogen and progestin compared to a placebo.[60] Not only did HRT raise breast cancer risk, the cancers were more difficult to detect on mammograms and were diagnosed at a more advanced stage.[61] In addition, use of continuous combined hormones raised women's risk of ovarian cancer.[62] Nor was HRT associated with improvement on health-related quality of life measures, including general health and vitality, mental health, sexual satisfaction, or cognitive abilities.[63] One small benefit compared to the use of a placebo was decreased hot flashes, and an associated small improvement in sleep, among women ages fifty to fifty-four years with moderate to severe symptoms. And, although relatively short-term use of hormones was associated with lowered risk of colon and rectal cancer, these tumors, as with breast cancer, were diagnosed at a more advanced stage.[64] Regarding HRT's value in lowering risk of osteoporosis and bone fractures, the study's results led the researchers to conclude, "When considering the effects of hormone therapy on other important disease outcomes . . . there was no net benefit, even in women considered to be at high risk of fracture."[65] And finally, a suggestion that HRT might protect cognitive abilities and lower women's risk of developing Alzheimer's disease or other dementias proved false. To the contrary, rather than protect or improve cognitive abilities (as measured by the Modified Mini-Mental State Examination) or prevent mild cognitive impairment, women receiving HRT were slightly more likely to experience cognitive decline.[66] Even more stunning, women age sixty-five years or older taking the combined hormone therapy were more likely to be diagnosed with probable dementia—a nearly double risk, though still small in number of women affected.[67] Given an additional finding of a 31 percent increase in stroke risk, explanation of the cognitive results, especially regarding dementias, may involve an increased incidence of vascular disease and silent stroke.[68] In 2004, WHI researchers canceled the remaining ongoing studies of estrogen only (for women with a previous hysterectomy), citing a similar pattern of risks and advising against this form of estrogen replacement for chronic disease prevention.[69]

Hormone replacement illustrates well how the blur of advertisements with glowing, exaggerated if not outright false claims, and finely printed or hastily uttered warnings can deftly obfuscate evaluation of health benefits and risks, proven and potential. The most successful promotional campaigns may even result, as with HRT, in blanket prescription of a medication grown popular with doctors and patients alike. During the 1960s large numbers of women began taking estrogen pills, brand-named Premarin, initially promoted as a way to prevent unwanted cosmetic and sexual consequences of the drop in estrogen at menopause. Promotional efforts of Premarin's manufacturer were aided in no small measure by the popular writings of a New York gynecologist, Dr. Robert Wilson. If women could not prevent aging itself, they could at least prevent what he considered disastrous signs of menopause (which he labeled a galloping catastrophe). Women could avoid becoming dull, unattractive, and unpleasant to live with. They could remain, as the title of his 1966 book declared, *Feminine Forever,* a book underwritten by Premarin's manufacturer, as were the doctor's lecture tours and research. Although scientists knew of estrogen's carcinogenic properties, a major risk for women taking estrogen—increased rates of uterine cancer—would not become apparent until the next decade. Only then did further study show that adding a second hormone, a progesterone (progestins are its synthetic versions), could eliminate the uterine cancer risk; the combination became standard hormone replacement therapy, reigning as the country's most widely prescribed drug treatment over many years. Yet those years also brought the confusing riddle of risks and benefits as preliminary data expanded into larger studies. In light of so much contradictory evidence, doctors and women commonly chose HRT, assuming benefits overall would likely outweigh risks—until the Women's Health Initiative data compelled researchers, doctors, and their patients to conclude, for most postmenopausal women, just the opposite.

If by 2003 the newly reported data constituted a triumph for systematic research and for consumer health advocates long critical of HRT's broad use, health-care momentum appeared more generally to favor the pharmaceutical industry. Much to the consternation of academic medical researchers, for instance, advertising agencies previously involved only in promoting a product were taking on an entirely different role: identifying potentially profitable new drugs, then financing, designing, and conducting studies required for their approval. A drug manufacturer's marketing and sales effort thus reached back to initial development stages, melding promotion with generation of knowledge about the safety and efficacy of the promoted product.[70] Ad agencies could then return to business as usual: ghostwriting medical articles about manufacturer-financed studies for well-compensated physician-authors while wining, dining, and further educating doctors about the drug. As troubling as Madison Avenue's inroads are, the drug industry also advances its interests more directly and substantially through a well-financed and powerful presence in the country's political processes.

POLITICS

The 1990s demonstrated in no uncertain terms the pharmaceutical industry's political muscle. During the battle that overwhelmed the Clinton administration's proposal for universal health insurance in 1993–94, and throughout the managed-care shakeout that followed, drug manufacturers exhibited more broadly the influence they exert regularly within the medical community. By the Clinton administration's end, the president's goal—and drug industry's target—had narrowed to revising Medicare, including the program's most glaring omission, coverage for recipients' prescription medications. The threat to drug makers underlying this popular and seemingly more possible goal: adding drug benefits to Medicare would mean direct government involvement, including, most likely, establishing price limits in order to control the government's prescription costs.

As obvious as the need for prescription drug coverage for older Americans appeared by the year 2000, medications played a less prominent, everyday role when Medicare was established in 1965. In the political give-and-take that shaped this landmark federal health insurance program, legislative priorities centered on treatment of acute illness, including hospitalization—the major medical emphasis and financial threat for individuals at the time. Thirty years later, a burgeoning number of medications had taken over a continually enlarging portion of health care and costs for the also enlarging population of older adults. Doctors were increasingly prescribing daily drug regimens to treat such chronic ailments as arthritis, heart disease, and high blood pressure and to lower a patient's risk for suffering the acute, life-threatening heart attack or stroke. This trend, consistent with efforts to lower health-care costs by reducing hospitalizations, promises to continue well into the twenty-first century, as a maturing biotechnology provides new generations of drugs to the aging generations of baby boomers.

By the mid 1990s, changes in demographics and medicine highlighted inadequacies built into Medicare. Much of the cost burden of prescription medications fell on individuals. Beyond Medicare recipients with no drug coverage throughout that decade, those who had insurance tapped varying sources and received differing, often inadequate, benefits. While 25 percent of this insured group received drug benefits through employer-based insurance, including retirement plans, less than 10 percent purchased supplemental drug insurance as individuals, the most expensive Medi-gap policies. The remaining recipients either enrolled in a Medicare HMO offering at least partial prescription drug payment or qualified to obtain medications through federal and state government health insurance programs for the poor.[71] In some states such use of Medicaid did lead to a legal fight. Drug manufacturers sued states to halt expansion of eligibility for more people to gain Medicaid drug benefits, programs for which individual states can impose restrictions on drugs available in order to control pharmaceutical costs.[72] Even as the industry lobbied at the state level against Medicaid price controls, more specific battles arose over particular medications, as manufacturers fought to assure their share of the large state-paid market.

In 1999 President Clinton proposed a major legislative initiative that would add prescription drug coverage to Medicare, starting in 2002. This most heralded of the basic changes, intended to ensure Medicare's longevity, could serve as a coda for the twentieth century and his presidency. A *New York Times* report provides a telling depiction of the context for his proposal and an eerie prophesy of the drug benefit's prospects: "The economic context . . . could hardly be better, with a vibrant economy generating a windfall of federal revenue. The White House said . . . it foresaw surpluses totaling nearly $3 trillion over the next decade. One in eight of those dollars would go to shore up Medicare under the President's plan." Announcing his plan, the president declared, "In a nation bursting with prosperity, no senior should have to choose between buying food and buying medicine."[73] Having learned his health-care lessons years earlier, the president's prescription drug proposal was quite limited and came nowhere near government-mandated price controls. Rather, private benefit management companies could negotiate discounts for Medicare recipients from drug manufacturers and pharmacies.

For an industry staunchly opposed to government regulation that might erode the $100 billion a year drug market, any price discounts within Medicare represented the much loathed top of a slippery slope. With the 2000 election looming, prescription drug costs for older Americans became a highly visible, politically charged issue. Drug manufacturers poured resources into lobbying against legislation that would add drug coverage to the existing Medicare program (nearly three hundred Washington lobbyists, about half of the industry's total force, focused specifically on this most immediate threat), as well as into supporting candidates sympathetic to the industry's stance. In a reprise of tactics successful against Clinton's universal health insurance plan, the pharmaceutical trade association, the industry's official lobby, launched television, radio and newspaper advertisements. As the seniors' organization AARP noted, in many instances the industry funneled money through nonprofit groups—such as United Seniors Association or Seniors Coalition—purporting to advocate for older Americans.[74] This time the advertisements featured not Harry and Louise, a worried media couple who helped sink Clinton's earlier plan ("The government may force us to choose from a few health plans designed by government bureaucrats"), but Flo, a concerned older arthritis sufferer exclaiming, "I don't want big government in my medicine cabinet." Even so, some manner of help paying for older Americans' prescription drugs seemed likely, whatever the election's final outcome.

By the time of Clinton's proposed startup date, the nation's economic bubble had burst, and a Republican administration was at midterm. Yet nothing—recession, tax cuts, a federal budget surplus vanished into a staggering record deficit, or the Bush administration's focus on responding to the September 11, 2001 terrorist attack and on building up toward war against Iraq—could alter what Clinton had rightly stated:

that older Americans should not have to choose between food and medicine. At least nominally, prescription drug coverage remained on the legislative table. Democrats and Republicans lined up behind proposals reflecting their usual role-of-government divide, though even some Republicans supported measures to encourage use of generic drugs and discourage drug advertising to consumers as ways to control soaring costs of prescription medications. Retirees with drug coverage from their former employer faced the prospect of less generous benefits under a Medicare plan. The likelihood of co-payments posed potential hardship for Medicare's lower-income recipients. Prescription drug prices continued to rise, and doctors continued to prescribe more drugs. Many HMOs terminated their once touted plans for Medicare recipients, and employers cut back sharply or ceased offering drug coverage to retirees as well as to current employees. A remedy for prescription prices paid by Americans age sixty-five and over, along with broader modernization of Medicare's basic health insurance coverage, faded into an uncertain future. Following the 2002 midterm elections, the same *New York Times* reporter, Robert Pear, so optimistic just two years earlier, painted a drastically altered picture: "Having spent more than $30 million to help elect their allies to Congress, the major drug companies are devising ways to capitalize on their electoral success by securing favorable new legislation and countering the pressure that lawmakers in both parties feel to lower the cost of prescription drugs. . . . The industry's hand appears stronger now than at any time in recent years." Describing a postelection strategy meeting of company executives, Pear and a coauthor summarized major industry concerns: to block legislation that could reduce profits through drug price controls or increased access to less expensive generic drugs, no matter the customer's age, and to shape legislation ultimately proposed by Democrats and Republicans adding prescription drugs to Medicare coverage.[75]

The strategy session proved fruitful. Less than a year before the 2004 presidential election, hundreds of pharmaceutical industry lobbyists ensured that a Republican-dominated Congress pushed through, following an acrimonious House and Senate vote, an essentially Republican-written (with generous industry input) prescription drug benefit, the largest Medicare revision since the program's inception. Embedded within a much broader Medicare bill, the legislation carved out health and social policy only a drug manufacturer or private insurance corporation could love. Not only would the pharmaceutical industry remain free of government-imposed price controls, Congress forbids the government from even negotiating price discounts, as it does on drugs within the Departments of Defense and Veterans Affairs (resulting in prices 60 percent lower than retail), and as do other large but private purchasers—including such insurance middlemen as pharmaceutical benefit managers, HMOs, and AARP, which has long offered Medi-gap prescription coverage. The legislation also maintains the ban on re-importing American-manufactured drugs from Canada, where that country's government, as the only payer in a national health insurance program, does negotiate cheaper, regulated prices from the same manu-facturers. One concession to the spiraling expense of prescription med-ications: the Medicare bill trims certain strategies that brand-name drug makers have used to delay introduction of cheaper generics.

The prescription drug benefit itself is a feat of gerrymandered cover-age, with a void at its center. Medicare will partially cover very low pre-scription costs. Coverage reappears for much higher costs, leaving a breach within which individuals pay completely out of pocket. On top of premiums and deductibles this coverage gap will force lower- and middle-income moderately ill recipients to pay substantial drug costs, or perhaps cut back on medications, until they grow sick enough to gain further Medicare protection from catastrophic prescription costs.[76] Re-publican congressional leaders promised a ten-year $400 billion maxi-mum government expenditure, prying votes needed in down-to-the-wire and exceptionally contentious passage of the Medicare bill. Two months later the Bush administration revised this estimate upward by a third (to approximately $534 billion over ten years). Not long after that, Medicare's chief actuary, Robert S. Foster, revealed that he had re-ported this higher sum to administration officials months before the vote—only to be warned by Medicare's chief administrator not to com-municate his cost estimates to Congress, where they would likely have doomed or substantially changed the prescription drug benefit. Accord-ing to various calculations, the revised budget would reimburse about a fourth to a third of recipients' total drug costs. In February 2005 the government's estimated ten-year total costs swelled to between $724 billion and $1.2 trillion, depending on finer details of calculation.[77]

Among retirees who maintain drug coverage through their former employer, a third face the prospect of once-generous benefits reduced to levels comparable to Medicare's or eliminated altogether. Indeed, ana-lysts predict that employers will eliminate the drug benefit for close to three million people, given the new excuse of available Medicare cover-age, regardless of subsidies the bill offers businesses to maintain their retiree plans. Medicare will likely cover fewer drugs than have people's Medi-gap policies. Yet the legislation prohibits individuals who choose a Medicare drug benefit from purchasing supplemental policies to cover their own costs or additional medications.[78] The rationale, once again, is to encourage consumers, through payment requirements, to purchase drugs in a more cost-conscious manner. With state-federal Medicaid drug coverage subsumed into Medicare, many of the poorest of the old and disabled will see restrictions on their medications. Moreover, the bill prohibits state Medicaid programs from filling low-income residents' coverage gaps. And some previous recipients will lose eligibility for government drug subsidies, forcing even more people into hospital emergency rooms when a resulting health crisis hits, thus worsening an already terrible situation (which I discuss in chapter 4).

Even more far-reaching and ominous, this newly added prescription drug benefit serves as the vehicle steering recipients out of traditional Medicare into private health insurance plans. Unlike Canada's insurance program or traditional Medicare's reimbursement to doctors and hospitals, as a single payer, the new benefit inserts the private insurance market. Although the Bush administration sought initially to require Medicare recipients to enroll in a commercial health plan in order to obtain drug coverage—that is, to leave the traditional Medicare program—strong and immediate opposition, including from some Republicans, forced a modification. For the startup in 2006, government funds will subsidize (or "bribe," in the words of Senator Edward Kennedy) commercial insurers who provide prescription coverage to Medicare recipients through either a stand-alone drug benefit or a more comprehensive managed-care package. In 2010, the government's traditional Medicare program must begin competing fully with private health insurers for all benefits offered to enrollees, at first as pilot projects to test the model in six metropolitan areas (this latter limitation a last minute Republican concession during legislative negotiations). If Medicare's costs are higher than competing private plans, its recipients will pay more.

The ultimate goal remains consistent: lure Medicare recipients into commercial HMOs and preferred provider plans with attractive benefits and lower costs, a market competition skewed from the outset through government subsidies and, in years to come, through limits Congress can impose on how much government monies the Medicare program spends. Labeled a Trojan horse by critics, including most visibly and vocally Senator Kennedy, prescription drug coverage represents the initial foray of a grander assault intended to dismantle the Medicare program. Rather than lead the United States down the slippery slope of price control feared by drug makers, the 2003 legislation retreats in a blatantly regressive direction, toward privatization of the country's only universal, government-insured, and generally successful single-payer health plan.

As if current policy has no history, the prescription drug legislation ignores the refusal of commercial for-profit companies, before enactment of Medicare, to insure older and disabled Americans who brought preexisting conditions and/or too little ability to pay. This major social and health problem, for which the universal government program finally became the solution, currently threatens increasing numbers of the country's middle-aged. Perhaps more surprising, the very recent Medicare HMO experience demonstrates the private market's failure when it comes to health care for older Americans. People with prescription costs exceeding a yearly cap, similar to the new benefit gap, cut back on medications, including ongoing treatments for chronic illness.[79] Although private plans used various methods of selective enrollment to attract the healthiest individuals needing fewest services, a cherry-picking process certain to occur also with the new prescription drug benefit, these private plans could neither lower costs nor expand coverage. In short order, for-profit insurers abandoned such plans and their enrollees en masse. Now the most sick and frail, with greatest costs, are more likely to choose traditional Medicare, where at least they maintain choice of doctors and good hospitalization coverage, and soon the expense of choosing the government-run plan will become prohibitive.

In the wake of the Medicare bill's passage, analysts of all persuasions generally agree on the big winners. First is the pharmaceutical industry, which avoided encroachments on its prices and profits, even as market demand promises to grow larger. With no controls included in the legislation, prices will continue to rise, borne largely by recipients through direct out-of-pocket drug costs, premiums, and deductibles. Second, the private insurance industry wins a huge population of new customers, initially subsidized, assuming these corporations are not too shell-shocked from the 1990s HMO era to reenter the Medicare fray. Other middlemen, managers of the various prescription drug plans, gain customers as well. Engineered not to begin until 2006 (safely beyond Bush's reelection campaign), the legislation's real impact, and people's reactions to it, will be correspondingly delayed. An interim measure, voluntary discount cards available for Medicare recipients to purchase, did not bode well. With 73 different Medicare-approved private insurers, pharmacy management companies, and drugstore chains offering 73 different cards allowing myriad different discounts for approximately 60,000 medications, confusion and low participation prevailed. Commented one pharmacy management executive about this preliminary step and with reference to the overall drug benefit in 2006: "You can take this market confusion [over discount cards] and cube it."[80] Moreover, whatever savings the discount cards promised were already dissipating into an accelerated rise in drug prices. Whether intentional on the part of drug makers or not, a Families USA report warned: "Like used car buyers drawn by the promise of a rebate—only to find that the base price has risen dramatically—seniors purchasing a new drug discount card may succumb to 'sticker shock.'"[81]

Years may pass before Medicare recipients, including those newly arrived at age sixty-five, can identify and voice dissatisfactions, years before retirees know their gains and losses, before the middle-income moderately ill can calculate their medication costs. The 2004 election outcome gives a more firmly ensconced Bush administration and Republican-dominated Congress more years to redefine Medicare's future, including the drug benefit. With amendments to the Medicare bill possible before the startup date, it is too soon for older Americans, and their middle-aged offspring, to determine whether travels to Mexico and Canada still provide the better deal.

Now that prescription medications and their makers have become a more public topic than ever before, the dominance of concerns about cost over questions about health is particularly striking. Most directly, of course, cost involves amounts consumers pay, profits drug manufacturers and insurers make, the role of government in monitoring, regulating, and spending within this market relationship. While discussion needs to focus on medical questions—to determine appropriate prescribing of currently available drugs and identify safer, more effective medications that help prevent or manage illness and disability—it is all about cost. For many patients, treatment decisions revolve around a medication's expense and whether they have insurance that covers prescription drugs, rather than on medical assessment of their individual risks and benefits. Too often patients avoid costly medications regardless of whether, medically speaking, they can afford *not* to take a particular drug.

Although the pharmaceutical industry contends that free markets provide a regulatory force, the prescription drug market is not free.

Through exclusive patent rights and unchallenged price setting, makers of brand-name drugs vigilantly guard their highly profitable monopolies. Drug manufacturers command vast resources to convince potential customers in a topsy-turvy dynamic of (high-priced) supply creating demand, at times by making false or misleading claims about their products. Customers purchasing prescribed medications have not only limited or inaccurate information about these products but essentially limited freedom not to buy drugs they believe they need. Drug manufacturers fight all manner of price controls, while customers live with uncompromising financial limits. Even more basic, the overriding commercial goal of ensuring profit for investors, an attribute carried over from truly free markets, continues to trump people's health and well-being in this country and throughout the developing world.[82] As a result, the task of sorting out already complex and contradictory medical patterns of overtreatment and undertreatment with newer and older drugs remains that much more difficult.

MEDICAL KNOWLEDGE, ITS SOURCES AND USE

Summarizing the role and tactics of major drug manufacturers, Dr. Marcia Angell, former editor-in-chief of the *New England Journal of Medicine,* describes an industry far removed from "its original high purpose of discovering and producing useful new drugs. Now primarily a marketing machine to sell drugs of dubious benefit, this industry uses its wealth and power to co-opt every institution that might stand in its way, including the U.S. Congress, the FDA, academic medical centers, and the medical profession itself."[83] Indeed, at each stage drug company interests and influences compromise the search for medical answers to delineate appropriate, beneficial prescribing. For example, who needs to be taking cholesterol-lowering or bone-strengthening medications, taking on the risks in order to gain proven benefits? Is a subgroup of patients especially likely to experience harmful side effects? And which formulation provides the best balance of safety and efficacy? For which arthritis sufferers, including those with other health problems (say, cardiovascular disease), do benefits of new prescription medications, alone or in combination with over-the-counter drugs, outweigh risks; and which patients are better off taking over-the-counter drugs alone?

More broadly, under the Bush administration, scientific inquiry and policy decisions within several government agencies mandated to protect public health—among them the FDA, the Department of Health and Human Services, the Environmental Protection Agency, and the Department of Agriculture—have suffered untenable compromise. So much so that in 2004 sixty of the most prominent American scientists publicly delineated unprecedented "manipulation, suppression, and misrepresentation of science by the Bush administration." The scientists' investigation of policy decisions revealed "a well-established pattern of suppression and distortion of scientific findings by high-ranking . . . political appointees across numerous federal agencies [with] consequences for human health, public safety, and community well-being." Misrepresenting scientific knowledge and misleading the public about policy implications, they said, occur in a manner far more systematic and widespread than in previous administrations. The scientists described "case after case" of scientific knowledge and policy making "being censored and distorted" to achieve partisan political objectives, asserting that "the public deserves rational decision-making based on the best scientific advice about what is likely to happen, not what political entities might wish to happen."[84]

Almost simultaneously, an editorial in the British journal *Lancet* cited "a climate of fear and intimidation" experienced by scientists in the United States studying sex and sexually transmitted disease, birth control, drug use, AIDS—an atmosphere created, at its core, by political and ideological battles.[85] As if to illustrate, a few weeks later in the *New England Journal of Medicine,* a member of the President's Council on Bioethics described her disturbing experience involving this advisory group's deliberations on embryonic stem cell research. Alarmed by what she considers a biased report that failed to incorporate the best scientific information, as reviewed by council members, this molecular biologist states, "When prominent scientists must fear that descriptions of their research will be misrepresented and misused by their government to advance political ends, something is deeply wrong." And, she adds, with skewed membership of scientific advisory groups (her services were no longer needed, she had recently learned), and through delay and misrepresentation within reports, "something has changed. The healthy skepticism of scientists has turned to cynicism. There is a growing sense that scientific research—which, after all, is defined by the quest for truth—is being manipulated for political ends."[86]

Safeguarding medical knowledge—for instance, ensuring that research data and pharmaceutical information are trustworthy and complete—requires scientific investigation and educational dissemination with no reason to fudge (financial gain, political or religious ideology, to name a few possible reasons). Most reliable in the case of medications would be data from sources unconnected to the drug's manufacturer. Independent, not-for-profit research institutions could conduct studies on the efficacy, side effects, and costs of competing drugs. Unlike pharmaceutical industry research that the FDA must hold confidential (including negative test results that show no benefit), the methods and raw data, statistical analyses, and results from these studies would be available to all. (And FDA officials could not attempt to suppress their own investigators' data, as claimed during the Vioxx/Celebrex revelations.) A current case in point: the need for independent studies of drugs prescribed for Alzheimer's and other dementias, in order to sort out manufacturers' questionable claims and identify the most promising types of treatment. At the least, all clinical studies of drugs' safety and efficacy should be listed in a public registry, so that the scientific and medical community, along with the general public, can review all data and know all results. Moving toward such a goal, editors of eleven major medical journals worldwide (with support from the American Medical Association) announced in September 2004 that these journals will publish studies only if entered, at the outset, into a public registry under nonprofit management, with set requirements for reporting study methods, data, and results.[87]

Safeguarding people's health—for instance, ensuring that they can obtain needed medications—requires deliberate social policy. Yet the unbridled power of pharmaceutical giants, and especially the expense of their products in the United States, now determines whether individuals have access to them. With regard to prescription drugs, most older Americans have long joined the country's un- or underinsured, caught up in a daily if implicit cost rationing of medical treatment. Medicare's new prescription drug benefit, as written, will not likely improve substantially that status. Today's middle-aged, perhaps protected now through employer-insured co-payments and modest prescription drug needs, can no longer count on the prosperity that gilded the 1990s. Whether their protection will extend when they reach Medicare age, retire from jobs, and need medication to control blood pressure or arthritis pain, prevent heart attacks or stroke, preserve mental abilities—using bioengineered wonder drugs soon to come—remains, in the early 2000s, anyone's guess. Already, among people ages fifty-one to sixty-four who report fair to poor health, 37 percent also report taking less medication than a doctor prescribed because of its cost; 21 percent report reducing such necessities as food and heat in order to buy medications.[88]

In the decades after the baby boom generations reach their sixty-fifth birthday (assuming the Medicare age is not delayed, a revision suggested by Federal Reserve chief Alan Greenspan, among others, in 2004), the fallout from privatized Medicare drug coverage may well extend beyond their medications, enveloping all health insurance coverage post-2010 for older and disabled Americans. The most immediate effect may be on the type of employer-based retiree prescription-drug and health insurance plans available, if any. In the longer run, the rollback of Medicare, the one government-guaranteed health insurance program through which all older Americans are eligible for the same basic benefits at the same cost, brings additional profound, if less tangible consequences. Call it erosion of social solidarity or social ethic, however inadequate that already was, call it refusal to share cost and responsibility across society for its members. The pattern fits within a broad tableau. Certainly, proponents of this newly accomplished Medicare shift have long eyed privatization of Social Security, for example through individual tax incentives and retirement account investment, a radical change pushed strongly by the second Bush administration. After the baby boomers' parents have died, the younger old may not feel a serious direct impact until they in turn grow more old and sick, more in need of medications and other care—a stage in life that could last for a very long and difficult time.

To whatever extent cost rationing of prescription medications presently occurs, it signals a more comprehensive rationing of health care for people of all ages in this country. The next chapter considers this process as a fundamental force defining what manner of care sees people through their adult years.

4

Health-Care Rationing
Taking It Personally

The fact that middle-aged and older Americans are doing without prescribed medication because drugs cost too much would seem outrageous. Yet limiting medical treatment by cost, as noted in the last chapter, reflects a far more pervasive rationing of Americans' health care. This chapter expands the view of such limitations, outlining the broader array of health services subject to sometimes hidden forms of rationing. The discussion turns first to additional limits on available medications, then explores the larger context of cost rationing, calling attention to ways everyone, including people with health insurance, experience restrictions on care. As a major locus for rationing, hospitals nationwide deal with ever-growing numbers of people in our communities without insurance. Underscoring the critical impact of this population, the chapter describes one explicit health-care policy linking the uninsured and rationing—Oregon's Medicaid program. Discussion turns next to rationing by age beginning with Medicare HMOs offered by private health insurers, attempting to manage both costs and care for older Americans. The focus then shifts to age itself as a criterion for denying potentially beneficial medical treatment and considers the uneasy borderland between restrictions on care by chronological age and limitations appropriate to end-of-life care. Surely, health-care rationing is here to stay, and everyone will feel it in a variety of ways more and less visible, direct, and personal. The overriding question is what criteria for imposing limits on care—what manner of rationing—would be better than what Americans face now?

THE PHARMACY AND BEYOND

Every day, doctors are prescribing medications their patients cannot afford, especially the patent-protected brand-name drugs discussed in chapter 3. Many of these newer medications target the chronic ailments, depressions, and dementias suffered by an increasing number of increasingly older customers. In addition to setting prices for these medications, drug manufacturers determine supply. Certain rare diseases fail to spark drug makers' interest in research and development that bring no prospect of a profitable product. The relatively small number of individuals suffering these conditions—the orphan diseases no drug company wants—face severe, even life-threatening limitations on medically necessary treatment.[1] All the while, drug manufacturers rush to develop and market competing brands of remedies for less threatening ailments, no better illustration than the flurry of advertisements pitting Viagra against Levitra against Cialis. The larger American population faces periodic shortages of vaccines for common pneumonia, tetanus, and certain childhood diseases that will never contribute much to a pharmaceutical bottom line. More publicly, recent years have brought questions about supply and cost manipulation for yearly influenza vaccines recommended for older adults and other susceptible individuals of any age. The 2004 shortage, predicted by public health experts, revealed the dangers of inadequate government oversight—especially the absence of mandates for enough manufacturers, in order to ensure the needed supply. Even the availability of the antibiotic Cipro, sought during the 2001 anthrax scare, remained subject to the patent-holder Bayer Company's dictate, given the government's refusal to order, during this time of national emergency, more rapid production by other willing manufacturers.

Obtaining prescription drugs as enrollees in some variant of managed-care plan, as most insured Americans do before age sixty-five, does not eliminate restrictions on medications they take. To the contrary, health plans have established lists, or *formularies*, of the specific medications they will co-pay. Under certain plans, members can choose off-list medications only by paying considerably higher, often total, out-of-pocket costs. Increasingly common are tiered formularies, which create a financial incentive for enrollees to purchase less expensive choices—medications the health plan (though not necessarily the doctor or patient) prefers because they are cost-effective for that insurer. In place of a flat $5 or smaller co-pay for any prescribed medication, as in past years, 86 percent of American workers with prescription drug coverage in 2003 participated in a health plan with a tiered formulary.[2] In the most common type, a three-tier co-payment scheme (for about 60 percent of insured workers), the lowest enrollee co-payment buys generic drugs, the next higher the health plan's preferred brand-name drugs; the highest co-pay applies when the enrollee chooses a nonpreferred brand-name drug.[3] Similar financial incentive–based coverage appears likely under the new Medicare prescription benefit as well.

While insurers can calculate the cost-effectiveness of their particular tier arrangement, determining the health consequences of consumers' cost-conscious selections is more difficult. To the extent that drug winnowing and cost saving by insurers result in more appropriate and economical use of generic and less expensive brand-name drugs, these limitations constitute a reasonable step, given market conditions as they exist. However, in addition to shifting a greater portion of drug expenditures to consumers, this trend also shifts health risks and benefits. In some instances, as indicated in the previous chapter, using an older drug because it is cheaper can also mean patients must tolerate greater, even dangerous side effects. For example, new generation antipsychotic medications (such as the brands Zyprexa or Risperdol) appear to have fewer adverse side effects than earlier types (say, Haldol) when treating certain dementia symptoms in the old; but an HMO may cover only the cheaper alternative or strongly encourage its selection through a tiered formulary. A similar pattern arises with newer and older forms of antidepressants. Moreover, introducing incentive-based pricing may lead some patients not only to choose less expensive drugs but to stop purchasing a medication altogether, an outcome particularly worrisome for individuals needing ongoing treatment for chronic illness.[4]

More generally for health-plan members, the selection of drugs co-paid by their plan may depend less on medical qualities than on whether a drug's manufacturer offers the insurer a large enough discount in exchange for including its product on the formulary as a preferred drug. Yet information about such agreements, formulary expenditures and savings, insurer and drug company profits remain industry secrets, unavailable for public assessment. All in all, beyond the question of serious health consequences from cost-conscious drug shopping, no immediate saving on a particular drug's cost outweighs the severe deficiencies in health care quality that are endemic to rationing within the health-care system. Whether regarding their prescription medications, a hospitalization, or coverage for specific diagnostic or treatment procedures, patients find themselves pulled into wider battles among stakeholders: drug manufacturers, insurers, hospitals, pharmacies, physician management networks, physicians, and, of course, politicians establishing policy.

GATEKEEPERS AND GAG RULES

Notice of our family's own potentially disrupted care caused by stakeholder battles arrived in two letters. The first came from our longtime primary care doctor explaining that her three-woman practice could no longer afford the low fees and administrative costs of managed-care plans. It would no longer participate on any HMO or preferred provider list; patients would have to pay up front, at the office (generally at a higher rate than before), then submit their own reimbursement claims. Or they could choose another doctor. The second letter arrived a while later from our University of California health plan assigning us a doctor from its revised list, a doctor whose name we had never heard. Our doctor was just a bit ahead of her time. The next years would see significant numbers of doctors, emboldened by low reimbursements and the managed-care backlash more generally, refusing to take HMO members or even patients from the less restricted but still discounted preferred provider organizations. In 1998, as one example, more than four hundred Dallas physicians dissatisfied with contract negotiations cut ties with the area's Aetna HMO, uprooting health-care arrangements for thirty thousand patients. The poor, patients insured by the state and federal governments' Medicaid program, were no longer the only ones to experience difficulty finding a doctor.

To whatever extent diminishing fees threatened the lifestyle to which doctors had grown accustomed (or even their ability to break even), managed care interfered more deeply with decisions about the care doctors thought best for patients, jeopardizing patients' trust that their best interests remained foremost. Most onerous and notorious were insurers' denials of diagnostic tests, treatments, referral to specialists, hospitalizations, even emergency room visits—rationing health care through the requirement for prior approval. Patients might not even hear a full array of diagnostic or treatment options, as some managed-care plans were imposing gag rules on doctors. Such contractual agreements prohibited doctors not only from informing patients of options not covered by their health plan, but also from revealing their own contract-bound silence, a particularly insidious form of limiting care, for how can patients make well-considered decisions among choices they do not even know exist? Managed-care bureaucrats further restricted and angered physicians through a process called utilization review, keeping tabs on the procedures each doctor ordered and the costs incurred in order to bring future numbers down.

Withholding useless tests and treatments, thereby reducing the quantity of unnecessary services and inappropriate medication use, would not mean reducing the quality of patients' health care. In fact, for older patients with serious chronic illness, providing less hospital-based care, when coupled with easier access to primary care, does not appear to be harmful to their health and may in fact improve it.[5] If managed care managed initially to wring from American health care inappropriate medical procedures, hospitalizations, and other excessive spending, however, observers during the early 1990s predicted that within ten years, cost-cutting measures would be eating into needed, beneficial care. By mid-decade, insurers were refusing to cover not only case-by-case procedures but also categories of care, such as mental health. People with health conditions an insurer defined as preexisting were becoming essentially uninsurable. Denials of care became the subject of media and medical journal reports and television dramas; even a major motion picture cast HMOs as villains. Initial rumblings of consumer protection began evolving toward state regulations and, in the U.S. Congress, a patient's bill of rights for members of managed-care plans. In their own defense, managed-care plans began pulling back on restrictions as well, for instance as reported in the *New York Times* under a headline capturing the oddity health care had become: "Big HMO to give decisions on care back to doctors."[6] By decade's end, health-care costs were again accelerating, picking up speed into the new century.[7] As predicted, studies indicated serious shortcomings in care for HMO patients, especially within investor-owned as compared to not-for-profit plans.[8]

Everyone had or knew someone with a frightening tale. Consider, for example, this story from Fresno, California, a flat, midsized city sprawling into its vast agricultural surroundings in the San Joaquin Valley. A front-page story in the *Fresno Bee*'s Sunday business section—headlined

"A doctor says no to his HMO"—reports that one of the region's busiest oncologists will no longer work with one of the state's largest health plans, PacifiCare. His final straw: new limits, negotiated by the physician management organization's middleman, on reimbursements to doctors for chemotherapies and for drugs that alleviate the debilitating side effects of these cancer treatments. The health plan will now pay doctors according to a preset monthly fee rather than reimburse for costs as before. And PacifiCare offers an added incentive for lowering costs: the insurer will share savings from this new policy with the plan's participating doctors. The Fresno oncologist considers this proposal "unconscionable." Only by providing fewer and cheaper, but less effective, treatment options for patients could he stay within budget, let alone reap shared savings. Reports the *Bee*, the oncologist "tells the story of a patient suffering from a rare cancer. The patient was saved with an aggressive course of chemotherapy and radiation. The treatment, in all likelihood, would have forever damaged his teeth and taken away his ability to produce saliva."[9]

I know this story well. His patient, my brother, was barely past fifty years old when, out of nowhere, a tumor suddenly threatened his life. Just as a skilled surgeon had taken care to preserve his facial nerves when excising the cancerous salivary gland, the oncologist insisted that the best care for my brother included a drug that would protect his ability to eat normally—a prescription not likely to fit within the allotted monthly budget, but crucial for the quality of a life they were fighting to keep long. Now hundreds of the oncologist's current patients, in the midst of cancer treatment, must scramble to either change doctors—finding an oncologist still on the health plan's list—or change health plans.

In 2000, no lesser forum than the U.S. Supreme Court described explicitly and bluntly the elephant in doctors' offices and hospitals: managed care means rationed care. The ruling *(Pegram v. Hedrich 2000)* zeroed in on the financial incentives through which HMOs encouraged doctors to lower costs by limiting care; in this case a woman's appendix burst following her HMO's eight-day delay in allowing the needed diagnostic test. Writing for a unanimous Court, Justice David Souter declared, "No H.M.O. organization could survive without some incentive connecting physician reward with treatment rationing." As the Supreme Court saw it, rationing of beneficial care is inherent to managed care, as are inducements for doctors to do the rationing. The incentive of financial profit reflects "the very point of any H.M.O. scheme."[10]

To have the Supreme Court state the reality of lessened care was more dramatic and immediate than the actual ruling that this patient could not sue her HMO in a federal court. The legal remedy for patients, Justice Souter indicated, must derive from congressional legislation of minimal HMO standards, including HMO members' right to file a lawsuit in their state's court system. Adding to the decision's significance was the reality that managed care had become a fact of every American's life. If initially the wealthier sidestepped HMOs, exorbitant hikes in the most liberal health-plan premiums forced most people into some form of managed care, subject to limitations on pills, procedures, and choice of doctors. Not that the wealthier could ever avoid the country's health-care reality altogether. Not if they needed emergency care.

THE NOT-FOR-TV ER

As my parents drifted deep into old age, I found myself learning more than I ever wanted to know about emergency room staffing and its lack, and about triage of its continually arriving clientele. Here, in the city's only ER, the sheer volume of patients strained the hospital's capacity to handle medical emergencies. As in other ERs throughout the country, the growing number of people with no health insurance could find here a doctor who, by law, must at least stabilize their condition. Typically, that illness or injury had grown increasingly serious from lack of earlier care because the individual could not afford a doctor's office visit or care at a clinic offering sliding-scale fees. Now I sat with one parent or the other beside the uninsured, waiting: a wheezing, suffocating asthma attack; soaring blood pressure; uncontrolled diabetes; a festering wound infection; miserable vomiting from food poisoning or alcohol abuse, a drug overdose, or influenza; the heavy, juicy cough of a possible pneumonia or even the resurgent tuberculosis then worrying public health officials in Berkeley, as elsewhere throughout the country. Among those waiting were people suffering mental illness, needing far more sustained and comprehensive care than any ER could provide, people who would return to life on the streets because there was nowhere else for them to go. The staff labeled some patients frequent-flyers, showing up fifty and more times per year; others, a solitary man or woman brought by ambulance from a parking lot's edge or a downtown doorway, the paramedics described simply as found-down.

Unless wheeled through the ER doors on an ambulance gurney, patients began with a wait for the triage nurse whose task was to distinguish the critical from urgent, extreme pain from merely sick, assigning each case its place on an expansive list of priorities. Insurance questions followed close behind. And then the real wait: the large nondescript room with its barely watched television, endless and unchangeable, babbling from high on the wall next to the clock, above a sign about using a face mask if coughing. Sometimes, if able, someone would leave in frustration. It took but a visit or two before I dreaded another. And when that next decision point arose, I resisted the ordeal for my parent and myself, a self-imposed care delay perhaps longer than was wise.

My parents, at least, were Medicare patients, obviously so; the hospital could count on some amount of the payment due, albeit a steadily diminishing portion. Patients younger than sixty-five were questionable. During the 1990s, even those insured patients might include one whose HMO refused later to define this visit as an emergency or this hospital as allowable or refused to authorize treatment on the spot when ER staff called (as some plans required) and patients waited. This latter practice finally prompted a federal government advisory late in 1998, reported under another notable *New York Times* headline seeming to announce what should be obvious: "Hospitals told not to delay emergency room treatment."[11] Such an advisory, of course, would not help patients whose HMO required their own triage-by-telephone, patients who called their HMO as instructed, then stayed home, as instructed, waiting until morning, a wait that in many instances proved to be too long.

Perhaps our local ER does not display the grim chaos of a big city hospital. There may be fewer stab or gunshot wounds, fewer homeless ill than in New York or Chicago. Berkeley's ER undoubtedly experiences less time when it is so overcrowded that it is forced to divert ambulances to a different hospital farther away. In cities throughout the country, however, increased demand combined with cost-cutting ER closures have even forced ambulances to circle, at times, with paramedics working on their passenger while the driver seeks a place to land. Before 1996, for example, San Francisco General Hospital diverted ambulances for a few hours during two or three days out of a month. By 2000, ER staff hoped for one day each month with no diversions. During months of greatest demand, of winter flu and pneumonia, this ER—site of the city's renowned and only trauma unit—turned ambulances away nearly 50 percent of the time.[12] Yet for smaller communities, like Berkeley, the one hospital's ER is the only game in town; it feels particularly unsettling to know ambulances cannot alight, all the more so when the same condition prevails simultaneously at the next closest ER, the next town over. Within the fewer ERs throughout the country, moreover, an absence of specialists, neurosurgeons for instance, might rob critically ill and injured patients of lifesaving care.[13] And in 2003, further aggravating an already dismal situation, the Bush administration weakened the 1986 law requiring physicians to at least stabilize the medical condition of anyone arriving at a hospital, including those who could not afford to pay for such care.[14]

The critical function and alarming state of an emergency room concentrate the threat to health care more generally: if many Americans face restrictions by reason of cost, all experience limits on access and quality. I could not know why an ER doctor discharged my mother in the wee hours of the morning after what began as an early evening visit (described in the introduction) rather than admit her to the hospital and monitor her condition the remainder of the night; but I certainly could not feel confident he made this decision with an eye toward most prudently safeguarding her fragile health. Reducing hospitalizations was, by then, a well known economizing strategy. To my surprise, moreover, I learned there might not have been a bed available for my mother that cold and rainy night, primarily because too few nurses were already assigned too many patients, an outcome of prior cutbacks in staff and services. The reason, then, might not have been a doctor's concern about the number of patients he admitted. Perhaps there was just no room at the inn.

HOSPITALS AS A LOCUS OF LIMITS

"If you are in the hospital and being told to leave, press 1 now"—this telephone-answering menu selection verbalized succinctly the fact that emergency rooms dramatize but one dimension of rationed hospital care. Fortunately, my call to the organization designated to investigate appeals and complaints about health-care services for Medicare patients was less urgent (I was phoning to initiate a formal review of my mother's recent ER experience). Other callers were obviously in the throes of a conflict requiring immediate response, attempting to avoid what they considered untimely eviction from a hospital.

"Quicker and sicker" is the characterization critics use to describe the way hospitals now send patients home. The cost-cutting policy enlarges not only need for care at home but also chances for costly readmission to the hospital because of recovery complications. Quicker and sicker discharge poses risk especially for older adults with complex multiple health problems and little physiological reserves, the approximately 25 percent of Medicare recipients who require a lion's share of the program's spending. This approach poses all the more danger given inadequate resources for individualized discharge planning, case coordination and follow-up contacts, not to mention cutbacks in Medicare's already meager home-care coverage. An analysis of hospital discharge for Medicare patients with congestive heart failure, for instance, indicates that comprehensive discharge planning with follow-up care (such as case coordination of home visits, medications, diet, exercise, social services) results in patients' lowered hospital readmission rates and improved outcomes, without raising costs.[15] Instead, a greater care burden for sicker convalescents shifts primarily to family members over a longer stretch of time, at least for patients fortunate enough to have such informal care available at home. Yet over the years Medicare has wrongfully denied home health benefits for significant numbers of eligible frail homebound elders, reimbursing their payments for formal care only after a lengthy appeal. In 2003, the Bush administration initiated steps to curtail such appeals, thereby reducing government safeguards and legitimizing denial of payment for what the reviewing judges considered "reasonable and necessary care," care that meets the longstanding legal standard for Medicare coverage.[16]

For older patients without even inadequate home care available, earlier hospital discharge may deliver the final push into a nursing home. Similarly, residents of assisted living, who maintain some degree of independence before a hospitalization, may emerge too sick, requiring too much care to return to the residence they left. Most of these discharged patients will face rationed care in its final form, within a skilled nursing facility. Notoriously understaffed, the most troublesome and persistent limit on a nursing home's necessary care is not sophisticated medical technology but the number of hours each day a resident receives hands-on attention from a sufficient number of trained, qualified nurses and aides. These are the people who administer medications, monitor and manage ongoing health problems, help residents eat and toilet, bathe them, get them out of bed or turn them in it. A lengthy study of skilled nursing facilities during the 1990s, requested by Congress (the first DHHS report appeared in 2000; see chapter 1), documented the critical shortage of nursing home staff, resulting in malnutrition, severe bedsores, infections, pneumonia, and other avoidable life-threatening conditions.

Abbreviated hospital stays, and their adverse health repercussions, have not been limited to the old. Managed care's mid-1990s heyday brought Americans "drive-through" labor and deliveries, mastectomies, and other surgical procedures as health insurers rushed their hospitalized customers in and out. Even with the most egregious such HMO practices curtailed, the rationing of hospital care diminishes more than the count of days. For some patients, health plans deny essential types of care—for instance, rehabilitative care following brain injury due to an accident or stroke. Whatever a person's age, regaining speech, mobility, or other physical abilities can depend on timely and appropriate rehabilitation in a specialized unit, often within a hospital site, extending at least throughout initial post-acute stages. Unfortunately, insurers may define even such medically necessary care as transitional, which they do not cover, unlike the immediate acute hospital care, which they do. Further rehabilitative services at home, especially physical and occupational therapies during the first post-stroke year, improve patients' abilities as well.[17] Indeed, middle-aged Americans are well advised to follow enough preventive health measures that they avoid suffering a stroke before reaching Medicare age; only after age sixty-five can they count on at least minimal rehabilitative transitional and home care before the cost comes out of their own pocket.

Individuals admitted to a hospital, insured or not, can find there a managed stinginess of care from day one. Most prominent is a dearth of nurses and aides. Patients wait for medications, bedpans, sponge baths, for an answer to their call, even as nurses circulate nonstop, perhaps armed with a cell phone, trying to cover their assigned patients' basic needs and periodic crises. Fatigued nurses less often catch a mistaken medication before the patient receives it. Nurses and doctors know these deeper limitations, these pervasive aspects of lesser care. Writing in the *New England Journal of Medicine* in 1998, a physician outlined deficiencies, errors, and frustrations rendering hospital care, in his view, mediocre. Unsafe nurse-patient ratios and overly long work shifts are common, sapping nurses' mental and physical abilities. Nurses, always rushed and in some instances with insufficient training, may fail to document in the patients' charts ongoing clinical status—vital signs, medications, intravenous infusions, changes in mental state—the key source of information for doctors and other staff. Moreover, hospitals hire lower-wage, lower-skilled nurse assistants to accomplish nursing tasks, resulting in errors and omissions that delay diagnosis and appropriate treatment, with "grave consequences for the overall quality of care."[18]

Two studies reported in 2002 quantified the consequences. The first analyzed discharge records of more than six million patients in nearly eight hundred hospitals. The results demonstrated consistently better care for patients in hospitals with a higher proportion of care from registered nurses, rather than less trained nurses and aides, as well as more hours of registered nurses' care.[19] Better outcomes included lower rates of urinary tract infections, upper gastrointestinal bleeding, pneumonia, shock, or cardiac arrest; in addition, patients' length of hospital stay was shorter. The highest rates of poor outcome entailed *failure to rescue,* defined as patients' death from one of five life-threatening complications that develop during hospitalizations—pneumonia, shock or cardiac arrest, upper gastrointestinal bleeding, uncontrollable infection, deep vein thrombosis (blood clots)—and that all require early identification for rescue to succeed. The second study linked data from nurses' surveys with records of surgery patients at 169 Pennsylvania hospitals. In hospitals with a higher nurse-patient ratio (each nurse is responsible for more patients), nurses' dissatisfaction and burnout were higher; patients' death rates from surgery and from failure to rescue were higher as well. In addition, hospitals in which nurses had higher levels of education (a college BA or more, with comparably higher salary) experienced lower patients' death rates from surgery and failure to rescue.[20]

And there is more: rushed, poorly paid, and poorly trained technicians fail to properly obtain and process a doctor's laboratory orders, resulting in repeated vein-sticks to draw blood (each puncture painful and likely to bruise the fragile veins and skin of many older patients; also difficult for the very young) and delays in reporting results; patients are discharged at midnight so that insurers avoid another day's costs; discharged patients require at-home intravenous medications and laboratory tests as well as daily care; hospitals employ fewer dieticians, meal-deliverers, supply clerks, pharmacists, and housekeepers to clean up the mess.

Another form of limits on hospital care essentially rations a primary care doctor's availability and time. That is, in increasing numbers of hospitals, patients will never see their own doctor. A new breed of physician, descriptively dubbed a *hospitalist,* sees patients of many different primary care doctors but only in the hospital, providing the general medical care and supervision of individual patients that were previously facets of their own doctor's practice; the latter sees patients only at the office. And increasingly, if the hospitalist determines a patient needs intensive care, an *intensivist* will be in charge. The goal of such in-house physicians is to minimize the length of a patient's stay and the use of consultants, thereby accomplishing a more cost-effective hospitalization. Granted, these new specialists provide expertise with sophisticated technologies available in hospitals for diagnosis and treatment. The data are not yet in, however, on the way cost-effectiveness, as calculated by hospitals and insurance companies, translates into the quality of patients' experiences in the hospital or their health outcomes. The immediate side effect for patients can be a more bewildering and helpless experience allowing them little involvement in medical decisions. Though perhaps more efficient, the trend denies what the alarmed physician cited previously defines as "a central tenet of primary care: continuity of care," even when individuals are hospitalized.[21]

For patients and their families, this recently developed restriction threatens more than the loss of a familiar physician's face, important as that can be, especially for many older hospitalized patients who, beyond feeling sick and vulnerable, become disoriented or even delirious (to the point that some hospitals with too few staff use physical restraints, essentially tying patients to the bed). A hospitalist disrupts an ongoing dialogue between patients and their primary care doctor, a long-term relationship in which this hospitalization is but the latest episode of a health history far more extensive than any patient's chart. That more comprehensive history includes understandings and compatibilities built over time about approaches to, and wishes regarding, various types of medical intervention. An in-house physician may be more available physically during daytime hours to see hospitalized patients and, perhaps, to talk with family members. And even if a hospitalist or intensivist consults the primary care physician, this availability may be of limited value, especially now that health-care economics plays such a prominent role in decisions about testing and treatment, hospital discharge, and subsequent needs for skilled nursing and rehabilitative care.

These concerns become particularly weighty as individuals age, develop more complex health problems, and eventually approach the time when difficult, highly personal decisions about aggressiveness of treatment may in fact come into play.[22] The primary care physician will more likely know family members, perceive their reactions and needs, and be better able to provide them needed advice and support. Less likely, finally, will be experiences similar to the case of a seventy-seven-year-old woman suffering chronic but rapidly worsening lung disease, as her family decided about mechanical ventilation. Reported in the *Journal of the American Medical Association,* the story illustrates a troubling disconnect: although a hospitalist "perceived [the patient's] family to be comfortable and satisfied with limitations on life support . . . the family's experience was quite different. Despite [that doctor's] careful attention, he does not appear to have been aware of the depth of [the son's] grief."[23] Reality does not usually meet ideal conditions, in which a patient not only has previously written directives, particularly conveying wishes about end-of-life care, but someone actually brings this document to the hospital (I discuss this and related issues in chapter 5). Moreover, even with an advance directive on hand, many written wishes will not quite fit the actual, often acute and unforeseen situation. Reaching a treatment decision that respects the patient's wishes and autonomy, made in that individual's best interest, while tending also to family members involved, is hard enough for the primary care doctor, let alone a stranger.

Throughout managed care's reign, hospitals have remained at the center of broader health-care rationing, primarily through lessened access to them. One threat to access arises directly from negotiations between managed care's largest players—especially insurers and hospitals—seeking the best deal they can muster. When these stakeholders reach an impasse over the amount of reimbursement, the people insured by a negotiating health plan may lose services of their area's hospital. In northern California, for instance, the highly regarded Oakland Children's Hospital terminated its agreement in 2002 with a major insurer, Blue Shield, after a year of unsuccessful fee negotiations. Plan members would no longer have access to a hospital known for the excellence of its programs for childhood cancers and blood disorders, of its emergency room and other surgical and medical services, and of the region's only child trauma center. Two years earlier the state's largest HMO, Blue Cross, informed its San Francisco Bay Area members that the health insurer would no longer cover care at any of the nearest hospitals, all owned by the same corporation, whether for treatment of a life-threatening condition or delivery of a new baby. Though the most immediate factor was failed contract negotiations with the regional hospital network, the potential for this deadlock had grown over the years: just as emergency rooms closed, so too had hospitals merged, cut back on available services, or gone out of business, leaving the public, via its insurers, fewer hospitals from which to chose.

Beyond the elimination of excess resulting from pre-1990s hospital overbuilding, these business decisions—which mergers and closures are—diminish access for many Americans to important resources for medically necessary and beneficial health care. Small community hospitals disappear, forcing nearby residents to travel great distances for hospital care. Hospitals connected to medical schools and universities suffer as well. As centers for medical research and training, these academic hospitals have long provided diagnostic and treatment expertise for people with unusual or mysterious conditions, as well as experimental therapies that become the last hope for intractable illness or disability. In many of the country's large cities, the urban poor living in the shadows of an academic medical center find their only source of health care in its clinics and ER.[24] Moreover, declining government reimbursement to these hospitals undermines not only today's medical care but also the training of doctors for the years ahead, for all segments of society.

And finally, repercussions of limits established during the past decade of managed care threaten our future health and well-being in a different but now undeniable way. The mysterious outbreak of anthrax immediately following the World Trade Center and Pentagon attacks in September 2001 raised public alarm not only about this treatable disease but also about potentially more devastating illness—of known or unknown origin. The anthrax scare alarmed even more profoundly public health physicians and administrators. They are aware that managed care, and profit-driven health-care policies more generally, have decimated this country's capacity to safeguard the public. Cutting off services in order to recoup financial loss targets the public hospitals and clinics that should be prepared for key roles in a large-scale emergency. Also severely trimmed are city, county, and state health departments responsible for monitoring health and illness in their communities, responding quickly and efficiently to disease outbreaks, and ensuring whatever preventive measures are possible. American health care has been stripped down in the name of cost-effectiveness, left with no margin of error should the unforeseen threat materialize. Even a particularly severe influenza outbreak would worsen dangerously with so many uninsured adults and children unable to afford early care or a preventive vaccine (if available). The health-care rationing now well established for people's everyday ordinary ailments and injuries will seem a luxury in light of the rude awakening to come: there are too few doctors, nurses, and facilities in place that everyone must share, whatever the extraordinary public health emergency.[25]

INTERDEPENDENCE AT MANY LEVELS

As I expected, the official complaint about my mother's ER visit—what I perceived as unhealthy rationing of overnight hospital care—caused not a ripple. How could it when the process is a review by physician colleagues, and the doctor involved decides whether to reveal to the patient what that review determined? Anyway, I knew this protest provided mainly a salve for my own frustration. In whatever manner a well-intentioned but overwhelmed ER staff implicitly rationed my mother's care, it was a single, minute event within a fundamentally malformed, malfunctioning system of interdependent, interacting parts.

Just as the health and care of older individuals entail complex interactions, the overall health-care system straining now to accommodate an aging population reflects intertwined social policies' pressures. Even during the economic boom of the Clinton years, health-care costs continued to rise (albeit more slowly), as did the number of people unable to afford the corresponding increase in the expense of insurance. Health care for these uninsured, in turn, required increasing the financial subsidy—for example, of ER and hospitalization costs—through higher prices charged to insured Americans, prices reflected in higher premiums, co-pays, and deductibles. With certain excesses of traditional fee-for-service medicine trimmed, a reescalation of expense guaranteed a correspondingly greater burden of care for so many uninsured. In 2001, the government's annual report of health-care spending revealed an increase sharper than during any year of the 1990s. Along with increasingly sophisticated and costly medical technologies, persistent excesses of expense attached especially to unregulated drug prices (up 15.7 percent, the fastest rise and accelerating) and hospital costs, a pattern repeated in subsequent years.[26] Overall, the country's upward pattern also reflects health-care needs of an aging population and the considerable costs of having approximately 2,500 private, for-profit health insurance plans mediate and manage everyone's care.

By the century's turn, it was no secret that managed care was not solving problems with the cost or the quality of care. With all the rising expense lavished on medical interventions, broad nationwide studies revealed that adults received, on average, only about 40–50 percent of recommended standard care for common acute and chronic illness and important preventive measures.[27] Private insurers began reversing course, eliminating many of the most unpopular health-plan restrictions and providing more flexible options, with the greater choices and expense shifting to insurance purchasers.[28] Yet the managed-care era's most profound failure remained the uninsured, whose numbers were climbing past forty-one million. The trade association representing insurance companies trotted out once again the same two characters— Harry and Louise—who had helped smother Clinton's proposal for universal health insurance just a few years earlier. Now, however, this familiar media couple lamented the plight of uninsured Americans and advocated the industry's own plan—a combination of government subsidies that would, no surprise, make it easier for workers and small employers to purchase private insurance. Two years later, with conditions worsening, the health-insurers' association would join a new and unusual coalition (including the U.S. Chamber of Commerce, AFL-CIO, Service Employees International Union, Families USA, AARP, and other organizations). The coalition's aim: to publicize the worsening threat to every American's health following the largest one-year increase of uninsured in nearly ten years, an estimated two million people during 2001, a majority of whom worked at full-time jobs.[29]

In 2002 the record fell again, with an increase of 2.4 million that brought the total to 43.6 million uninsured Americans, 15.2 percent of the population. More than 80 percent lived in a family that included one or more jobholders.[30] The numbers were, in fact, even grimmer, as the coalition cited above demonstrated to the American public through media advertisements and activities nationwide. While the usual annual statistic of uninsured reflects a U.S. Census Bureau estimate of how many people lacked health insurance over the entire previous year, it ignores all the people uninsured for some portion of a year. Analysis of census data spanning 2001 and 2002 revealed nearly 75 million people under the age of sixty-five (30.7 percent)—not yet eligible for government-insured Medicare—who were uninsured for all or part of the two-year span.[31] A full 90 percent lacked health insurance for three months or more, 65 percent for six months or more, and 24 percent throughout the entire twenty-four months. Nationwide, 70.7 percent of uninsured adults were employed as of December 2002 (with no coverage offered or employee premiums unaffordable), and nearly 10 percent more were actively seeking a job.

The next year's report revealed clearly the direction Americans' health insurance situation was moving. The total uninsured for all or part of 2002–03 rose to 81.8 million, one person out of three. Over half were uninsured for at least nine months. In fourteen states the proportion exceeded one-third (up from nine states), including the large states of Texas (43.4 percent of the state's residents uninsured, 8.5 million people), California (37.1 percent, 11.9 million), New York (33.4 percent, 5.6 million), and even Florida, with its large Medicare population (34.8 percent, 4.8 million people). By December 2003, nearly eight of every ten uninsured adults (78.8 percent) were employed, along with one in every twenty (5.7 percent) actively looking. With so many Americans, including children, experiencing insurance gaps year-to-year, if not all year, the failure of tying health insurance to employment is evident. Moreover, the statistics no longer affect primarily the working and unemployed poor: for instance, among people with an annual income between $55,980 and $74,640 (for a family of four), more than one-fourth were uninsured at some point during the previous two years.[32]

Initially, the well-insured middle class felt the impact of the uninsured indirectly, through various implicit forms of health-care rationing discussed earlier—emergency room waits, declining quality of hospital care, as well as higher out-of-pocket costs. Yet these mounting indirect effects were fast becoming a major social and economic burden. Especially prominent in the employment-centered health insurance system, working people consistently paid more to receive the same, if not reduced, health benefits, as employers increasingly shifted health-care costs to employees through larger insurance premiums, co-payments, and deductibles and cut back on benefits provided. The Kaiser Family Foundation's survey for 2002 found that 56 percent of large companies (200 or more employees) increased the amount of premiums employees pay. The next year, more than 60 percent raised employees' contributions, with nearly 80 percent of the companies anticipating increases for 2004. People insured through their employer were paying 48 percent more of their own health-care costs than they paid three years earlier. Among all businesses, 17 percent provided fewer health-care benefits in 2002, compared to a 7 percent decrease in 2000.[33] Beyond tiered prescription drug co-payments described above, some health plans were introducing tiered hospital co-payments, a troubling proposition, for how well can laypeople, let alone health-care analysts, evaluate and choose among hospitals that vary in cost and quality?[34]

By January 2003 employees' dissatisfaction focused increasingly and more vocally on inadequate and overly expensive health insurance benefits rather than wages or working conditions. For example, General Electric workers called a two-day nationwide strike, their first in more than thirty years, protesting the company's decision to raise by hundreds of dollars their yearly share of health insurance costs. This pattern would repeat throughout other industries—for instance, a lengthy and bitter strike of southern California supermarket employees, a four-day strike in 2004 of SBC Communications employees.

The new century's economic recession compounded people's serious concerns about unaffordable health insurance. Retirees counting on health-care benefits through a former employer faced changes similar to those still employed: the lucky ones must pay higher out-of-pocket costs for reduced coverage; the unlucky lost retirees' health insurance altogether. In 2004, 79 percent of large businesses that provide benefits raised their retirees' premium contribution, and 85 percent expected to do so in 2005.[35] Somewhere in between, a new trend limited retirees to access-only health plans. That is, individuals could obtain the company's group retiree insurance but must pay the full costs. Loss of an expected employer's subsidy created a particularly onerous burden for retirees not yet eligible for Medicare (whether or not the promise of continued health insurance had influenced them to retire early). Close to 50 percent of companies that still provide retirees' health plans are likely to follow the access-only route before this decade's end. Newly hired employees are less likely than in years past to be offered retirement benefits, a prospect that ties some people to jobs they would otherwise leave. By 2025, predicts the Princeton health economist Uwe Reinhardt, retirees' health insurance will be history.[36]

Furthermore, with nearly two-thirds of the under-sixty-five population insured through an employer, layoffs posed a direct threat to workers' health insurance; after all, a decade earlier, during the recession of 1990–92, half of the people who lost their jobs also lost their health insurance. As described above, however, you certainly do not need to be unemployed in twenty-first-century America to join the ranks of the uninsured or seriously underinsured. With premiums skyrocketing, fewer employers and employees, especially in smaller companies, can afford even to share the expense of providing health insurance benefits.

The loss of a job and its health insurance benefit is particularly worrisome for the middle-aged. In the first place, women and men in their fifties and early sixties who lose a job are unlikely to easily find new employment, especially a job that assures affordable health care. And in yet another display of interdependence in the vicious cycle American health care has become, many employers have refrained from filling vacancies or creating jobs that would include health insurance (premium costs rose 11.2 percent in 2004), no small reason for the jobless and sluggish recovery from recession, and for persistently rising numbers of uninsured. Moreover, people lacking health insurance for whatever reason at midlife are more likely than insured age-mates, and of course than younger adults, to experience a noticeable decline in health.[37]

RATIONING UNVEILED

Throughout the 1990s, most Americans experienced limits on their health care, the types and amount generally reflecting income level and insurance status. Given the limitations on resources, the state of Oregon decided on rationing of health-care services as explicit public policy— but only for the poor. Recognizing that people were going without basic health care and, further, that a large uninsured population undermines the quality of care for everyone, the state attempted to devise a more fair and adequate distribution of health services for its low-income population. In order to include more uninsured residents in Oregon's Medicaid program, in 1991 a state health commission, with public input, drew up a prioritized list of hundreds of diagnoses and treatments. It designated a cut-off line intended to eliminate only ineffective, futile, or nonessential medical services, allowing the state to use its limited resources for basic, effective care of more low-income people. The state would pay for treatments prioritized higher than the cut-off line. So, for instance, Medicaid would not cover certain organ transplants—with high expense but low success—nor in vitro fertilization (same reason), or cosmetic stripping of varicose veins; instead, the state's health insurance program would enroll more uninsured pregnant women and provide their prenatal care. The Oregon experiment reflected a classic instance of half-empty–half-full. Critics argued, in principle, against rationing, that is, denying services, only for the poor. Proponents focused on the state's effort to recognize a right to health care and assure nearly all low-income residents, including those not eligible for standard federal-state Medicaid insurance, a package of basic services.

Whatever the pros and cons of Oregon's program, its rationing experiment has been burdened, in practice, by the same nationwide realities of soaring costs. By 2000 the priorities cut-off for treatments covered became more restrictive, yet still the state's budget could not cover all of the eligible treatments for all residents who would otherwise be uninsured. By spring 2003 Oregon Health Plan officials announced a major setback: the program could no longer cover such necessary services as prescription drugs for all of its recipients.[38] A few months later, months filled with pharmaceutical lobbying, the setback changed form. Instead of cutting back on prescription drugs, the program would take an alternative approach to lowering costs, dropping thousands of enrollees from insurance eligibility.[39]

Other states too were cutting back Medicaid programs in response to rising costs and declining revenues—narrowing eligibility criteria, reducing benefits provided, increasing co-payments, and decreasing payments to health-care providers.[40] As throughout American health care, the most rapidly rising expense was prescription drugs. And no medications were more problematic than the newest, most expensive generation of antipsychotics used to treat mental illnesses, including dementia symptoms in the old. Just as private insurers established formularies that favor lower-priced medications, state health insurance programs for the poor have designated preferred medications Medicaid will cover. One antipsychotic brand—Zyprexa, a $10 per day drug whose monthly tab for my father so shocked me—has been the focus of particular controversy.[41] As the top moneymaker for Eli Lilly in 2002, and with most sales going to government programs, primarily Medicaid, its manufacturer fights hard to maintain this market. Although drug companies have been largely successful over the years in preventing states from restricting drugs for mental illness—as of 2003, twenty-eight states exempted them from restrictions of preferred medication formularies— Zyprexa's excessive expense pushed the limits. With a similar medication (Risperdol) available at close to half the cost, a few states sought to limit Medicaid coverage for Zyprexa in order to provide this type of medication to more of their low-income residents. So, for example, a state would require Medicaid recipients treated for mental illness to begin with Risperdol, switching to the Lilly brand only in cases where the first, less expensive medication proved unsuccessful.

Eli Lilly Company, a suddenly outraged champion of the poor, rallied in support of these patients' needs—that is, for the same choice of new drugs available to everyone else in the state, regardless of ability to pay. Denials of medication choices are unfair to the poor, Lilly spokespersons insisted, and interfere with a doctor's medical decisions. In addition to the manufacturer's own intense lobbying, Lilly orchestrated broader campaigns to avert state Medicaid restrictions on Zyprexa, funding consumer advocacy groups for the mentally ill to mount protests and ghostwriting newspaper articles in the local press (minor variations of marketing strategies described in chapter 3). Neither Eli Lilly nor other drug manufacturers, however, demonstrated similar concern when suing states that attempted to regulate Medicaid drug prices in order to provide drug coverage for more low-income residents.[42] Nor is the pharmaceutical industry concerned about far wider unfairness and harmful consequences of the high prices it sets, pushing certain medications completely out of reach of patients who are poor and, in many instances, creating financial burden for all but the wealthy.

More generally, by the early twenty-first century rationing was no longer unmentionable. Joining the Supreme Court's earlier utterance, for instance, was another major national institution, the *Wall Street Journal*. Its series "Who Gets Health Care? Rationing in an Age of Rising Costs" reported an array of limits not only on care for the poor, but for all Americans, insured (including regional variation in Medicare-paid services) or not: on diagnostic and treatment procedures, days in an intensive-care unit, home health care, as well as expensive medications like Zyprexa.[43] Adding to the unfairness and illogic of American health care, while many people are losing access to needed medical care, others undergo expensive procedures based not on medical rationale and data, but on the strength of commercial interests in concert with prevailing payment incentives.

If on a smaller scale than the pharmaceutical and insurance industries, other corporate players shape treatments patients are more or less likely to receive. A good example: medical device makers reward doctors—through consultant fees, research grants, expense-paid conferences in desirable locales—for performing and promoting surgeries that use their devices. This industry also influences health plans, with Medicare the largest payer, to maintain generous coverage. Thus, surgeons and hospitals receive much higher reimbursements for spinal fusion surgery that employs metal screws and rods than for a simpler procedure that does not use such hardware; yet no scientific evidence indicates that the former reduces back pain more effectively than the latter, except in a very limited number of very limited conditions. This surgery does significantly increase costs and medical complications. Some surgeons assert that most fusion procedures performed in the United States are unnecessary and urge greater FDA testing and surveillance of the hardware, even as others join medical hardware makers lobbying legislators and government officials who make health policy, in order to secure the procedure's financial support. More broadly, as mentioned in the previous chapter, most treatments of very common back pain may be unnecessary.[44]

The struggle of Oregon and other states to pay for health services under Medicaid, including prescription drugs and various surgeries, does make explicit one answer to questions of whose health care is rationed, on what basis. At least one significant state expense—pharmaceutical costs for older adults who are poor—is expected to become the federal government's problem in 2006 when the new Medicare prescription benefit replaces Medicaid for everyone sixty-five and older (58 percent of Medicaid drug expenditures have covered prescription costs of Medicare recipients who fall below a set poverty line). With private, for-profit insurers providing the coverage, analysts predict that low-income older adults who formerly obtained medications through their state's Medicaid program will likely face a more restricted list of available drugs.

Another answer about targets of rationing nationwide applies to everyone who lives long enough: limits on medical treatments for the old. More hushed and hidden than rationing health care by income, rationing by age is in many ways less clear-cut, especially with patients nearing the end of life. Withholding medical interventions from the old may reflect inadequate practice and unjustified rationing—medical ageism—or appropriate, humane, and respectful end-of-life care. On the one hand, physicians may underestimate benefits of certain treatments, giving up on older patients prematurely; on the other hand, aggressive and futile medical interventions for frail and elderly patients can, in the words of one geriatrician, "border on assault."[45]

Few doctors or hospitals state a policy for limiting care to older patients as bluntly as one memorandum circulated at a London hospital during the mid-1960s: "The following are not to be resuscitated: very frail elderly, over sixty-five years. The top of the yellow treatment card is to be marked NTBR [not to be resuscitated]."[46] This directive, issued in the context of budgetary restraints, caused a furor, and the age of sixty-five now sounds disturbingly young. In the United States, with no national health service comparable to the United Kingdom's, budgets and age loom nevertheless as a worrisome combination.

MANAGED CARE MEETS OLDER AGE

Physicians treating aged patients no doubt reach decisions shaped by implicit, even subconscious views of life quality, life expectancy, death, and the reasonable allocation of medical resources between young and old. As discussed earlier, however, this country's lurch into managed care demonstrated a less personal influence on the type and amount of medical treatment people of any age receive: financial incentives underlying payments to doctors and hospitals. Before managed care, fee-for-service payment—reimbursing costs of every visit and procedure—pushed in the direction of excess medical intervention. Managed-care plans reversed the financial incentives. Most prominently, insurers pay doctors a preset fee for each enrolled member, called *capitation,* or paying per head, regardless of the amount and type of treatment a member receives. Less treatment means greater savings for participating physicians. During the early years, insurance bureaucrats guarded the purse; payments to doctors depended on stringent requirements for authorization of each proposed test, treatment, or hospitalization. Forced by patients' and doctors' dissatisfaction to modify their role, insurers instead left to doctors the unwelcome business, as well as financial risk, of budgeting and administering reimbursement fees. If insured patients wanted more flexible plans, they paid more in premiums, deductibles, and co-pays.

The old occupy a particularly vulnerable and shifting niche within this financial incentives scheme. Although traditional Medicare maintains its fee-for-service structure, the actual amount the federal government pays for each service has fallen low enough, over the last dozen years, that doctors and hospitals no longer view older patients as a more steady, reliable source of income than younger patients. Rather, Medicare recipients have become yet another financial drain. By 2002, more and more doctors were simply refusing to accept new Medicare patients, a problem not only for people over sixty-five but also for many middle-aged daughters and sons intent on moving parents to a new location. (In some instances doctors even referred out longtime patients to another physician.) Medicare patients who had no primary care doctor or needed a specialist were more often becoming an added emergency room problem, further straining already exhausted resources—arriving like the uninsured, more sick and needing care more costly than it would have been if they had seen a doctor earlier.

Older Americans did have an alternate route into a doctor's office. Federal legislation had forged a direct link between managed care and Medicare, allowing recipients to opt for a Medicare HMO, offered by private insurers. During the mid-1990s commercial health insurance companies heavily promoted this new product, as they refer to it, targeting seniors through media advertisements, direct mail appeals, free meals with promotional pitches at local restaurants, speakers at residential facilities. These burgeoning senior plans promised lower out-of-pocket costs yet more comprehensive health services than traditional Medicare. To enroll, individuals need only sign over their government Medicare funds to the commercial insurer, which would manage the monies more efficiently even while providing benefits Medicare did not—for example, prescription drug coverage, preventive screening and health education, services for vision and hearing, chiropractic, and dental care.

My own parents avoided the HMO route, despite the barrage of advertisements touting various local plans. In fact, solicitations confused them, requiring an understanding not only of Medicare's parts A and B, but also of the comparable costs and benefits of the several managed-care alternatives. My father's questions to me, his request for a daughter's advice, had marked a first. Perhaps his mental capacities were in early decline, and perhaps he alone noticed; my mother had never involved herself in such matters. Neither could make an adequately informed decision. Fortunately, they could afford to stay with what they had: traditional Medicare and supplementary private insurance, especially to cover my mother's medications. In their confusion they were not alone. How many other Medicare recipients felt similarly uncertain what it all meant and what to do?

Many senior plans would have avoided my parents anyway. Contrary to federal regulations, these HMOs enrolled selectively, developing marketing tactics that skewed membership toward younger, healthier Medicare recipients. Among the more notorious examples: advertising at gymnasiums, emphasizing exercise classes as a benefit, signing up members in offices inaccessible to the frail and disabled. If less-fit individuals slipped in, the plans could, as one analyst put it, "encourage the sickest people to go elsewhere by giving them poor service."[47] (Critics of the 2003 Medicare legislation foresee similar tactics by private insurers offering prescription drug coverage or a broader health plan, leaving the population most in need of costly care within traditional Medicare.) There are reported instances of patients at the other extreme, receiving minimal end-of-life custodial care as noncompetent, even comatose nursing home residents who somehow became enrolled in a Medicare HMO without the knowledge, let alone agreement, of family members.

In sum, through such efforts HMOs were undermining the very principle of insurance, which spreads financial risk as traditional Medicare does across the full gamut of a population, healthier and sicker, in order to protect individuals who incur large expense. Indeed, before Congress established this government insurance program in the mid-1960s, half of the people sixty-five and older were uninsured and uninsurable, rejected because of preexisting health conditions and other restrictions imposed by commercial insurance companies.

If prospects for Medicare HMOs initially sounded bright, the track record has not been. High-profile marketing gave way in just a few years in the face of a different form of media attention. Month after month, reports revealed health maintenance organizations were raising costs for enrollees of senior plans and eliminating once-promised services. Among the most important of disappearing benefits was coverage for at least a portion of prescription drugs, the benefit most costly for individuals and insurers alike, the very benefit luring many Medicare recipients to HMOs in the first place. By the twentieth century's end, major managed-care companies were discontinuing their Medicare plans altogether— essentially dumping their enrollees—having determined that people older than sixty-five, even the cherry-picked, were not profitable after all. Suddenly thrust into health insurance limbo, millions of Medicare-age patients either had to find a different, comparable HMO—an increasingly difficult task—or return to traditional Medicare and find a doctor willing to accept them (also increasingly difficult), still with no prescription drug coverage. Frequently, a supplemental Medigap plan they had dropped in order to join a less expensive HMO was no longer available or affordable: if not rejected by the plan altogether, they now found its premiums and co-pays prohibitive.

And there was more bad news for people still enrolled in a Medicare HMO. Evidence began accumulating that, overall, managed-care plans provided lower-quality care resulting in poorer health outcomes than traditional Medicare, especially for the acutely sick or chronically ill— just the individuals requiring extensive high-quality care. For instance, HMO members less often received health care at home following a hospitalization, although such home care can improve outcomes and reduce hospital readmissions.[48] Following a stroke, HMO members more often landed in a nursing home for custodial care rather than in a specialized rehabilitation facility, although the latter improves chances of recovering at least some former abilities, even more so when followed by rehabilitative therapy at home.[49] More broadly, a comparison of physical health measures indicated greater deterioration over four years among Medicare HMO members than their non-HMO counterparts.[50] Additional studies suggested substantial underuse of medically necessary care in the private managed-care plans, with poorer health outcomes likely.[51] Interviews of patients during 2000–2001 found that although HMO patients reported receiving more preventive services (e.g., flu and pneumonia immunizations), which traditional Medicare did not cover, patients in the traditional program experienced easier access to care and better communication with their doctors.[52] Nor would traditional Medicare fee-for-service patients necessarily remain untouched by the HMO spread: like secondhand smoke, in the geographical areas with the greatest proportion of managed-care enrollment, everyone—non-managed-care patients included—received fewer, less intensive health services than in areas maintaining greater fee-for-service dominance.[53]

In the failed experiment of Medicare HMOs—the supremacy of cost and profit ending with so many elderly patients denied needed services, if not dumped—my parents' generation has been the guinea pig. This attempt crystallizes the spirit infusing for-profit managed care across all ages: packaging health and well-being as a product to promote and sell, an enterprise wrongheaded and lacking in humane social concern, if not mean-spirited at its core. Someday Americans may look back on the turn of this century, pre-Medicare prescription drug coverage and pre-universal health care more generally, the way people now can hardly imagine a time of no Medicare and Social Security. Until then, especially given efforts to force these government insurance programs into the private corporate marketplace, today's middle-aged might do well to see today's old also as canaries in the mine, alerting us to the dangers of allowing market competition and economic means to determine the health-care services people do and do not receive, particularly as they age.

AGE AS THE LIMIT ON CARE

As suggested earlier, the financial incentives of managed care are not the only factor raising fears that doctors and institutions may skimp on care for the old. Age itself has long been a consideration in treatment decisions, even while fee-for-service payments reigned supreme. Whether at a specific age or less precise cut-off, patients have been designated as too old, and thereby ineligible, for certain medical interventions. Although systematic studies were rare, many physicians assumed, for example, heart surgery or cancer treatment to be ineffective or of marginal benefit compared to risks for older patients. Regarding treatments with limited availability and high cost, such as organ transplants, and other increasingly sophisticated and expensive medical technologies, estimates of time to live that individuals will gain, as well as their future contributions to society, favor the young.[54]

The old continue to face the double bind of overly aggressive, futile treatment on the one hand, and arbitrary age cut-offs on the other. Certainly, estimates of a treatment's effects on life expectancy and life quality are crucial for reaching medical decisions. Such evaluations, however, need to arise from solid data and call for appropriate application to individual patients. Addressing one dimension of this task, researchers are presently attempting to assess more systematically the usefulness of screening tests to guide treatment decisions as people age. Such assessments analyze quantitative population statistics while also incorporating individual doctors' qualitative clinical judgments and patients' views of the benefits and risks of a test and the potential treatment. Bone density screening, for example, can help identify women most likely to benefit from long-term medication use, rather than exercise and dietary measures alone, although improved treatment guidelines await greater understanding of what the test measures and the relation of the range of density results to bone fracture. In cancer screening and treatment, one puzzling question is the extent to which screening identifies cancers that would never progress to cause symptoms during the patients' remaining lifetime, let alone contribute to death—most prominently, prostate tumors in men, and breast ductal carcinoma in situ identified through mammograms in women.[55] More qualitative questions involve the psychological distress that screening causes individuals, and, importantly, whether they would in fact consider undergoing treatment if a malignancy were detected.

Presently, individual doctors and their older patients may discuss views about medical intervention in various existing or potential circumstances, especially toward the end of life, but such conversations remain more the exception than the rule. Rationing by age proceeds in the absence of adequate data, based primarily on implicit, unstated, unformulated, and perhaps not fully conscious beliefs. Clearly, the impact of patients' age on medical outcomes requires documentation, along with public awareness and discussion of this relation. People need to know the extent to which limited resources and physicians' conceptions currently restrict health care provided the old. Medical concerns—regarding treatment's efficacy or futility during late decades of life, especially in cases with questionable prognosis—need to be identified and distinguished from cost concerns. Criteria used when allocating limited technologies, related to high expense or low availability (e.g., transplantable hearts and livers), need to be made explicit.

One outspoken medical ethicist identified with the notion of rationing by age has long argued the folly of directing health-care resources toward efforts that may add a few extra months or even years to an already long life. American medicine, Daniel Callahan asserts, perceives no tolerable cause of death. Too often doctors employ aggressive interventions aimed at curing whatever ailments afflict an aged patient, attempting to fight off death in cases where benefits are marginal at best, the interventions themselves barely tolerable, any added time likely of poor quality. While commonly accused of ageism, Callahan's arguments for redirecting resources into younger years aim at improving the quality of people's lives within a span that already extends toward their mideighties. Preventive public health and individual measures, supported by equitable distribution of health-care resources, would form the core of a lifelong medical approach directed at reducing sickness, disability, and premature death throughout the population. As people aged, their inseparable social, economic, and health needs would translate into policies that would ensure financial security, bolster independent living, and provide, if needed, long-term home or institutional care. Rather than striving always for cures—medicalizing old age in order to extend it—Callahan argues for efforts at improving quality at the end of life, with a goal of comfort and palliative measures, as embodied most fully in hospice care. He criticizes Medicare policies that cover heroic rescue medicine in hospital intensive care units while failing to provide home care for frail elders and the chronically ill; he proposes altered goals and expectations for health care at different stages of life, including limits on the pursuit of ever-increased longevity.[56]

In advocating a more general medical philosophy and orientation for the country's overall health-care enterprise, Callahan paints in broad strokes important principles and goals—even if rationing by age does sound harsh. Indeed, the limits he proposes may feel most harsh when individuals face difficult medical decisions about specific tests and treatments for an aged parent or spouse, or for themselves: How to respect a person's unique life and autonomy? How to accommodate family wishes? How to deny what could be the only, even if minimal, chance to live—when this individual may be one of those few who do turn out to benefit? While many people would agree about limits in the most extreme cases—for instance, resuscitating an extremely old, frail individual suffering heart and kidney failure—chronology alone is not generally decisive. The next chapter will focus on the types of care and care limits that are appropriate and compassionate as people pass through their life's end. The present concern is the less certain gray zones, the commonly occurring, uncommonly difficult situations when neither doctor nor patient and family know which medical path to follow.

As the population ages, its heterogeneity is becoming all the more apparent. Studies are beginning to identify not only important characteristics distinguishing the younger old from the older, but also the variability of physical and mental capacities regardless of chronological age. Researchers are attempting to sort out differences in the condition of older patients and to develop health profiles and histories that portend outcomes that are positive or poor. For instance, among Americans age sixty-five and older, researchers describe approximately one-third as vulnerable elders, with greatest likelihood of severe impairment or death within two years.[57] These individuals need health care that focuses on such geriatric conditions as incontinence, falls, pressure wounds, delirium, dementia, and end-of-life care, in addition to more general medical conditions (diabetes, heart failure, acute disease). Another useful example distinguishes between four categories among the old: the robust elderly, the frail, the demented, and the dying.[58] In this scheme, the goal of medical treatment for the old centers on maintaining or improving the quality of daily life. For individuals who are basically healthy and strong, the reason for heart valve replacement or bypass surgery or for treatment of certain cancers is not primarily to add on months at the end of an already old age, but to avert a slow decline into extended frailty. Individuals who are frail, even if chronologically younger, do not have the physiological reserve and resilience of the robust and therefore bring a different balance of risks and benefits to medical treatment decisions. Here the goal includes avoiding burdensome interventions with little chance of improving their quality of life. The same treatment helpful for the robust patient may well be futile and harmful for someone suffering multiple chronic health problems who already has little strength or energy or resistance to infection, or who has a weakened heart; in fact, for the frail, a troubling cascade of uncontrollable complications frequently follows medical interventions, particularly those involving hospitalization.[59]

Frailty among the old, of course, is a matter of degree. So too is dementia, a condition receiving increased attention due to increasing numbers, especially of those living into advanced stages, suffering severe symptoms. Health professionals and the public are gaining awareness that Alzheimer's and other dementias progress from early through intermediate stages and, especially for individuals with relatively few additional physical problems, into a final stage. Such awareness requires corresponding attention to the appropriateness of care that patients receive at differing points along the course of their dementia.

While medications and environmental interventions can benefit people during earlier phases of dementia, late stages with severe impairments can pose more vexing dilemmas. How aggressively to treat them for conditions such as pneumonia or cancer is but one decision that may arise. Other health-care decisions involve their daily existence. Advanced dementia often entails loss of physiological capacities. In addition to incontinence, swallowing becomes difficult during the last stage, and patients lose interest in eating. The common medical response, particularly in America's nursing homes and hospitals, is insertion of a feeding tube through the abdominal wall; surveys indicate that more than a third of nursing home residents with severe dementia undergo this surgical procedure.[60] However, the woman or man with severe dementia cannot understand what is happening, may become terribly frightened, and often attempts to pull the tube out. The risk of infection is high, the gain from any extended time with severe dementia hard to imagine. Arguments for limiting such intervention are growing. As one geriatrician explains, "There is a pervasive failure—by both physicians and the public—to view advanced dementia as a terminal illness, and there is strong conviction that technology can be used to delay death. The first step in changing these attitudes is for physicians to acknowledge that feeding tubes are generally ineffective in prolonging life, preventing aspiration [food particles sucked into the lung to cause pneumonia], and even providing adequate nourishment . . . and that they can have adverse consequences—principally the need for restraints [to prevent patients from pulling out the tube]."[61]

Such medical considerations are not the sole factors, and too frequently not even prominent ones in determining the use of feeding tubes. A study of nursing homes throughout the United States revealed the institution's logistics and budget to be the most significant factors—not residents' medical needs or wishes. This method of providing nutrition and preventing dehydration is less labor intensive, and therefore cheaper, than the alternative type of care: a trained staff person feeding patients by hand. As the researchers put it, more bluntly, "The staff's time required for feeding residents by hand is expensive."[62] In many states, moreover, government Medicaid payments per day are larger for residents with feeding tubes than for those without. In fact, this study found greater use of feeding tubes within for-profit nursing homes compared to not-for-profit facilities, a finding the investigators describe as "among the most notable observations . . . consistent with the notion . . . that feeding tube use among patients with advanced cognitive impairment may be used by nursing homes as a means of cost-saving." Also consistent with bottom-line concerns—and in contrast to calls for limits on medically aggressive interventions—is greater use of feeding tubes in larger facilities (more than a hundred beds), in nursing homes with no nurse practitioner or physician-assistant on staff, and in those with no special dementia-care units (their greater use also characterized nursing homes in which fewer residents had written health-care directives stating their wishes; see chapter 5).

For people suffering advanced dementia, inappropriate rationing replaces hands-on, individual care with a more technological, invasive, but cost-saving method. For many older patients with another age-associated disease, cancer, the rationing of more aggressive medical interventions may not be warranted. Physicians are more able than in the past to manage cancer as a chronic rather than imminently fatal illness, marked by periods of remission if not cure. Rather than withhold treatment only because patients are beyond a particular age, they now consider medical intervention to be appropriate for otherwise robust older adults, especially as treatments develop that bring less debilitating side effects. Physicians assess each individual's overall physical and cognitive health, and ability to tolerate the side effects, along with the quality as well as quantity of life likely to result from medical treatment.[63] Again, between relatively clear-cut extremes are all the grays, shaded not only by medical assessments but, importantly, by an individual's wishes about her own life at this age, especially whether she wants a cancer treatment or its side effects to be any part of it.

Identifying unjustified restrictions on care based on chronological age does not solve the problems of rationing by cost discussed earlier in this chapter, through which people's inability to pay imposes the limits. Paying for tests and treatments determined to be appropriate and necessary for older adults requires parallel changes in Medicare coverage. Until 2002, for instance, Medicare automatically denied reimbursement for services if patients' primary diagnosis was Alzheimer's disease or other irreversible dementia.[64] Surprising as this lack might seem, given public and professional concern and the burden of dementia on patients and their family, the rationale throughout previous years centered on efficacy: Medicare refused to pay for health care that had no positive impact on a disease's progression. Finally, policy began catching up with the epidemiology and the personal costs. Though surely not able to cure or reverse most dementias, certain measures—mental health services; physical, occupational, and speech therapies; home health care—can at least temporarily improve an individual's ability to function safely and comfortably in the world, maintain greater independence, and postpone or avert the need for institutional care during the average ten years beyond initial diagnosis. Acknowledging such benefits, policy makers added these services to Medicare coverage (see figure 15).

Medicare revisions passed in 2003 did include new coverage for a recipient's initial doctor's appointment, some minimal preventive services, disease screening, and case coordination for chronic diseases—even as the legislation posed a fundamental threat, through privatization, to the government insurance program's long-term survival. Moreover, given the prescription drug benefit's convoluted and inadequate dimensions, people with Alzheimer's and other dementias, as well as people suffering other chronic health problems, may find that the intervention with greatest potential for lessening and, perhaps, slowing relentless symptoms—newly developed and therefore patented, costly brand-name medications—will remain, like most drugs, largely at the patients' own expense. The Medicare-eligible population will more than double in thirty years from 35 to 75 million (from 12.4 percent of the population to 20.6 percent).[65] With ever more sophisticated drugs, surgeries, medical technologies and devices, motorized wheelchairs and other assistance, along with consistent need for better preventive and health-promoting care, the broader question of what Medicare will and will not cover—that is, how health services will be rationed—looms as an inescapable factor in determining the health

15. HEALTH-CARE SERVICES NEWLY AVAILABLE TO PEOPLE WITH ALZHEIMER'S DISEASE—2002

PHYSICAL THERAPY

Balance problems

Unsteady gait

Hip fracture rehabilitation

OCCUPATIONAL THERAPY

Fall prevention

Memory loss aids

Continued independence in daily activities

SPEECH THERAPY

Difficulties with chewing and swallowing

Caregiver's training—e.g., communicating with impaired individual

COUNSELING

Anxiety and depression

Health-care planning

Legal/financial arrangements

Caregiver's stress

Based on *Focus on Health Aging* (October 2002).

and well-being of aging Americans and the longevity of the Medicare program itself.[66]

■ ■ ■

In the midst of my work on this chapter, my father struggles to die. I write of health-care rationing as distinguished from appropriate end-of-life care, and I talk with his visiting nurse about comfort care and relief from pain. His one kidney, she tells me, appears to be failing (the other, with its malignant tumor, removed many years ago), along with his heart and lungs (minus one-half, removed with its tumor a few years later). I read a medical journal article analyzing the ethics of "withdrawing very low burden interventions in chronically ill patients" with advanced or end-stage disease.[67] The case described sounds eerily like my father's. The question posed: should doctors, with family agreement, deactivate a heart pacemaker in an aged man suffering severe dementia, the man's combativeness, agitation, hallucinations refractory to medications intended to improve his daily interactions. Until recently, my father, like this patient, was in otherwise "fairly good physical health." Just three years ago, my father's cardiologist replaced the worn pacemaker batteries, a minor surgical procedure that made sense at the time. Some months ago, I chose a more passive deactivation than that in the journal's case report: I gave up on the periodic computer monitoring intended to detect any glitch. A malprogrammed, malfunctioning, or simply aging pacemaker may eventually fail to keep my father alive.

We have already lost whatever frayed thread held him to us, a tenuous, intermittent contact through familiar names, recognizable furniture, memories from his childhood and mine. I can no longer recognize what time or place he inhabits, as when he calmly and enjoyably reminisced, with me as his sister, remembering my advice that he should marry his girlfriend, my mother. Or the nights my mother was his mother in the childhood bedroom shared with his brother. We have watched him sink, as into quicksand, flailing. We all live now the anger and agitation that animate what remains, though I can't help wondering if attempts to medicate the sharpest flares do not sometimes become the most immediate cause of the next ones.

His body has remained stubbornly tenacious. A few weeks back, when I told him to use the walker, he swung his cane at me, barely missing. Last night, though greatly weakened, he kicked at a hired aide who was trying to bring him inside the house; then, gathering a last ounce of strength by force of utter frustration, he threw his walker across the front porch. It is not easy, keeping some individuals at home. And we are the lucky ones, with money to hire health aides and buy expensive medications, with family to coordinate care and fill in gaps and run to the pharmacy for every new medical mix, with a patient whose particular physical condition renders him eligible for continued Medicare-paid visits from a nurse who is superb. But I must begin calling skilled nursing facilities that accept people with an agitated dementia, just in case, and it will feel like a defeat. And that assumes they would have him.

The hired help at home covering each day and night of a week includes now five women, all African American, and one Ukrainian man, Vladimir, whose clearest English sentences are "You have big problem" and "This is life." All of us caregivers, formal and family alike, feel the strain, and all of us feel exhausted. My mother continues to withdraw. How bad is this for her, keeping him at home? The balance of risks and benefits, for two, grows all the more perplexing in that he insists now from morning to night, angrily, that he wants to leave this place, to go home, no longer recognizing ever—as he did from time to time—that he is at home, and growing angrier still if we tell him.

Should it take so much effort, energy, and money? What alternatives exist for him and for us, not to mention for other families with fewer resources? Dying at home does not necessarily mean peacefully in sleep. Labor-, money-, and emotion-intensive, the process can be difficult to accomplish without considerable help. Loosely defined, the experience may span weeks, and even months, with many moments far from serene.

It is not easy at all. And in this lack of options—the country's poverty of affordable and desirable alternatives for long-term and end-of-life care—looms the final form of health-care rationing.

5

End of Life

Looking back, I can better see that my father entered and passed through a time of dying. His body for the first time thin and frail, his dementia severe, he had left robust far behind. White gauze swaddled his bruised, mottled purple arms, holding together wounds that refused to heal, his skin too fragile for emergency room stitches or staples. With scabbed nose and a bandaged brow, scraped open by the latest bump or fall, he looked the picture of abuse.[1] As he moved from cane to walker to wheelchair, my father's last weeks sped like a too-fast home movie, yet with each hour agonizingly slow. To my surprise, he welcomed the wheelchair, exhausted, no doubt, from fighting to stay on his own two feet. He seemed not to notice the seatbelt we kept buckled, as a nurse instructed us, in case he tried to walk. Like residents I saw in nursing homes, he would sit there, strapped in, looking small.

There was no clear moment that announced the need for end-of-life care. The rented hospital bed seemed almost to belong in the living room, fit snuggly into the piano's curve. The raised side railings seemed almost superfluous, as he hardly moved. Mentally, he was no longer in our world, ever. No family names or familiar objects, no distant memory of place could even momentarily pull him back. Now my father talked to people no one else could see. He kept sinking deeper into his own chaotic jumble, unable to summon, finally, the strength to climb out. With his body failing quickly, as if in sudden decline, the nurse and I skirted indistinct boundaries of treatment and comfort care, of enough medication to ensure no pain or distress, an amount that might, however, fatally suppress his ability to breathe. "This is not what he would want," I told her, "this" meaning his current existence. She repeated the statement back, as if to confirm.

This chapter examines the last stage of life, indeterminate in length of time and varying in condition of health, for people who have grown old. The discussion moves away from the previous chapter's concern with limiting medical tests and treatments in order to lower costs, based on patients' wealth, insurance status, or age. Here the focus is on rationing's more humane side: limiting medical interventions in order to avoid the overly aggressive, while still providing appropriate end-of-life care. Perhaps the topic need not be grim, if approached ahead of time, with the security of having options and support. Moreover, attention to this stage of life is imperative simply because everyone sees more of it now. Late life extends longer for more people—with an array of medical methods available to prolong the time—than during past decades when the norm was a quicker, earlier death.

Many women and men of my generation are participating in the final life stage of their parents, other relatives, or friends, an experience frequently cluttered with doctor's appointments, medications organized by weeks, days, and hours, emergency room visits, hospital stays, and perhaps a skilled nursing facility. For me, this chapter is a way to stop and reflect on an experience just completed and certain to come again, perhaps sooner than later. The discussion looks beyond efforts at successful aging to the desire for a good death. Just as rationing displays the tremendous impact of our broader health-care system on Americans' health and well-being, so too does a presently inadequate care system determine the fate of many people's end-of-life wishes and decisions. Observing life endings, the middle-aged are old enough to think forward and then begin working backward, asking what choices they want available during their own last years. Then comes the more difficult task: taking steps that can help ensure that those choices exist.

AGGRESSIVE MEDICAL TREATMENTS: TRIALS AND TRAPS

The end of life is hard to do well in this country, as doctors sometimes attest when describing their own parents.[2] Ironically, for people with access to state-of-the-art medicine, the greatest threat to fulfilling their wishes may arise in the most advanced hospitals, where technologies and doctors may descend on patients who had hoped for a peaceful end. Yet individual choices about life's end vary widely, from insisting doctors "do everything they can" to fight and delay impending death, to requesting that a doctor hasten it. Whether for a parent, friend, or themselves, the most prominent wishes cluster around freedom from pain and suffering, both physical and psychological. People want to maintain personal dignity, as well as some control over what is, after all, still their life. A wish commonly expressed is that they not linger, unable to enjoy life, a financial, physical, and emotional burden on family; they do not want to be "kept alive" by machines.[3]

Until the late twentieth century the option to remain alive, at least technically, did not exist. As the medical ability advanced, more and more stories emerged of the old languishing in hospitals and nursing homes; people began wondering whether new medical treatments and technologies—mechanical ventilators, feeding tubes, surgical and intensive care—were best described as extending life or prolonging death. With greater use of such medical interventions came observations that certain of these efforts seemed futile.

With medical interventions growing increasingly sophisticated and common throughout the 1990s, the dilemma of medical futility enlarged apace.[4] Health-care providers and ethicists debated criteria for determining when, if ever, a medical treatment should be considered futile, a debate continuing to this day. Some definitions center on a number—for instance, on less than 1 percent likelihood of adequate recovery after treatment. Critics of this concept consider the number arbitrary, impossible to determine, and dependent on a doctor's assertion rather than discussion with a patient or family of potential outcomes and probabilities.[5] Although basic disagreements remain, the definition of futility generally encompasses interventions when there is no reasonable likelihood of curing a patient's underlying condition or extending what the individual considers a satisfactory life, and when treatment cannot improve the quality of life through reduced pain or other distressing symptoms.[6] More simply put, the treatment dilemma for an individual patient—often seeming impossible to decide—is knowing when to stop.

Questions of medical futility involve crucial matters of professional ethics and patients' rights. Beyond precise definitions and legal disagreements, several key considerations complicate efforts to attain appropriate care yet avoid futile, overly aggressive medical intervention at the end of life.

- Futility may become apparent only in retrospect. A medical intervention helpful for some individuals will not be for others; neither doctor nor patient and family can know unless they try it. A trial-of-treatment with explicit, planned reassessments can provide greater certainty, though deciding to withdraw or discontinue an intervention can feel more difficult than never starting it at all.[7]

- Doctors and patients alike tend to overestimate the amount of time a treatment will gain, a piece of information that may be important in considering whether a treatment is futile. And it is often difficult to predict how long individuals will live without treatment, especially with many cancers or heart disease. More generally, research suggests that seriously ill patients foresee overly optimistic treatment outcomes, if that treatment does keep them alive; informed that severe cognitive or functional impairment is likely, they more frequently decide against treatment, essentially considering such outcomes a fate worse than death.[8]

- Managed care's efforts to limit costs can leave a patient and family wondering whether an unfamiliar doctor's recommendation against treatment truly reflects the best information available about medical outcomes, probabilities, and uncertainties interpreted in light of that patient's wishes and best interests. Such concerns arise particularly among vulnerable populations without economic resources or, in many cases, health-care savvy—the poor, minorities, and the old, the latter often isolated and weakened physically and mentally.

- Chronic disease and disability characterized by gradual deterioration are more common than acute life-threatening crises as people grow older.[9] The burden of medical treatment may render it futile for some individuals if a longer life brings only extended pain, depression, dementia, anxiety. For example, implanted cardiac defibrillators, which internally jolt an erratically beating heart that may otherwise stop altogether, cause some chronic heart disease patients continual physical and psychological distress; particularly for the very frail, averting sudden death from heart failure may not (or no longer) be a health-care goal.[10]

Chemotherapies that may hold cancer temporarily at bay in some instances bring extra months dominated by side effects at least as miserable as the disease symptoms themselves.

Unlike medical rationing of potentially beneficial care, eliminating futile treatment does not sacrifice desired quantity or quality of life. Like so much else in health care, however, determining whether treatment is futile requires a balance between competing concerns—in this case, acknowledging limits on aggressive care as a legitimate consideration, yet recognizing the finality of decisions that result in a life's end. Physicians have identified some of the extreme conditions for which medical intervention is most certainly futile in the very old—for example, during the final stage of terminal illness with multiple organ system failures, or in cases of irreversible coma following a stroke. More recently, as mentioned in the last chapter, geriatric specialists have begun discouraging tube feeding for patients with end-stage dementia, an invasive procedure that "seldom achieves the intended medical aims and that rather than prevent suffering, can cause it."[11] In fact, providing nutrition and liquids to the dying may in most cases be detrimental.[12] Short of extremes, the perception of medical futility rests, to varying degrees, in the eye of the beholder: the doctor, patient, or family; a hospital ethics committee. People will not always agree. The dominant precept that should guide medical decisions whenever possible remains a patient's autonomy—that is, in matters of my own life and death, my choice among existing possibilities prevails.

PROLONGING LIFE

A brief history of an apparently simple procedure—*cardiopulmonary resuscitation,* widely known as CPR—allows better understanding of the complexities surrounding treatment decisions as people near the end of life. Today's public may be unaware that the ability to restore a patient's heartbeat, blood circulation, and breathing through CPR developed as recently as the 1960s. Initial use of this procedure targeted patients who had just suffered a heart attack, landing them in the hospital—especially within a cardiac-care unit, another new medical advance at the time. If a patient's heart stopped beating, a hospital team could immediately begin resuscitation efforts. Doctors soon discovered that CPR could also successfully revive many patients suffering cardiac

16. EXAMPLES OF PROCEDURES PATIENTS MUST REJECT TO FORGO LIFE SUPPORT

Mask to mouth resuscitation without intubation
External chest compression
Electrical ventricular defibrillation
Chemical ventricular defibrillation
Intubation without mechanical ventilation
Intubation with mechanical ventilation

If a patient desires any one or more of the above, cardiac arrest code must be called, with the following procedures requiring consent or rejection:

Inotropic and vasoactive support
Electrical cardioversion for atrial tachyarrhythmia
Transfer to ICU
Dialysis
Transfusion
IV support
IV hyperalimentation
Antibiotics
Enteral nutrition
Chemotherapy
Radiation therapy
Radiology/Laboratory studies

List from St. Francis Hospital, Pittsburgh PA, mid-1990s; based on Rafkin and Rainy 1997, 30.

arrest caused by a drug overdose or severe reaction to anesthesia during surgery.

As is typical of new medical practices, CPR did not remain simple or specifically targeted for long. While people may picture the mouth-to-mouth procedure and external chest compression taught to scouts, lifeguards, teachers, and new parents, they are only the layperson's everyday hands-on version. Far more sophisticated methods not only monitor and restart an arrested heart but also keep hospitalized patients alive through increasingly technological physiological support, known in the health-care world as the medical armamentarium (see figure 16). Moreover, within hospitals and nursing homes CPR became the rapid, automatic code response for patients of all ages and conditions, including the very old and frail and terminally ill, though with far less positive outcomes.

With life-sustaining techniques proliferating throughout the 1970s, this newfound ability also began generating disagreement about appropriate use—most pointedly, when not to attempt CPR or other life support. Not only might an individual's resuscitation be brief, gaining only a few extra days or weeks of added pain, but a distressing number of patients were revived yet severely disabled or irreversibly comatose, an outcome that might drag on not weeks but months and years. Some physicians began arguing the need to pull back, to discriminate, in the medically appropriate sense, between patients for whom CPR held some reasonable chance of benefit and those for whom the effort made no sense.

The era of increasingly widespread CPR, then, engendered the advent of DNRs—the Do Not Resuscitate orders—and arguments about when such orders are justified and legal. Furthermore, with the traditional paternalism of doctors weakening, disagreement also centered on questions about who decides: Who decides whether to initiate and continue life-sustaining efforts—doctors, patients and family, a health-care proxy? Who determines the chances considered reasonable, the attempt worth trying? Indeed, controversy spilled into public view with agonizing cases, turned legal battles, of a patient or family asserting the right to reject or withdraw medical life support—insisting, that is, on a patient's right to choose a natural death rather than attempting through medical technology to remain technically alive. Among the landmark cases were *In re Quinlan* (1976), a New Jersey Supreme Court decision allowing the parents of a comatose patient, Karen Ann Quinlan, to withdraw life support, implementing a decision they asserted she would make if able; *Bouvia v. Superior Court* (1986), a U.S. Appeals Court ruling that Elizabeth Bouvia, severely disabled, maintained the right to starve herself, disallowing forced feeding; *Cruzan v. Director, Missouri Department of Health* (1990), in which the U.S. Supreme Court affirmed a competent adult's right to refuse any medical treatment, including artificial nutrition, with procedural safeguards established by states, especially regarding health-care proxies for patients who are not mentally competent.[13]

During the twentieth century's last decade, conflict between a patient's autonomy and a doctor's professional autonomy reappeared, but in reverse. Now the power struggle over ultimate medical decisions—who initiates life support and who pulls the plug?—found doctors seeking to curtail treatment that, in their medical judgment, is futile, even harmful and, in some cases, an unjustified use of limited resources. Fighting this conclusion were patients and families insisting on CPR and more. Here were cases in which a patient's autonomy should perhaps not prevail. In some instances, doctors asserted, professional ethics should gain supremacy, precepts that proscribe unnecessary treatments and, especially, that demand a doctor do no harm. Few courts have tackled this dilemma, leaving to future legislation the crafting of a legal framework that can resolve impasses between the autonomy of patient and doctor.

In October 2003 a highly publicized conflict demonstrated just how entangled end-of-life medical decisions can become. This case of a thirty-nine-year-old woman in her thirteenth year of a persistent vegetative state (similar to Ms. Cruzan) pitted husband against parents and state legislature against judiciary, with religiously conservative groups and politicians part of the mix. Based on the testimony of medical experts about her condition and prognosis, Florida courts ruled in favor of the spouse (her legal guardian, and the usual default proxy in the absence of a patient's directives), who wanted a life-sustaining feeding tube removed so his wife could die, an action he claimed was consistent with views she had previously stated to him. Her parents, supported by noisy and visible right-to-life demonstrators outside the hospice caring for their daughter, remained bitterly opposed, insisting she showed signs of a life that could someday more fully revive. Six days after medical staff removed the tube, the Florida legislature nullified the court decision by granting Governor Jeb Bush (brother of the president) authority to order the feeding tube reinserted, an order he gave in time to prevent her death. In May 2004 a state circuit court judge declared that legislation unconstitutional, a ruling Governor Bush immediately appealed. After losing this appeal in the Florida Supreme Court, the governor moved on to the U.S. Supreme Court, which in January 2005 refused to hear that appeal. On March 18, despite last-minute efforts by a handful of U.S. congressmen to intervene (through subpoenas critics denounced as illegitimate intrusion), doctors removed the tube. An extraordinary congressional response—passage after midnight Sunday of emergency legislation, signed immediately by President Bush—forced the disturbing battle into a federal court, prolonging this personal-turned-political ordeal.

PRESERVING AUTONOMY

For most older Americans and for their families, the predominant fear remains that they will end up where they do not want to be—in a hospital, perhaps an intensive-care unit—hooked to machines, with no control over the high-technology surroundings or care. Medical studies of end-of-life care discuss similar concerns, noting for instance a frequent perception among family members that the individual did linger, with pain and other distress, undergoing unwanted medical interventions that only made matters worse.[14] Or such reports describe conflict, especially among family members or within the health-care team, including disagreement with the patient's wishes, if known.

Why, then, are autonomy and choice so difficult to attain? Most commonly, patients never conveyed wishes about life-sustaining medical treatments to a doctor or to family members, at least not in a clear and explicit way that could override not only family conflict but also the legal and ethical obligations of ambulance paramedics, doctors, and other hospital staff to provide treatment aimed at keeping their patients alive. People also fail to designate an individual who will make medical decisions reflecting what care they would want, if unable to do so themselves, the person to whom doctors will turn when attempting to determine their patients' best interests and wishes (in some states called a health-care proxy or power of attorney, often designating an adult daughter or son, if not a spouse). By the time such wishes are at issue, patients may not be fully conscious or able to consent to or reject treatment. Some cases are obvious and abrupt medical emergencies: a stroke that seriously impairs communication or cognitive abilities, cardiac arrest, or loss of consciousness, whatever the cause. In other instances, the ability to understand and decide may erode gradually, along with mental capacity more generally. With age, the individual might already have developed substantial cognitive impairments and no longer be competent to understand fully and decide.[15]

Regarding such uncertainties and conflicts as well as end-of-life treatments overall, the generic advice from doctors, lawyers, medical ethicists, and patient advocates is twofold. First, complete written instructions, most commonly known as advance directives or living wills, stating explicitly your wishes about life-sustaining medical interventions, including CPR, mechanical ventilation, tube feeding, and hydration. That is, under what circumstances would you want such efforts started and stopped? With what physical and cognitive conditions would you want to be allowed to die? Also in advance, appoint a trusted health-care proxy who understands your views and will make decisions about medical treatment, consistent with your wishes, if you are unable.

Only 15–20 percent of American adults have completed written advance directives.[16] And unfortunately, such documents aren't foolproof. Even directives written in advance have limitations in real life and death. Although all states have passed legislation supporting a patient's advance directives, various legal strictures introduce limits that can result in individual wishes not being followed. For instance, states differ in defining the circumstances in which patients' directives to withhold, withdraw, or provide treatment are legally binding on doctors, hospitals, and nursing homes. State laws vary on who serves as proxy if an incompetent patient did not choose one earlier (a default proxy or surrogate), and in the limitations they place on any proxy's decisions. States differ also in defining the legal rights of doctors or nursing home personnel to issue orders not to resuscitate a patient, in the absence of clearly stated wishes or consent. At a more practical level, while advance directives should be part of a patient's medical file, a copy of the document may simply not be available when needed. For example, if an individual is rushed to a hospital's emergency room or intensive-care unit, treatment will begin. If written instructions are available at a hospital or nursing home, doctors and other staff may consider them either too general or too specific and inflexible when facing that patient's actual immediate condition, available treatment alternatives, and shifting probabilities of potential outcomes.[17] Ambulance paramedics responding to an emergency call must, in some states, see a specific *pre*hospital DNR order or resuscitation efforts will begin, continuing on arrival at a hospital—including on a very old, sick, and frail individual who wants to avoid hospitalization and ultimately to die at home. Calling 911 is tantamount to "calling in the Marines," as one nurse described it to me; in pacific Berkeley, this lead force does an excellent job of rescue, delivering its patient, in some instances time and again, to the hospital's full array of medical weapons. In fact, if an individual wishes to avoid a hospital, including the emergency room and intensive care, family and caregivers may need to discipline themselves *not* to call 911.

Beyond such concrete instances, moreover, are obstacles inherent to the process and goal of writing treatment wishes and designating a health-care proxy. First, people may resist focusing ahead on the end of life, particularly while still healthy, mentally competent, and relatively young. They may avoid discussing such matters with their family and doctor as well. Their doctor in turn may never initiate such discussion or encourage patients to complete advance directives. Trained to cure disease by employing medical technology and prescribing drugs, most doctors are neither comfortable with, nor educated about, helping patients shape and experience the end of life, or providing palliative care, including social and emotional support.[18] With none of the participants eager to plan ahead for dying, written directives are easy to put off until the advance time has passed.

Preserving autonomy and choice for individuals suffering dementia can be especially difficult and frustrating. Before observing dementia close at hand, people may have difficulty imagining the disintegration of mental abilities, the bizarre rearrangement of thought and subtle changes that creep into another individual's everyday perceptions and tasks. With loss of mental competence impossible to pinpoint, you turn around and realize not only that it is gone, but how inscrutable that person's thinking has become. Although my father designated me as healthcare proxy just in time, before dementia engulfed his thoughts—and although I felt confident I understood his end-of-life wishes at the time—I became less certain, nearing the true end, that I knew or could decipher what, at any present moment, he wanted. When his visiting nurse asked my father if he was still able to enjoy life—his food, his music—I seemed the only one of us three surprised when he responded, "Sure," his tone familiar and, at least for that moment, convincing. Perhaps his own existence then, his internal experience of life's quality, was not as utterly deplorable as I perceived it.

Studies focusing on medical interventions toward the end of life often occur within a hospital intensive-care unit. Among patients suffering chronic illness who die in a hospital, about half receive intensive care within three days of their death, and a third spend at least ten days in an ICU.[19] Approximately three-fourths of treatment decisions within this setting involve initiating, withholding, or discontinuing life-sustaining measures (e.g., mechanical ventilation). A study of European ICUs finds limitations on life support to be common, though medical actions intended to shorten the dying process are rare.[20] However, considerable geographic variation in current ICU practices highlights an ad hoc character to many such decisions and care. That is, medical decisions, patients' and families' experiences, and outcomes constitute a fluid set of circumstances swayed by cultural and religious views. In the United States particularly, ICU patterns relate more to the local supply of specialist physicians than to patients' illnesses or an overall medical consensus about appropriate care.[21] In this country, clinical researchers are seeking a delicate equilibrium that averts futile treatment, whether patient- or doctor-inspired, while resolving disagreements and fulfilling the patient's health-care wishes. A trial program of ICU ethics consultations, for instance, resulted in less conflict over treatment decisions between family and medical team, or within either group, than did usual care. In cases where a bioethics consultant, the patient (if possible), family members, and the health-care team discussed explicit end-of-life concerns, the patient spent fewer days in the ICU and underwent fewer nonbeneficial or unwanted treatments.[22]

A study of ICU doctors' decisions about withdrawing mechanical ventilation in anticipation of a patient's death demonstrates the complexity of this scenario, and the need for more systematic analysis and development of best practices.[23] Along with assessments of the likelihood of a patient's survival and consequent cognitive condition, doctors' perceptions of the patient's wishes were an important consideration. However, the investigators raise troubling questions about the source and accuracy of the doctors' views. Commonly, hospital physicians (hospitalists, intensivists) do not know their patients, let alone their desires about starting or stopping life-support measures. With a patient's preferences unknown or undocumented, doctors rely primarily on family members; yet their wishes "are often at odds with" the patient's. These researchers conclude, "It remains questionable whether patients' preferences will be optimally represented in crucial life-support decisions in the absence of clear and detailed advance care plans" (Cook et al., 1131). Moreover, the prognosis a doctor conveys to patients and their families greatly affects their decisions. Commenting on this study, one ICU doctor notes significant changes in the nature of a doctor's advice over his thirty years in medicine: "In the 1970s there was less medical technology I could use . . . but I usually knew my patients, their families, and their mutual wishes. In [the ICU nowadays], it is rare for me to have a true understanding of how patients and their families have faced, emotionally, what could be a terminal illness."[24] He emphasizes the profound impact these unfamiliar doctors have on what patients and families decide—"the near impossibility of conveying their predictions to patients' families without, in part, influencing the outcome."

Certainly, advance instructions provide crucial information about what health care people want and serve as nonfinancial insurance in case, in the future, they can no longer make decisions or give informed consent. Yet perceptions and wishes may change as people grow older, and as disease or disability progresses. Some individuals cling more tenaciously than they earlier imagined to whatever chance medical intervention offers to continue living. Other individuals' priorities and goals diverge from the strong medical current attempting to cure disease and extend life, toward maintaining abilities and enjoyment of a perhaps shorter stretch of time.[25]

Aside from explicit revision of a directive, can doctors, family, a designated or default proxy always, or even most of the time, know an individual's present experience, especially whether life remains worth attempting to live? How can involved observers best interpret and act on what an individual says and does as the end of life nears? A search for answers in the medical literature reveals no special knowledge. Most strikingly, medical reports and ethical debates about heroic medical interventions, life-sustaining technologies, and the conundrum of treatment futility boil down to such terms as communication, explanation, dialogue and discussion, individualized care. As one analysis focused on withdrawing life support describes, in classic understatement, "Unfortunately, skill in communications is not a universal strength of critical care practice."[26] Concludes another report, a European study that includes deaths that occur at home, "The dying process typically involves less than optimum communication between [medical] caregivers and terminally ill patients."[27] And, although the medical literature increasingly includes examples of ways doctors could better talk with their patients, previous educational efforts to improve doctors' communication about and response to end of life wishes have not generally achieved significant change.[28]

That people should be talking with their doctor seems such a simple concept in a technologically sophisticated medical world—such common sense, as patients age, to discuss openly various decisions that may shape the care they receive during later years. As one Harvard University Medical School geriatrician remarks, "Advance care planning involves more than naming a proxy or filling out a form."[29] Conversation about wishes for the last stage of life cannot wait for a bedside crisis. Rather, the process begins before a patient faces acute illness or disabling impairment, as a doctor helps the patient articulate health-care priorities and treatment goals and explore the potential benefits and hazards of each differing medical path. This exchange serves to ensure the most fundamental goal—to maintain the patient's autonomy and self-determination—and to prepare for the difficult decisions that may ultimately arise. And if the patient becomes unable to decide or declare his wishes regarding a specific medical intervention, the conversation gives the doctor and the patient's proxy a crucial context for defining and honoring those wishes.

Questions about the care appropriate for any individual have no set answers but carry vital, and then final, consequences. Yet the ongoing communication and discussion needed to sort through medical information and personal values rarely occur in doctor-patient relationships today. Even as increased medical options have enlarged the need for such exchanges, as patients' rights and autonomy have gained legal support and doctors' paternalism has lessened, other characteristics of contemporary health care work against efforts to nurture communication between a patient and primary care physician who knows that individual: the pressures of time and productivity, the trend in hospitals toward in-house specialists, and the focus of medical training on skills demanded by technology and cost-effectiveness.

CONVERSATIONS

Much of Berkeley's high-quality health care in the last stage of life occurs at a community clinic serving the city's most vulnerable residents, people who are not only old and often frail but have little money and are disproportionately nonwhite. As the medical director of the Over 60 Health Center, Dr. Floyd Huen, put it, "The end of life and dying are what we do here." Low-key but high-energy, Dr. Huen speaks rapidly, as if cramming in more sentences will keep him moving through the overly filled days. A thick, unruly swatch of hair keeps flopping over his forehead, and he keeps flopping it back. This doctor's involvement with social and political issues is longstanding: as a university student in Berkeley three decades earlier he helped establish an Asian American studies department; before coming to Over 60 he headed the medical staff at Highland Hospital, the county hospital notorious, like so many others, for its chronic underfunding and ongoing difficulties in serving the poor and uninsured. His own father, an Over 60 patient, died recently after deciding, with support from his family, to stop the frequent and difficult kidney dialysis needed to keep him alive.

Dr. Huen's statement tells only part of the Over 60 story. Here the goal is to provide end-of-life care that concludes smoothly, without disruption, a health-care approach aimed at helping individuals remain as active and independent as possible throughout the last decades of their lives. Central to attaining this goal are deliberate efforts to develop with each patient an advance plan, a baseline conversation open to revision with the passage of time. Unlike most doctors, who generally focus on treating single diseases as they arise—on asking a patient, "What hurts?"—doctors at Over 60 try to talk with each patient about what that individual wants to be able to do late in life, how the patient wants to live. If the patient's main recreation is, like that of one of Dr. Huen's patients, frequenting the local racetrack, a specific but prominent goal of his care will be to maintain his ability to do so. Another longtime Over 60 doctor, Helena Lainer, tries to determine with each patient what health problems "can be fixed, and what that patient can settle for." Especially, how can doctor and patient prevent or at least slow the progress of an individual's particular chronic ailments or disabilities? Dr. Lainer's vocation also reaches back to the early 1970s, when she volunteered at the Berkeley Free Clinic. Encouraged by a supportive group of women who met regularly, she pursued a long-deferred ambition of applying to medical school. Now, with silver hair and velvety complexion, she juggles care for her patients with long-distance care of her ninety-year-old mother, as well as with the immediate demands of an adolescent daughter.

All of the physicians and other staff attempt to implement as basic care what geriatricians recognize is essential, though often difficult to achieve: to take time with patients over a span of time. During a patient's initial three visits, the physicians attempt to discuss and establish a care plan. Rather than focus on specific medical treatments or written advance directives alone—and long before an individual's acute health crisis or chronic illness or cognitive decline leave patient and doctor less able to engage in this ongoing conversation—their exchange centers on goals of health care and the quality of life over time.[30]

Weekly team meetings of social workers, psychologists, nurses, and doctors form a core of the Over 60 approach. Unlike a typical physicians' practice, this multidisciplinary group discusses together patients' problems and progress, devising next steps in light of their specific health and living conditions. At one lunch hour meeting, for example, a social worker presents a case for which she is the care coordinator: a ninety-year-old woman with severe asthma who lives alone. During a recent visit to the client's home, the social worker noted that the stairs to her second-floor apartment are finally fixed. But the woman does not go out much now and seems mildly depressed. Her asthma is generally under control, although it flares at times of increased stress, as does her borderline hypertension. Her adult daughter seems to be one source of stress, but a granddaughter does help out, shopping at the market and drugstore as well as checking in on the grandmother several days a week. Although the woman said she eats two meals a day, the kitchen looked quite barren. The team discusses ordering Meals on Wheels, and debates the pros and cons of adding blood pressure medication.

A team meeting might identify the need for other types of care available at the Over 60 clinic: education, support, and treatment groups (for diabetes, smoking cessation); dental work, not only to avoid infections and pain, but to allow patients to eat nutritious foods; a podiatry appointment for someone who cannot see or reach overgrown toenails or painful bunions, a simple measure that can maintain a person's ability to stand and to walk on her own two feet. The team may decide a social worker will coordinate referral of a patient to an appropriate daycare program. For each patient the team seeks ways of obtaining help with expenses beyond what Medicare covers. In addition to identifying patients who qualify for certain state-federal MediCal benefits (California's Medicaid program for low-income and disabled state residents), a social worker will check a family caregiver's eligibility for county funds, if needed, or for gas and electricity rate discounts. (Help with costs becomes an even larger task for patients not yet sixty-five.)

Cost concerns arise most consistently when the team discusses current or potential medications. Since Medicare has not covered prescription drugs, and with patients' cost-sharing requirements under the new Medicare benefit starting in 2006, ongoing care for many patients requires subsidizing their purchase of needed medications. Beyond expense, doctors at Over 60 have other reasons for thinking twice, at least, before prescribing medications. In fact, one request to new patients is that they bring to their first appointment all prescription and over-the-counter drugs they are taking. The purpose is to see whether patients can eliminate or take less of a medication and avoid many of the drug-related problems cited in previous chapters.

Finally, just as the quality of a patient's life is a dominant health-care focus, so too is the quality of their death. Reviewing together each death, Over 60 doctors not only assess specific medical procedures and effects on the patient's course of illness, they also ask such questions as: Did I help reduce this patient's physical and psychological suffering, and the stress for family members? Did I help him spend meaningful time at home? Am I helping her maintain a sense of control?[31] That is, they attempt to evaluate whether they helped the patient and family attain the life ending they desired, a health-care goal varying in specifics, and in how successfully it is achieved, from one patient to the next.

In sum, throughout their patients' later years, the multidisciplinary team approach described here aims at supporting individuals in living daily life at home and adapting it, as needed, toward the end. For one patient, a sturdy cane and psychological counseling may lessen a paralyzing fear of falls that overly restricts that individual's activities. For a patient similar to my father, who never feared falls quite enough, a social worker's home visit may result in alterations of the physical surroundings, reducing the likelihood or frequency of falls, and the resulting injury. For aged couples, the team tries to stave off the too common cycle of one ailing spouse dragging down the other, though in some instances the staff feel sadly they can only watch, just as I watched my parents' decline. More generally, of course, Over 60 patients will not be immune from accidents, acute illness, or other health crises people experience as they age. Then the physicians must not only provide appropriate medical treatment but also, in many cases, become the patient's advocate within the larger health-care system. For a patient diagnosed with cancer, the doctor may help convey to an oncologist that this individual does not wish to pursue aggressive and debilitating chemotherapy; for a patient approaching death, the doctor may need to "sweat the conversation with family," in Dr. Lainer's words, to ensure end-of-life treatment and care decisions that reflect what the patient wants, while attending also to the family's concerns and emotions.

At the same time, there are trends the doctors must resist for all Over 60 patients. Unlike many primary care physicians, to cite one example, they continue hospital rounds each morning so that patients see not an unknown hospitalist but a doctor who is familiar, who knows them and their immediate family, their history and their wishes. One aim of this time-consuming practice is to avoid such "geriatric nightmares" (again Dr. Lainer's words) as having the on-duty hospitalist move a patient to intensive care, initiating a medical intervention that progresses inexorably toward just the kind of life ending that individual did not want, dominated not only by technology but by the patient's disorientation or delirium, and perhaps subjection to physical restraints. Such nightmares are no secret to doctors and are by no means exclusive to hospitalists or intensive-care units. They occur under any doctor's watch when a test or treatment that may in itself represent a reasonable medical intervention initiates for an aged hospital patient a series of complications, the treatment of which may gain for that patient only a prolonged and miserable hospital death.

Certainly, many aspects of a patient's daily environment remain largely beyond the efforts of even the broad social services characterizing Over 60 care. An individual's family dynamics or network of friends can greatly affect her health and well-being, as can the physical surroundings, particularly as they reflect the country's socioeconomic inequalities. However, the achievements of this clinic's multidisciplinary team suggest there is more that most people's health care providers should know and do, especially with patients who are old. Recalling that long winter night in the emergency room with my mother and driving her home at 2:30 A.M. through empty rain-soaked streets, described in the introduction, I wonder how many doctors know who, if anyone, an old person has to help with care at home. Should primary care doctors know if there is food in a sick person's refrigerator, meals prepared, hot soup or juice, cups of tea? Should they know whether a patient can afford the medications prescribed, know if someone can go to the pharmacy and assure that the patient takes the drug properly? Should doctors make efforts, as a standard of care, to determine if a medication they prescribed is causing unacceptable side effects, requiring a change in medication or dosage? And should a doctor once in a while make a house call, to see a homebound patient in her home?

Health care in this country leaves many people—patients, doctors, nurses—unhappy with its impersonal and rushed nature, and with its expense. Many people cannot afford to become patients at all. As a community clinic serving a predominantly low income clientele, Over 60 requires constant effort to maintain adequate financial support, and an overworked staff struggles daily with cost pressures linked to productivity and to time, that especially essential resource for patients who are old. The physicians barely manage to maintain the hospital rounds that run so counter to the current flow. Yet Dr. Huen perceives a "luxury" in Over 60's geriatric team focus, of caring for older adults the way it should be done. Ironically, the country's wealthier adults do not generally enjoy such luxury when they ultimately join one category of vulnerable patients—the old and frail. Their doctor may not be attuned, as patients reach old age, to the goal of helping individuals define and attain their particular way of living final years; most doctors do not help older patients compose the last clause of a care plan that chooses among self-determined endings. Finally, their doctor may not be knowledgeable, when it comes to dying, about an approach slowly gaining medical recognition and momentum—a *low*-technology cutting edge.

NEARING THE END

A health-care directive written in advance, even a proxy authorized to make decisions, can accomplish only so much if few options exist at life's end. In fact, these declarations of individual wishes pertain primarily to cases involving refusal or withdrawal of life-prolonging medical interventions. Patients' autonomy and choice are circumscribed not only by the overwhelming thrust of medical technology and training, but also by the accompanying lack of care systems, social policies, and legal framework to support alternatives. Heroic medical cures still attract status, honors, and resources; yet small groups of doctors and nurses throughout the country are creating a quiet counterculture of care for very ill and very old patients needing more than state-of-the-art curative efforts can offer—a forefront of care noticeable for its success and for its lack of medical glamour.

PALLIATIVE CARE

Designed primarily for patients with life-threatening illness unlikely to be significantly slowed or arrested by medical treatment, palliative care (also known as comfort care) aims to relieve or, even better, prevent pain and suffering—both physical and psychological—even if the underlying cause cannot be successfully treated. Although patients generally die within one year, palliative care ideally begins early in what doctors think is a terminal illness, or as a patient declines into the frailty of long-standing chronic disease. The doctor's role is to ensure comfort as the underlying condition progresses toward death, care that in every state is a patient's legal right. Such care often follows aggressive attempts for a cure—for example, chemotherapy or surgery. A patient need not, however, reject further treatments of the disease or of complications that may arise, such as pneumonia and other infections.

Comprehensive care of greatest benefit to patients combines appropriate life-prolonging treatments with relief of distressing symptoms, rehabilitation, and support for caregivers.[32] Palliative care can be crucial for people who choose to stop medical treatment that keeps a chronic disease in check, allowing them to remain alive. In most instances less dramatic than the artificial life support of mechanical respirators and tube feeding, discontinued interventions include dialysis to avert kidney failure and medications to control heart disorders or, in more recent years, certain cancers.[33] So too can doctors and other caregivers provide a range of pain control methods and personal care that reduce discomfort following a patient's less common decision to refuse food or liquids. This process of self-starvation can take up to two or three weeks and can be difficult for some individuals to complete. And late stages of Alzheimer's disease or other dementias, which doctors and family members too rarely perceive as terminal illness, are conditions for which palliative care is far too rarely employed, robbing patients as well as family caregivers of its many benefits.[34]

Most importantly, regardless of specific diseases or time till death in the absence of life-sustaining treatment, the palliative approach does not mean doing nothing. Rather, a team of doctors, nurses, social workers, and clergy may aggressively employ various methods to reduce pain and other distressing physical symptoms often neglected in patients nearing death. In addition to nonpharmacological efforts that help people remain comfortable, medications may lessen nausea, improve appetite, ease insomnia, diminish hallucinations. Administering oxygen in appropriate cases can help relieve difficult breathing. A surgical procedure may lessen the pain a tumor creates. Palliative care focuses also on easing depression, anxiety, fear, and isolation, and attending to the emotional or spiritual needs patients and family members may feel.[35] Program staff and written materials inform those involved how the dying process may look during final weeks, days, and hours, helping to make patients' physical and emotional changes less surprising or frightening. Ideally, patients receive most of the needed care at home, coordinated and supported by program staff, throughout the illness leading to death. This ideal generally relies on family caregivers (and/or the financial ability to hire others) whose central health-care role includes reporting to physicians and nurses on a patient's condition; deciding when a professional should see the patient as well as whether the patient needs emergency room care; giving medications (and making judgments regarding "as needed" prescriptions for pain, anxiety, sleep, agitation); and in many cases attending to skin wounds, diarrhea, and incontinence.[36] In a few, mostly academic, medical centers, palliative-care programs include hospital in-patient services, allowing terminally ill individuals to check in and out as needed to keep symptoms under control; however, as of 2002, only 700 of the country's approximately 7,000 hospitals maintained any formal program of palliative care.[37] In the absence of programs and health-care teams that support and coordinate medical, psychological, and social services, few primary care physicians are able to provide comprehensive, ongoing, home-based palliative care. Nor does Medicare reimburse many types of services and equipment a patient may need, unless that patient enrolls in a hospice program.

HOSPICE CARE The most familiar and widespread variation within the broader palliative approach is hospice care.[38] Local hospices, run by a public agency or private home health organization, may differ in certain services and patients' eligibility requirements. However, they share prominent defining features. First, unlike with a broader palliative approach, a patient does forgo medical treatment aimed at curing the underlying disease or prolonging life, consenting only to interventions, coordinated by hospice staff, intended to relieve distressing symptoms and keep that individual comfortable. In addition, to enter a hospice program, the patient's prognosis, certified by a doctor, must be six months or less to live (individuals who discontinue a life-sustaining treatment often fit within this limit; obviously, no one is held to the six-month time frame though a patient may be discharged from hospice care if prospects brighten). And, very importantly for patients and for hospice organizations, Medicare (and in some states Medicaid) as well as some private health insurance plans pay for hospice-provided services, including medications; ongoing case coordination; home visits by nurses, social workers, counselors, physical therapists, and other staff; consultation with physicians. Hospice programs bring paid staff and volunteers into the home, supporting a patient's family and hired caregivers through the dying process, support that includes, for instance, skilled nursing; personal care for the dying individual (bathing, mouth care, incontinence care); doing the patient's laundry; preparing simple foods and liquids; sitting with the individual to talk, read, listen to music; and facilitating arrangements at the time of death and after. And hospice care extends into the months of bereavement that follow. In some locales, hospice works also with nursing home residents, and a very few freestanding hospice facilities exist where patients can stay while receiving end-of-life care.

Medical studies focused on the quality of end-of-life care confirm the value of hospice care, as reflected, for example, in greater satisfaction among the families of deceased hospice patients compared to those whose family member died in a nursing home, hospital, or with a home nursing service. Families report more frequently that home hospice care successfully met the patient's physical and emotional needs and provided greater support for family members.[39] Yet throughout the United

States, slightly more than a fourth of dying patients enroll in hospice, and many of these only when death is a matter of days, or perhaps hours away.[40] In comparison, approximately half of this country's Medicare recipients die in a hospital. Among the sick of all ages, the proportion of hospital deaths rises to six of every ten patients; one or two out of ten die in a nursing home.[41]

With increased doctors' referrals, more people could receive hospice care. The program does impose limits that restrict its patient population, however. Beyond requiring that patients forgo potentially curative or life-extending treatment, the six-month prognosis may disqualify many seriously ill people with a longer or uncertain life expectancy, who could benefit greatly from hospice-type care. For instance, while the greatest number of hospice patients are dying of cancer, most chronic illness late in life runs a less predictable course. People who are old and frail may live with severe disease and disability over a year or more.[42] Rather than reaching an identifiable terminal stage, individuals may decline steadily in their abilities even as they struggle to function, then experience a sudden acute complication and death. People suffering advanced dementia may also need care to alleviate pain and discomfort for longer than six months, yet they remain particularly neglected. Studies of nursing homes indicate not only the infrequency of hospice care for residents with severe dementia, but also an excess of aggressive medical interventions, such as feeding tubes, laboratory tests, and intravenous catheters requiring vein punctures and mechanical restraints. Use of antipsychotic medications may substitute for adequate control of pain and discomfort. In addition to economic factors cited earlier and lack of staff trained in providing palliative care, researchers note the difficulty of predicting how long individuals with dementia will live. In one study, only 1.1 percent of new residents with advanced dementia were considered likely to die within six months, yet 71 percent died.[43] Outside of nursing homes, even with a six months' prognosis, patients and family may not be able to arrange or afford caregivers at home needed to work with Medicare-covered hospice staff.

Whether through hospice or a broader version of palliative care, the patients (or closest family or other authorized proxy) are choosing in most cases to let death come when it will, preferably at home. Participating doctors, nurses, and other program staff are assuring patients they will receive treatment necessary to relieve suffering and keep them comfortable; neither dying patients nor family will be abandoned and alone. The old will not lose their dignity, as a medical student sorrowfully described, in pages of the *Journal of the American Medical Association,* her own grandmother, kept alive by doctors who failed to use the tools available for relief of suffering: "Reduced to a skeleton, curled up in her white hospital sheets and crying in pain," her grandmother's commode and adult diapers were "just the details" in the much deeper humiliation that was dying in avoidable agony.[44] While palliative care does not seek to hasten death, it also avoids attempts at delay. Rather, the approach reflects an individual's right to die rather than undergo life-prolonging efforts that can seem endless, until their failure, death itself. Most patients are able to maintain some control over the care they receive. For instance, some individuals will tolerate greater discomfort by taking less painkilling medication, in order to remain more mentally alert and able to talk with family, read, listen to music, even to remain aware that they are, in fact, dying.[45]

In certain difficult cases lines blur, often mercifully, between ensuring comfort and hastening death. Known as the double-effect (a term attributed to St. Thomas Aquinas), the type and amount of medication required to control pain and relieve suffering can depress breathing beyond a point that sustains that individual's life. Some individuals will pass into an unconscious state before discomfort can be alleviated. The morphine we dripped into my father's partially opened mouth to reduce his agitation and discomfort kept him, finally, sedated, in and out of consciousness. This practice, which I now know has a name—terminal sedation—could have shortened his life a day or two, perhaps more. For those delivering palliative care, and for the law, the crucial definition is a matter of intent. While the goal is not to cause death, or bring it sooner, they accept the reality and risk of their treatment's secondary but unintentional outcome in order to attain the overriding benefit of relief from suffering. Given palliative care's defining purpose, it remains distinct from—though its initial efforts may precede—a patient's more active assertion of the right to die sooner rather than later, by that individual's own hand, assisted if necessary by a physician.

PHYSICIAN-ASSISTED SUICIDE

During the early 1990s physician-assisted suicide burst into public view through the highly orchestrated and widely reported actions of Dr. Jack Kevorkian. Over a span of years, this Michigan pathologist helped several very ill individuals end their own lives, hastening a death that would otherwise have come only after months or years of further deterioration. Often sufferers of progressive neuromuscular disease, such as amyotrophic lateral sclerosis (also called Lou Gehrig's disease), which had already destroyed their ability to use their own hands in suicide, these patients turned to Dr. Kevorkian, in some instances employing a Rube Goldberg–like contraption the doctor provided to swallow lethal pills and potions. Acting initially in the absence of a law, then testing a new Michigan prohibition legislated to stop him and any other physician so inclined, the gaunt, intense physician invited media glare, pushing physician-assisted suicide into national awareness and eventually landing himself in jail. With his dramatic flare, Dr. Kevorkian would become, in caricature, the visible embodiment of a broader, unseen, and technically simpler action by physicians: providing patients, through the power of writing prescriptions, with a means to end their own lives. Also toning down the action, some supporters of physicians' assistance reject the term "suicide" as sounding too violent, too alone, and too detached from terminal illness. Rather, they emphasize the compassionate end to a dying process already well along its way, for individuals needing medical aid to accomplish that more humane death.[46] Whatever the terminology, the patient is the one who decides to hasten death, requests a prescription for needed pills, and takes them at the time, place, and in the manner of her or his choice.

As brazen as Dr. Kevorkian's demonstrations could be, materializing unpredictably from time to time, another physician's somber, equally intense, yet quietly dramatic statement confronted this broader phenomenon of assisted suicide. Writing in the *New England Journal of Medicine,* also in the early 1990s, Dr. Timothy Quill captured attention within the medical world by revealing the recent death of his patient—a middle-aged woman diagnosed with acute leukemia—following his decision to prescribe medication she requested in order to end her life. Dr. Quill described a series of conversations with his patient, Diane, that "stretch[ed] me profoundly," ultimately convincing him to cross the legal, professional, and philosophical divide.[47] A former hospice director, Dr. Quill felt disturbed initially by Diane's rejection of treatment, albeit a very difficult and painful chemotherapy, that brought 25 percent survival odds for her otherwise deadly cancer. However, after talking with his patient, who had previously undergone treatment for vaginal cancer, he came to believe strongly that as her doctor, he would be "setting her free to get the most out of the time she had left, and to maintain dignity and control on her own terms until her death" (1991, 693). Not despondent, not overwhelmed by untreated depression that could undermine her judgment, Diane was seeking the least painful and most peaceful, humane death. Dr. Quill's prescription would allow Diane, with the support of her husband and college-age son, to feel the security and relief of having enough medications available to ensure a safe death. Although Dr. Quill remained a strong advocate of palliative care, in his compelling case report he directly addressed the reality of suffering: "We have measures to help control pain and lessen suffering, [but] to think that people do not suffer in the process of dying is an illusion. Prolonged dying can occasionally be peaceful, but more often the role of the physician and family is limited to lessening but not eliminating severe suffering" (694).

Dr. Quill's admission, in print, of facilitating his patient's death caused an uproar within the profession and earned him a grand jury investigation (no charges resulted). Yet his concluding comments in 1991 posed two questions that persist to this day: "I wonder how many families and physicians secretly help patients over the edge into death in the face of such severe suffering. I wonder how many severely ill or dying patients secretly take their lives, dying alone in despair" (694). Certainly, the answer to both rhetorical questions is, then as now, More than anyone knows.

National surveys suggest that approximately 20 percent of physicians have been asked at least one time by a terminally ill patient to help bring on death. Between 3 and 18 percent report agreeing to the request.[48] One outcome of both Dr. Kevorkian's and Dr. Quill's actions has been increasingly available and improved palliative care, so that fewer dying patients need choose physician-assisted suicide. Interestingly, a survey of hospice nurses revealed a surprising frequency of terminally ill patients in their care choosing self-starvation, refusing to eat or drink—nearly twice the rate of physician-assisted suicide.[49] Moreover, for many such individuals who are not depressed and who receive adequate palliative care, this decision—an option that is legal—results in a death that is peaceful, with little suffering, a death family members can prepare for and accept. However, end-of-life options and care generally remain inadequate.

In their distinct ways, Drs. Kevorkian and Quill reflect the importance and complexity of patients' relationships with doctors during the last stage of life. At one extreme is the physician-for-hire, a stranger willing to defy legalities and professional norms to help desperately ill individuals end their lives. In stark contrast is a primary care physician agonizing over a patient he knows well, spending time over many months to talk honestly with her about living and dying, about her available care options and the impact of her choice on family members, then reaching a personally and professionally difficult decision that respects her wishes and autonomy, causing her the least harm. Most doctor-patient relationships fall in between, although the reduced choice of doctors in managed-care plans, or the need to change plans, may greatly affect where on the continuum patients find themselves.

Finally, Drs. Kevorkian and Quill force questions about the medical vow not to abandon patients, including throughout incurable illness and disability until death: Is nonabandonment better fulfilled by refusal to give up on sustaining life, by refusal even indirectly to help bring on a patient's death? Or is that refusal the true abandonment of patients who need their doctor to stay with them and to help hasten peacefully their chosen end? And what are the boundaries? What of the home-bound old with no terminal diagnosis—for example, the Over 60 patient whose family wrote in a letter after her death: "Can a person with no particular illness, no debilitating pain, who has lived a long, valuable and fulfilling life and who is facing a lessening of her ability to live with her sense of dignity decide that she has lived long enough?"

Whatever the deeply held and conflicting ethical views or legal prohibitions, the unclear and ad hoc boundaries, physician-assisted suicide does occur and will continue. However, with Dr. Kevorkian inhibited by a prison term, many of these deaths remain unseen and unspoken, outside any public policy realm, an unmonitored collaboration between individual doctors and patients. Their discussion and decision processes no doubt remain oblique in many instances, out of doctors' concerns about illegality and about disapproval from some colleagues. Except in Oregon.

MAKING IT LEGAL

Serving again as a test case for unorthodox health-care legislation, only Oregon has defined circumstances in which doctors can legally prescribe to certain terminally ill patients lethal medications for suicide (see figure 17). The circumstances are paired with safeguards aimed to ensure that an individual's judgment is not clouded by depression or other psychological disorder, and that she feels no coercion or undue influence in reaching this decision. More specifically, Oregon's law includes these provisions:

17. CRITERIA FOR DOCTORS CONSIDERING A PATIENT'S REQUEST FOR ASSISTANCE IN DYING

The patient clearly and repeatedly, of his or her own free will, requests to die rather than to continue suffering.

The patient's condition is incurable. It is associated with severe, unrelenting, intolerable suffering, and all reasonable means of relief have been fully explored.

The physician ensures that the patient's suffering and the request are not the results of inadequate comfort care.

Physician-assisted death is carried out only within the context of a meaningful doctor-patient relationship.

Consultation with an independent physician skilled in palliative care is required.

Clear documentation supporting each of the above conditions is required.

The patient's judgment is not distorted.

Based on Death with Dignity Alliance materials regarding development of Oregon's legislation, www.dwda.org.

- The patient, with a maximum prognosis of six months to live, makes a voluntary, fully informed decision.
- A second physician opinion is required.
- The patient must make two oral requests and one written, with set waiting periods in between; the patient can cancel the request at any time.
- The patient must be offered counseling.
- Oregon's Health Division must review each request.

In fact, the tortuous history of Oregon's statute, the Death with Dignity Act of 1997, demonstrates not only public and professional consensus that physician-assisted death should be legal in cases meeting strict criteria but also political threats to publicly approved legislated measures. Twice Oregon voters have approved a state law delineating the conditions under which physician-assisted suicides are allowed. Following an initial 1994 vote on a citizen's initiative, opponents (especially Catholic organizations and right-to-life groups) successfully blocked enactment of the law for three years, then introduced a ballot measure for outright repeal. Voters rejected that 1997 measure by a wide margin, affirming their support for the Death with Dignity Act.

Contrary to opponents' dire warnings that legalization would un-
leash a flood of suicides by prescription, the numbers have remained
small. Data required by law on all prescriptions for lethal medications,
along with additional studies, indicate a policy that serves Oregon residents well. During the statute's first two years (1998–99), doctors
agreed to requests from one out of six patients (for a total of 57 prescriptions out of 342 requests); forty-three of these individuals actually
took the pills. No patient a doctor evaluated as showing symptoms of
depression received a prescription.[50] By the fourth year, the total number of prescriptions rose to 140 (approximately 15 percent of 933 requests), the number of suicides to 91.[51] Compared to all deaths in Oregon, not even one in a thousand (6–9 of 10,000 deaths per year since
1997) could be attributed to physician-assisted suicide.[52] Moreover, the
demographics for patients receiving a prescription (age, gender, race, income level) show a population similar to all who died, allaying concerns
that vulnerable groups might be overrepresented; if anything, individuals choosing physician-assisted suicide tend to be more highly educated
than the general population.[53]

Not only are Oregon doctors complying with the law's safeguards
before providing a prescription, their greater attention to pain control
as well as to patients' other concerns appears to deter many people from
ending their own lives.[54] In fact, studies suggest that doctors are providing better palliative care more broadly in Oregon since legalization of
physician-assisted suicide. Medical and pharmacy records indicate that
doctors are employing more aggressive pain control methods and referring patients more frequently to hospice—36 percent of all deaths in
2000 compared to 20–25 percent throughout the United States. While
hospice care does not preclude suicide, patients' requests do receive
considerable review from a staff—including, importantly, nurses, social
workers, and clergy—focused on providing the best palliative options.
Overall, studies of the Oregon experience demonstrate that in most
cases, though not all, a dying patient's wishes—especially regarding
pain, control of circumstances, impact on family—can be fulfilled without a patient's feeling the need, finally, for physician-assisted suicide.[55]

Opponents have not been deterred by the Oregon public's will or by
evidence of a successful law, a policy with positive social and medical
impact. Perhaps more surprising, given the opposition's generally conservative political allegiance, is their forsaking of arguments that cite
states' rights and individual liberties. The definition and regulation of
medical practices have long fallen within state powers; freedom of indi-

viduals from government intrusion, especially as represented by laws limiting personal behaviors, has long stood as a goal shared by conservative Republicans and more adamant libertarians. Even so, rather than strange bedfellows, the affinities among those who reject physician-assisted suicide present familiar couplings: as in this country's ongoing abortion battle, regarding policies that conflict with their own religious and ideological beliefs, opponents would rather suspend states' authority and individuals' freedom of choice in favor of stronger federal government control.

As with abortion, efforts to eliminate physician-assisted suicide as a woman's or man's end-of-life option have materialized in various legislative and judicial arenas. In 1997, just before Oregon's second vote, the U.S. Supreme Court ruled unanimously, on cases from New York *(Quill v. Vacco)* and Washington *(Washington v. Glucksberg)*, that state laws prohibiting physician-assisted suicide do not violate an individual's rights as protected by the U.S. Constitution. While upholding such statutes in these two states, however, the Court did warn strongly that legal prohibitions must not obstruct palliative care, even if it unintentionally hastens death, including terminal sedation for the terminally ill. Furthermore, the decision left open the right of states to legalize physician-assisted suicide—to define as legitimate medical practice the prescribing of medications that patients could use to hasten their impending death.[56]

The next round moved to the federal Drug Enforcement Agency (DEA), whose director warned doctors, in Oregon and all other states, of the opposite: prescribing narcotics or barbiturates to enable a dying patient's suicide does not involve a legitimate medical purpose. State law notwithstanding, doctors could be prosecuted for violating the Controlled Substances Act, a federal law enacted in 1970 to fight abuse and trafficking of illicit drugs. In June 1998 the Clinton administration's attorney general, Janet Reno, overruled the DEA. The federal drug law, she determined, does not alter a state's authority to regulate the medical profession, including allowing doctors to prescribe medications for a dying patient's suicide, as established and regulated by Oregon's law.

Although the practice remained legal in Oregon, the DEA successfully chilled many doctors' willingness to prescribe lethal medications when requested. At the same time, opponents attempted a different strategy: if the existing Controlled Substances Act could not serve their purposes, they would have Congress amend this federal law. That amendment, introduced in 1999 as a bill benignly titled Pain Relief Promotion Act, would corral physicians in with major drug dealers and hard-core addicts, subject to twenty-year prison terms for the federal crime of prescribing controlled drugs in order to cause or assist in causing a patient's death. With a token bow to increased medical research and education on palliative care, the main purpose of the congressional act was to negate Oregon's legalization of physician-assisted suicide and avert similar laws in other states.[57]

In fact, many physicians warned, imprisonment or its threat would inhibit doctors from far more than the few instances of assisted suicide; the amended law would significantly impair palliative care more broadly by inhibiting aggressive pain control measures for terminal patients who are not seeking to end their own lives. Doctors would fear attempting new approaches for patients experiencing the most intractable suffering. Patients who did not respond to the usual treatments for pain, agitation, feelings of suffocation, and other difficult-to-control symptoms would never receive new palliative approaches that might, like terminal sedation with morphine or fentanyl, slip them into quicker death. Patients would be denied an additional positive outcome: the emotional comfort and security of knowing they have or can obtain legally medications needed for suicide, knowledge that helps many feel they need never use this last resort.

Most striking about efforts to criminalize physician-assisted suicide is the single-minded ideological manner of addressing complex and difficult end-of-life concerns—for example, trying to codify a clear distinction between permissible palliative care and illegal hastening of death. Writing in the *New England Journal of Medicine*, its former editor-in-chief Dr. Marcia Angell conveys the indistinct and often vanishing line between intent to ease suffering and intent to cause a quicker death. Citing "notoriously inadequate" treatment for pain in terminally ill patients, largely reflecting doctors' general apprehensions regarding legal scrutiny, she explains:

> When the suffering of a dying patient is prolonged and intractable, a doctor who administers or prescribes large doses of a controlled substance may well have mixed intentions. Just as family members often feel a sense of relief along with their grief when such patients finally die, so doctors often wish both to ease suffering and to hasten death. The balance of those desires may vary from hour to hour, depending on the patient's condition. . . . If all attempts at palliation fail, as they sometimes do, then the hope for an easier death may give way to the hope for a faster one. That is, the intent can shift. . . . It is absurd to imagine that doctors could be innocent in one hour, but deserving of 20 years in prison in the next, simply because the de-

sired outcome of treatment changed. What is important is whether doctors are doing their utmost to ease suffering in accord with their patients' wishes.[58]

The passage captures well distinctions grown irrelevant within my parents' home, intentions and hopes suffusing the living room around my father lying in his hospital bed those final days, hovering just short of intractable distress. However, the complexities Dr. Angell expressed failed to impress a majority within the U.S. House of Representatives, which passed the Pain Relief Promotion Act of 1999. The Senate never voted; with Oregon's Senator Ron Wyden threatening a filibuster (even though he personally opposes physician-assisted suicide), the bill died peacefully in December 2000.

Less than a year later, with the Bush administration in place, the new attorney general, John Ashcroft, reversed Janet Reno's ruling that Oregon's law involves a legitimate medical purpose, subject to state regulation. With the congressional route stymied, this attorney general revived efforts to outlaw physician-assisted suicide, in November 2001, by returning to the unamended Controlled Substances Act. He ordered the Drug Enforcement Agency to identify from Oregon records—and hold criminally liable—doctors who prescribed lethal drugs for patient suicide. Although Ashcroft's directive did not mandate prison terms for these doctors, he did authorize the DEA to suspend or revoke their license to prescribe any controlled drugs for any purpose, medically legitimate or not. An oncologist commenting on Ashcroft's order echoed Dr. Angell's earlier concerns:

> It is medically impossible to dissociate intentionally ameliorating a dying patient's agony from intentionally shortening the time left to live. . . . [The ruling] represents a striking lack of understanding of how physicians help patients to die, and it risks making the last days of the terminally ill a time of panic and pain rather than calm and comfort.[59]

Oregon's saga continued to play out back in federal court where, in April 2002, a U.S. District Court judge granted Oregon's request to block Ashcroft's directive, strongly criticizing him for attempting to usurp a state's authority over medical regulation. Ashcroft's rejoinder arrived that September in the Ninth Circuit Court of Appeals, in San Francisco, seeking to reverse the lower court's ruling and thereby nullify Oregon's law. That court ruled in May 2004: "The attorney general's unilateral attempt to regulate general medical practices historically entrusted to state lawmakers interferes with the democratic debate about physician-assisted suicide and far exceeds the scope of his authority under federal law." In July Ashcroft asked for a rehearing, a request denied that August. Undeterred, a new Bush administration, with a new attorney general, Alberto Gonzales, has appealed to the U.S. Supreme Court, which will hear the case (*Gonzales v. Oregon*, no. 04–623) in October 2005. A decision is expected in mid-2006.[60] At all levels—state and federal courts, state and national legislatures, in the attorney general's office, doctors' offices, and in the privacy of a patient's home—concerns regarding individual rights, professional ethics, the role of government policy revolve around a most basic question: Will individuals be able to determine and direct their own life's end? For above all, a life and its end are individual to the core, including the particular experience of pain and suffering, and of dying.

Asked the reasons for requesting a physician to facilitate suicide, patients and family members emphasize the individual's desire to control the circumstances of their own death, to maintain some degree of independence, to limit the loss of an essential self, a fundamental human dignity and community. They describe a poor quality of life, marked by disintegration of personal capacities, loss of social connection and support, a feeling of hopelessness and meaninglessness. They express the patients' readiness to die.[61] Physicians surveyed about their own past patients describe individuals close to death, suffering substantial pain and other distress. Many of these patients were bedridden, and the doctors had expected that many would die within a month of the request. Although nearly half of the patients, in the opinion of the doctors, were depressed, a doctor was significantly less likely to provide prescriptions for lethal medications for these individuals.[62]

Granting the legitimacy of a patient's wish to die more quickly, and the right of that individual to do so, there exists in equal measure need for strong protections enforced with vigilance. Those protections aim at averting suicide that should not occur because a less drastic and irreversible alternative can meet the individual's needs. Patients may need protection from other people who might influence them too strongly toward suicide—a family member exerting pressure, a doctor abusing, for whatever reason, her power. Patients may also need financial protection from mounting medical bills that they fear will burden terribly their family. And some individuals may need protection from themselves—if they act impulsively or are not mentally competent to make such a decision, or if they suffer physical or emotional pain that appropriate treatment could ease.[63] This latter group, terminally ill patients who are psychologically depressed when requesting assistance to die, present particularly difficult considerations for doctors and other health professionals. Distinguishing treatable depression from some normal span of sadness over impending death remains a philosophical and practical challenge. Whether depression necessarily interferes with a patient's competence in arriving at this request remains an unresolved question as well.

Certainly, in reaching a decision about hastening death, patients need accurate information about their medical condition and prognosis, information they can discuss thoroughly with knowledgeable and experienced doctors, counselors, and other health professionals. To avert suicides that need not occur, doctors will need better training to treat not only physical pain and distress, but also the emotional pain and despair patients may experience when facing death. Physicians need to develop skills to identify untoward family pressures on seriously ill individuals and to facilitate their patients' interactions with an experienced psychologist, psychiatrist, and, perhaps, a spiritual or religious counselor. Requests for physician-assisted suicide demand an exceptionally broad margin of safety, extending beyond the physician's response to include careful psychological evaluations and comprehensive palliative care by additional health professionals attempting to relieve their patients' suffering, whatever its origin and type.

The potential for physicians' error or even abuse in cases of assisted suicide will always exist. Rather than leave so consequential a process solely to one doctor's judgment, whether a Dr. Kevorkian or one less publicity-minded, to create a series of legal safeguards, as in Oregon, seems the more cautious approach. Regulations built into law, not prohibition of this medical response to a patient's request, can better protect patients. Prohibition cannot eliminate physician-assisted suicide, only the ability to monitor its safe and judicious use. Keeping the practice legally inaccessible more likely pushes it toward the equivalent of abortion's back alleys, where a less than scrupulous or competent physician need only write a prescription, or where some terminally ill individuals may ingest their own lethal concoction or attempt a more violent, difficult method of suicide—gun, razor, leap from a bridge or high building. Not only will such attempts in themselves be more painful, they may also fail, leaving the sufferers still terminally ill but most likely with greater debilitation and pain.

A doctor's role in hastening death does remain a particularly vexing proposition. For some critics of physician-assisted suicide, any such role is anathema to a doctor's mission, which is to heal. Others see the danger as an irreversible step down the slippery slope that crosses a next divide, beyond Oregon's law, to euthanasia.

EUTHANASIA

Sometimes called mercy killing, euthanasia expands a doctor's role. Instead of prescribing medications for a patient to obtain and take, a doctor more directly causes the patient's death, most often by lethal injection. In the United States, where assisted suicide remains contentious, the relatively few advocates of a more direct role for a doctor are represented primarily through the work of the Hemlock Society (renamed End-of-Life Choices in 2003) and the writings of Derek Humphry.[64] For them, euthanasia is but one method that should be available and may be necessary for the terminally ill to fulfill a basic human right: to choose the time and manner of their death. Euthanasia is not the mysterious homicidal killing periodically revealed in media accounts, mostly of elderly patients in a hospital or nursing home. Nor does euthanasia describe government-directed efforts, as in Nazi Germany, to eliminate undesirable beings. Rather, the crucial element is individual choice—a voluntary request, perhaps written in advance, perhaps expressed when pain becomes unbearable, asking a doctor to take an action that will result in death.

Euthanasia is not as extreme as it might initially seem. The continuum starting with unassisted suicide is quite fluid, distinctions in some cases fine enough to wash away. For patients physically unable to ingest lethal pills or liquids on their own, a Kevorkian contraption allows a charade that barely separates suicide—death by the patient's own hand—from euthanasia. That indistinct line dramatizes how difficult and problematic, practically and ethically, the process of dying and a doctor's role in it can be. Ironically, the reason some patients cannot physically take their own life, short of refusing to eat and drink, is that they waited too long, at least in part because no doctor would take the legal risk of assisting. Now, their condition having deteriorated too far, these patients are trapped. Absent the help of a doctor, what alternatives exist for a terminally ill woman or man who wishes to die but is unable to? Enlisting the aid of a family member or friend is fraught with ethical hazards, as well as with greater likelihood of an unsuccessful effort, resulting not only in extended physical pain and suffering for the ill individual but also in emotional anguish for both parties.

The dilemma of a doctor's role in hastening death becomes, more strongly put, a question about obligations. Most doctors recognize that for certain terminally ill patients, choosing to die reflects a reasonable, clearly stated, and persistent response to an insufferable existence. Granted the serious hesitations doctors feel at the thought of ending a life, what of their mission to seek an end to suffering, in these instances through a least painful and quicker death? Dr. Sherwin Nuland, the Yale University surgeon and medical historian well known for his book *How We Die,* written for laypeople, expresses the concern to colleagues in a *New England Journal of Medicine* editorial:

> If prevention and relief of suffering are the aims of medical interventions—and not only the preservation or prolongation of life—it seems imperative to rethink our profession's reluctance to participate in euthanasia or even be present during an assisted suicide without legal guarantees of protection. . . . Physicians who believe that it is a person's right to choose death when suffering cannot otherwise be relieved must turn to their consciences in deciding whether to provide help in such a situation. Once the decision to intervene has been made, the goal should be to ensure that death is as merciful and serene as possible.[65]

For some doctors, and for the U.S. Supreme Court, terminal sedation, intended to relieve pain and suffering, creates an acceptable middle ground. Yet with the ethical boundary of intent ephemeral, sedating a patient into unconsciousness, not to receive nutrition or water until death, may constitute prolonged euthanasia. One bioethicist notes that the Court's 1997 decision upholding state laws that prohibit physician-assisted suicide relied in part on considering terminal sedation a medical alternative for relief of intractable pain; the Court, he concludes, has rejected assisted suicide in those states "only by embracing what is essentially euthanasia."[66] He argues, moreover, that terminal sedation presents even greater risk of abuse than allowing doctors, in select cases of a voluntary request, to deliberately cause a patient's more immediate death. Unlike physician-assisted suicide, which requires some degree of the patient's active participation, or requested euthanasia, which retains some of the patient's control and choice, terminal sedation can occur without a patient's consenting or, if an individual's physical or mental condition slips beyond conscious awareness, even knowing. That is, any physically incapacitated or mentally incompetent patient can be subject to terminal sedation. (Perhaps the most frightening prospect involves patients who are aware but physically unable to refuse sedation.)

As with assisted suicide, there is no way to determine how often American doctors or nurses currently take the more active role defined as euthanasia, a number even more elusive given the medical cushion of terminal sedation. Legalized in the Netherlands in 2001, voluntary requested euthanasia has been quietly tolerated as an acceptable medical practice there and in other European countries over many years. In the Netherlands, nearly 40 percent of deaths follow medical decisions that "probably or certainly hastened" that death, although few cases involve a doctor's deliberate administration of lethal medications. In 2001, 2.6 percent of death certificates in the Netherlands indicated euthanasia as a cause of death.[67] Terminal sedation preceded death in approximately 20 percent of cases and is the only end-of-life decision on the rise in recent years, especially with patients over eighty years old. The rate of physician-assisted suicide and euthanasia has remained stable since last reported in 1995. A study of six European countries suggests that medical decisions about life-sustaining treatments, palliative care, physician-assisted suicide, and euthanasia become significant issues in approximately two-thirds of all deaths. The primary aim when reaching such decisions, in most cases, is to relieve patients' suffering.[68] In Europe, where throughout adulthood an individual's health care relies more heavily on a family doctor than in the United States, patient and doctor may be able to reach difficult end-of-life decisions with greater mutual knowledge and trust. Moreover, with universal government-paid health care, patients need not feel influenced in these ultimate decisions by looming medical bills they and their family cannot afford.

DON'T JUST DO SOMETHING, STAND THERE

My father entered hospice care by the skin of his teeth, one day before he died. Surely it could have been earlier. The delay may be testimony to a general underuse of hospice for the very old, but even more to a visiting nurse's valiant though unsuccessful effort to wrestle down symptoms resisting control—to gain him and us a time of shared calm. Two hospice staff, on their initial visit, heard his breathing change as we sat talking. I should call my brother sooner, they advised, rather than later. Then, for the first time, I watched a life end.

"The death we fear most," comments one geriatric researcher, "is dying in pain, unnoticed and isolated from loved ones."[69] My father avoided that fate, one too often describing a modern hospital or nursing home death. Yet dying at home does not promise dying peacefully or quickly. At times, it is not a pretty sight. My father's final decline, I now recognize, began around the time I called a skilled nursing facility, no longer confident we could keep him at home in the house he insisted was someplace else. Beyond his needs, I saw my mother, the couple's other half, being dragged down by his delusions, then hallucinations, his anger and agitation, as she made her way through each day. I called the morning after he refused to sleep another night in this place, demanding once again we take him home, then threw his walker as far as he was able. I made no further inquiries, however, as that night's outburst would be his last. The anger and volatility subsided in face of a more active dying. The intermittent panics, times he feared he would not live out the day, disappeared as well. We were all too busy now reaching the end.

It felt natural to avoid calling 911, the hospice way, as he drew raspy, then oddly spaced and suspended last breaths. This was not an emergency, it was a death. I am glad he remained living and dying at home and can only hope that in some way, at the end, he felt whatever being home meant to him. Too often during last weeks and months of life, people need to avoid, even fend off, unwanted medical interventions, while others find their health-care options limited primarily by cost and/or age. Too many people still face overuse of life-extending treatments and underuse of pain control. For women and men seeking a better death, in their own way, the same vocabulary from the 1990s, with attention newly focused on palliative care and assisted suicide, persists into the twenty-first century: choice, autonomy, control, comfort, and peace.

Maintaining the autonomy to choose among good options requires more than most people—patients or their doctors—can accomplish alone. While American medicine boasts its technological sophistication and heroic cures, it lacks a basic framework of care systems to support individuals in their chosen way of living late life. In Berkeley, calling 911 could land my aged parent in the emergency room (albeit an overcrowded one) any time, day or night, including weekends and holidays, and including X-rays, CT scans, perhaps ultimately the intensive care unit. And for that ability the community is fortunate. Far more difficult is setting up a sustained, comprehensive, and affordable caregiving environment for an older individual, at home if possible, where she can live safely, even if growing increasingly frail. The technology does not assure that she will receive nourishing meals, assistance with bathing and dressing and other personal care, company and conversation, physical therapy, needed medications properly taken (as well as filled, re-newed, and delivered, if needed)—even on weekends and holidays—along with continuing medical care from doctors and nurses who have developed a relationship with her over time.

It sounds like a lot. Yet these are the basic activities that sustain daily life until its end. Each person will differ in the type and amount of help required, in the length of time required, and in the degree to which family or friends can meet those needs. Each will differ in the extent of geri-atric conditions—falls and loss of mobility, incontinence, mood disor-ders and cognitive decline, skin wounds, nutritional needs—that few health-care providers treat adequately.[70] Some people will need hospital care; others will manage to stay away. Still missing from this picture, however, are medical training and rewards for doctors and other health-care providers to develop competence and ease with patients who are aging, then dying.[71] Planning for late-life care need not be relegated to a by-the-way experience haphazardly caught if at all, or ignored until moment-of-crisis decisions. Patients could feel comfortable knowing their doctor will honor a reasonable decision to reject last-ditch life-extending efforts, and doctors could know this choice does not mean giving up. Finally, patients need not be lying on their deathbed to qual-ify for palliative care. Relieved of distress by such care, fewer terminally ill patients would likely wish only for a quicker end. At the extremes, however, where suffering and pain will not be tamed, people would not be forced to wait patiently for death, forbidden to enlist aid from a fa-miliar and trusted doctor, and their doctor would not risk punishment and reproach by agreeing to help.

Any such picture remains a future possibility, given new generations of doctors, not only trained to achieve cures, but also educated to im-prove the quality of a person's aging and dying. Also essential: newly developed health policies. Currently, Medicare supports, through cold cash in diminishing reimbursements, very limited scenarios for older Americans. There is the hospital with its surgical suites and intensive care. Or individuals can choose hospice care during a final six months of life. But most older women and men fall outside the boundaries Medicare sets for care at home, categories marked by the forecast of a short time left to live or, for the homebound, specific physical needs (e.g., wound care, catheters) for a nurse. There are the many people with uncertain or less predictable futures: individuals who "might rea-sonably die in the coming year," as geriatricians describe them, people "sick enough that dying this year would not be a surprise," repeatedly in and out of emergency rooms and hospitals, people losing weight and lacking resilience, confused, and needing considerable personal care.[72] Among Medicare's population are even more people with chronic health conditions or disabilities who are not homebound yet cannot care for themselves completely. And so, a friend in her seventies survives open heart surgery that installs several bypasses and replaces valves, a successful heart operation but for one complication: during surgery she suffers a stroke, leaving half her body paralyzed, her prognosis uncertain but potentially long. Geriatric researchers present a not so different case study, noting that such an outcome is "not uncommon." They write, "at the point of [hospital] discharge, our system in effect abandons this patient and her family to their own inadequate resources."[73] The health of their patient, of my friend, and of a substantial proportion of other Medicare recipients with acute or chronic illness may fluctuate over time, moving them between hospital and home, hospital and rehabilitation or skilled nursing facility, and with luck again home, though once again on their own.

Today's middle-aged can feel certain that more sophisticated medical technologies, genetic tests, and bioengineered drugs will grace their old age. Yet they should be aware that medical voices are warning of urgent need to improve end-of-life care, referring explicitly to the baby boom generations.[74] With palliative care demonstrating cost savings at the end of life, hospital administrators and insurers are gaining interest, improving prospects that this option will expand. Already most of my generation know the feeling that suddenly our doctors are younger than we are, no longer the older wise men who knew best. Unfortunately, Americans cannot anticipate aging with the care of a doctor who knows them well, given care disruptions forced by the country's health insurance structure.

As baby boomers face the late life of their parents' generation, they can gain insight from the few older doctors sharing reflections on a career-full of patients and on the experience of their own parents, siblings, and friends. In *How We Die,* Sherwin Nuland casts a critical eye on the ways doctors, himself included, have responded to people who are seriously ill and dying. He conveys a medical mindset fixated on "the Riddle" posed by each patient's ailment—what has gone wrong and how can doctors correct it?—rather than focused on the quality of that patient's remaining life. Doctors' inability to give up their quest to solve the Riddle, he asserts, "will sometimes be at odds with our [patients'] best interests at the end of life."[75] This eternal quest shapes the advice they give patients to the point, he admits personally, of with-holding information in order to influence, or push, them toward bur-densome and often futile tests and treatments. Also shaping doctors' ad-vice is peer pressure from colleagues to do what they have been trained to do: in Nuland's specialty, to salvage a patient's survival, through sur-gery, whenever possible, regardless of a patient's wishes or the physical cost. Consistent with Daniel Callahan's critique, the prevailing credo—especially early in their medical career—is to never consider death an acceptable medical option.[76] Nuland castigates his profession, including his younger self, for "propell[ing] a dying person willy-nilly into a series of worsening miseries from which there is no extrication" (1993, 142), a medical venture particularly troublesome with patients who are old, and an apt description of Dr. Lainer's dreaded geriatric nightmare.

Finally, Nuland focuses on death itself. He minces no words in por-traying the physiological processes that culminate in death, a stark contrast to unrealistic expectations many patients hold of how the dying process will look and feel. Most pointedly, he criticizes the med-ical world for contributing to such expectations by always holding out one last surgery or drug that might save a patient, even with minus-cule chance for success but certain distress and suffering along the way. Reviving this hope, doctors deny the reality of dying, a process that more often than not, especially with hospitalized dying, is a "messy business," far from peaceful or serene. Doctors, so attracted to "the brilliance of rescue," too commonly abandon patients "when res-cue proves impossible" (265). The outcome: patients and their family are set up for disappointment and anguish that they have failed to achieve a good death. With this concept now reinforced in the popular culture, a culture already sold on successful aging, the dying and be-reaved are left blaming themselves and their doctors for somehow not doing it right.

Just as patients making treatment decisions wonder what a doctor would choose for his own parent, wife, or child, it is fair to ask how Dr. Nuland wishes to do his own end of life. "When my time comes," he writes, "I will seek hope in the knowledge that insofar as possible I will not be allowed to suffer or be subjected to needless attempts to main-tain life; I will seek it in the certainty that I will not be abandoned to die alone" (257). He adds that not suffering "unfortunately is not what I expect" (263). A "right death" may be beyond his or anyone's grasp. However, a realistic expectation is to reach decisions that avert the worst of the dying process, allowing people, himself included, to attain tranquility in the choices made and, thereby, in the actual death. If faced with serious illness, this doctor plans to seek the best medical advice from a skilled specialist, but he will not let that specialist "decide when to let go. . . . I will not die later than I should simply for the senseless reason that a highly skilled technological physician does not understand who I am" (266). For that understanding and support, he will turn to a "longtime medical friend." For most people, that medical friend may well be their primary care physician—if their health plan has allowed them to stay with their chosen doctor throughout extended phases of their adult lives.

Writing a decade ago, Nuland maintained hope that with greater knowledge of their own ailments, patients would develop more realistic expectations and decisions regarding the end of life. Certainly, the last dozen years have witnessed an explosion of medical information for the public through the media and Internet. As a context for their medical decisions, patients may also be gaining gradual awareness of the medical mindset Nuland describes—the Riddle and rescue orientation that is changing only in a slow and piecemeal fashion with, for example, greater attention to palliative care and at least some public discussion of physician-assisted suicide.

Just as certainly, even with greater knowledge and awareness, patients alone cannot accomplish substantial change in options available during the final stage of life. As another physician writes in 2004, "If I should find myself aged and failing physically and mentally, and if I sought relief from the 'pain' my life was causing me, I would hope that the physician I turn to for help has a good understanding of palliative care and end-of-life options, has the courage to act on my behalf, and has more merciful laws to protect the decisions we may make together about my end-of-life care."[77]

And once again, here is Dr. Timothy Quill, writing in *The New England Journal of Medicine* thirteen years after that initial revelation about his patient Diane:

> I recently helped my father to die. . . . Every effort was made to improve his quality of life with the use of modern treatments for dementia, as well as symptomatic treatments for his agitation and insomnia. But each of these treatments made his symptoms worse, rather than better. . . . Because my father had been very clear about his wishes while he was still mentally competent, and because our family understood how the system works and had the relevant knowledge and resources, we were able to use our fragmented health care system to provide him with comprehensive and humane end-of-life care. Most families are not so fortunate.

Again a case eerily like my father's; I can only conclude that the numbers out there must be large. Concerned that most people have no access to the type of excellent care identified since his original statement—individual treatment plans that include palliative care when severely ill, "seamless transition" into hospice care if desired, and "clarity about . . . last-resort options"—Quill concludes, "I hope that in the next 13 years, these pieces can be integrated into a coherent whole and made predictably available to all Americans as part of a universal health care plan."[78]

With the population of oldest old growing, the education and early experience of doctors may encourage an altered approach, a medical perspective that can accept and help patients through their time for dying. More difficult still for coming decades will be establishing the next generation of health policies and care systems to support our chosen ways of growing old and of securing a less bad death,[79] successfully averting the worst of dying while not expecting to go with a smile on our face.

■ ■ ■

Four weeks after my father dies, I find my mother sprawled on the dining room floor unable to move, her voluminous bathrobe fanned wide. She has fallen and broken a hip, or vice versa. Fortunately, my morning checks bring me across the street to her house soon after she is awake each day, after I see she has raised her bedroom shade. When I mention her injury to a doctor or nurse, shaking my head in disbelief at this bad fortune, they seem not all that surprised.

We enter the next round—surgery, rehabilitation, wheelchair, and walker, pain medications, arrangements for twenty-four-hour help when, or if, she returns home—and I am the one feeling punch drunk. The *if* arises from statistics. Among aged women who break a hip, half never fully recover their mobility and their ability to live at least somewhat independently at home. Surgery and hospitalization itself may leave them disoriented, irreversibly weakened, susceptible to infections they cannot overcome. For some individuals, the broken bone imposes a final decision, discharging them to some manner of residential institution. One woman out of four will die within a year.

My mother receives appropriate care, including transfer from the hospital to a skilled nursing facility that emphasizes rehabilitation centered around physical and occupational therapy. Medicare will cover this transition to home, but of course with limits: reaching therapy goals means Medicare will stop paying; and, as if in a geriatric Catch-22, not enough progress, suggesting the exercises and practice are ineffective, means the same. My mother's discharge reflects the latter. An overwhelming fatigue further weakens her depleted body. Her inability to endure walking an adequate number of steps down the busy hospital-like hallway, or up enough stairs that stop in midair, means she will be coming home.

Even as my mother regains a respectable degree of her former mobility and endurance at home—with Vladimir prodding her through the prescribed daily exercise regimen—she is receding in most other ways. Our Friday night dinners never mend. My father's absence, while gaping, is not the whole of it. Now it is her confusions we must untangle, questions and actions less agitated than his were, but mostly tied to him. When she manages an outing to the market, she buys for him. When she sits at her end of the long dining room table, she waits for him to appear across the way. When a burst of energy allows her to cook, she makes what he likes. Periodically she asks, with impatience, "So where *is* Dad?" Months pass before "What shall we have for dinner?" becomes "It's just me, isn't it?" She reports that someone brought Dad's clothes home from wherever he went, and a few days later asks, "What can we do to get Dad back?" She doesn't remember knowing, if fleetingly, that he died, and then she doesn't remember the several previous times she forgot.

My mother now represents, unhappily, the demographics. She is isolated far beyond the large empty house. She has outlived lifelong friends and made no new ones. Unable to drive, increasingly frail, she withdraws more persistently from social and recreational activities. Organizing thoughts to formulate full sentences, let alone engage in conversation, takes effort—becoming for her, it seems, more trouble than it's worth. With so much attention the last few years revolving around my father, her needs incidental to his drama, she appears now a cipher. With so much of the past six decades consumed by husband and children, she lacks the temperament, stamina, and mental energy to reshape her own life. She lacks the strength and perhaps the will to outlast two statistical truths: among the old, the death of a spouse raises significantly the survivor's risk of dying within one year; and a broken hip jeopardizes similarly the next year of life. Just four weeks after my father's death, then, my mother already has two strikes against her.

We have one last emergency room visit. Appearing fine on this spring morning, by afternoon my mother is feeling and looking ill. Vladimir and my son ease her into our car—a mistake, I realize, watching patients strapped to ambulance gurneys roll past us and the guard and the crowded waiting area before the triage nurse even looks at my mother. Vladimir, pacing, mumbles his supreme insult: "This hospital Ukraine."

Once inside, the ER is American health care at its best and worst. The best: well-trained, hard-working nurses and doctors, sophisticated tests and equipment, abundant medications. The worst: a thin, listless African American man whose age I can't guess, parked in a wheelchair against a hallway wall. Two shopping bags stuffed with belongings fill his lap. His ER visit apparently finished, a nurse tells him, "Roll yourself to that phone and call the shelter. See if you can find a bed."

Everyone tries to be gentle with my mother, but the mere squeeze of a blood pressure cuff leads to moans of discomfort. Finding a vein and threading in a needle—for blood tests, intravenous fluids, and antibiotics—makes her scream and leaves an arm bruised dark purple from wrist to elbow. She will be admitted this time, for this infection. I am relieved that, at least for now, we need not add acute illness to caring for her at home. As I leave the ER, hours after we arrived, knowing my mother is settled in for the night, there on a curb outside the entrance sits the same sick-looking man in the wheelchair with his bags—waiting for a ride, or for morning, or for his own Godot.

Over the next several days, the hospitalist manages my mother's care competently and efficiently. He lists for me the options, the explanations and discussion so oddly detached from any knowledge of who she is. She recovers enough to be moved, quicker and sicker, to the same skilled nursing facility she entered ten months before. There, physical therapists predict she will again climb the stairs of her house, sit in her garden, occasionally attend a performance at the senior center. I feel encouraged, especially when my mother declares, one morning, that she would love a chocolate milkshake (perhaps like those my father made for her each night when she was pregnant with my brother and then me), which my son and I bring later that day, and then again two days later. Her doctor sounds less optimistic. He poses the questions asked not so long before about my father: Do we want her to remain in a residential facility after this week of physical therapy? Are we able to care for her at home if she is bed-bound or perhaps can move only from bed to chair?

The physical and occupational therapists do what they can to build up my mother before sending her home. In fact, were we not able to afford two caregivers—Vladimir (the Ukrainian) every day, Mahnaz (a

woman from Iran) every night—and were they not extraordinarily de-
voted, we could not manage. On my mother's first morning home, however, she has a fever. Somewhere in that fragile, depleted body, infection
or inflammation or both have survived her medications. Or, I will learn
later, fluctuating temperature can reflect the dying process itself, as a
body shuts down. So too, I will learn, can specific cravings—say, for the
sweetness of a milkshake. Over the phone, my mother's doctor presents
tersely the revised list of options: the emergency room (i.e., dial 911),
first stage in doing all that modern medicine can do; no medical treatment, letting nature take its course until death; or a compromise, antibiotics at home.

He likely knows we will not choose the hospital route. Her prehospi-
tal Do Not Resuscitate form, which he signed, sits ready. During her recent hospital stay, we declined further invasive diagnostic tests (a scope
down her throat, for instance) or treatments. Yet we are not ready not
to try; being feverish and ill is not, after all, cardiac arrest. I ask him to
call in a prescription to the pharmacy while I consult with others in the
family. "I'm sorry," he says, as if final condolences were due.

During the next five days, my worry that antibiotics may only prolong her ordeal yields to fear of giving up too soon. But she does not
rally. We stop the medication, hoping to ease whatever discomfort it is
causing. Bed-bound, barely able to speak, she sometimes appears to
look at me with a puzzled, then questioning expression. Cutting
through the activity of care all around her—the sponge baths, the
changes of nightgown and sheets, the offers of juice and water, maybe a
piece of toast—she is trying to read my face. She is looking to find a
hint, or perhaps to confirm not a fear but a feeling, that this time it is serious and strange and unlike previous bouts of illness. She will hang on,
though not fight it, and wait to see what happens next. As with my father, she becomes a hospice patient, with no time to spare. Since offi-
cially Medicare coverage starts the following day, we will pay for morphine today, buying my mother twenty-four hours without pain—a
luxury, like the special mattress for her bed, like the paid caregivers,
that many people cannot afford.

My mother's life takes several days to finally die away. As the statistics predicted, less than a year since my father died, and less than ten
months after she broke her hip, I am once again dripping morphine under my parent's tongue, wondering if this breath will be the last. I study
my mother's aged, craggy face in the hope of never forgetting. If she
feels no pain, I surprise myself thinking, why blow out the last glimmer-

ings, why not wait, in reverence to some unknowable force of nature that sparks every life, disappearing when it will. And then, moments later, as her breathing grows louder, more congested and raspy, each irregular effort a jagged cut through the dark night, her comfort less certain, I know the wish to help her, with just the slightest extra puff, to be gone.

Soon after, I must have dozed, twenty minutes at most, until startled awake by her perfect and endless quiet.

6

Conclusions and a Look Ahead
Baby Boomers Take Stock

Across the street, my parents' house sits large and empty, in need of repair. Shortly after my mother's death a friend said, "You must be tired." With responsibility for parents ended, I recall with sorrow, nostalgia even, just months earlier when I allowed myself to say, in frustration over yet another crisis, "I'm tired of taking care of them." I was far more tired of watching them slowly die.

Across the country, my mother-in-law moves through her nineties. She no longer makes phone calls, so she speaks with my husband only when he calls her. During our last visit, she never quite grasped who I was. She still enjoys people in the present moment, and then again when the next moment comes. And fortunately her companion, a lovely woman from Guatemala, can still take her downstairs to sit on the Broadway bench to watch life in New York during seasons that are not too cold and icy, not humid and hot. She seems still to know her two sons, if not always which one is which, and her sister when she walks into the room. This younger sister, however, needs day and night help at home as soon as possible, and the long-distance phone calls between brothers now focus on finding caregivers for their aunt, a woman in her mid-eighties with no children of her own.

With Lillian I am gradually losing touch in every way. I visit less frequently and often find her near the nurses' station dozing, strapped into a wheelchair, her white sneakers spotless. She remains apparently content, though no longer able to walk in the garden, or anywhere else. She often seems not to recognize that I am someone familiar, even as I sit at the lunch table helping to guide food into her mouth. When I drive away from these visits, I imagine never showing up again. And yet the next time she greets me warmly, as if recognizing a face.

My brother remains healthy, his checkups showing him cancer-free. He might like to retire early but hesitates, because fortunately he does have a job that brings good health insurance (unlike many other middle-aged individuals, stranded without insurance because of its cost or because of a preexisting health condition until they reach Medicare age). Still, he is never free of worry that an unusual symptom or the next body scan will reveal lurking illness, his luck run out.

And the biweekly university-sponsored caregivers' group carries on. A few of us might now be considered emeritus members, a rank attained when the care receiver dies. Group participants continue sharing experiences with an unending stream of problems. One week a daughter cries describing her very frail mother, discharged from the hospital into its affiliated skilled nursing facility, an institution this daughter and her sisters would never have chosen. Finally, they pay out of their collective pockets to move their mother into a more pleasant, better-staffed facility. Another week, a daughter worries that she and her brother can afford too few hours of even a home health aide for their mother, in place of more hours of the skilled nursing care she needs.

In drawing conclusions about aging and health care, this chapter moves from people such as these to ask, in summary, what is the problem? What is missing for the presently old and for the wave of baby boom generations soon to replace them? Granting the need for limits on the overall cost of health care—through rationing, in one form or another—on what should restrictions depend? In addition to reviewing major concerns discussed throughout the book, this final chapter looks toward the task ahead, suggesting how individual experiences of today's old, and health-care wishes among those of us at midlife, might best translate into future scenarios of aging and health care, supported by national and local government policies. I delineate general principles and goals as well as cite, when possible, examples that may help point the way.

POLITICAL PHILOSOPHY MEETS HEALTH ECONOMICS

Of all the forms of inequality, injustice in health care is
the most shocking and inhumane.

Rev. Martin Luther King, Jr.

At the century's turn, with the 2000 presidential election approaching,
reports on American health care commonly described a system—or
nonsystem—in crisis, nearing collapse. With the population aging, concern about Medicare spread beyond the program's financial future, as
baby boom generations reached the age of sixty-five, to focus on its
most troublesome gaps: prescription drugs and long-term care. Among
people younger than sixty-five, the ranks with no health insurance or inadequate coverage continued to expand. The notion of a safety net—to
allow emergency rooms, public hospitals and clinics, state and federal
health insurance programs to catch individuals unable to afford even
standard medical fare—seemed wishful thinking. Rather, hospitals and
clinics closed, emergency care remained dangerously strained, health insurance programs for the poor whittled down eligibility and benefits.
Communities throughout the United States lost resources for insured
and uninsured alike, such as hospital specialty services, trauma units,
and emergency rooms, as well as public health programs responsible for
disease control and disaster preparedness. The insured continued to
subsidize medical care for the uninsured, through their taxes (an estimated 85 percent of the approximately $35 billion provided in 2001),
and through a shifting of costs to the rising expense of their own health
care.[1]

A striking dimension of this crisis, one difficult for politicians to
ignore, has been its direct impact on the country's middle-aged middle class. For increasing numbers of this population, unforeseen, perhaps hard-to-imagine events suddenly happened. At the drop of a lay-
off notice, income and health insurance disappeared, an especially rude
awakening for individuals accustomed to high technology- or Internet-
related salaries. Nor was job loss required. Individuals still working full
time might have an employer who significantly raised employees' contributions or discontinued health insurance altogether. Retirees lost coverage they relied on, and the next wave to retire could no longer count
on generous benefits in their future. Once financially secure families,
many with some health insurance but not enough, faced economic ruin

from medical bills resulting from relatively moderate, not catastrophic, illness or injury. Approximately half of personal bankruptcies filed in 1999 resulted primarily from the expense of such illness or injury, and in 2001 the number of such occurrences was twenty-three times higher than in 1981.[2]

One year before the election of 2000, two nationwide surveys and interviews with voters had identified health care as a dominant concern. Regardless of political party, their greatest single worry (from a list of fifty-one possibilities, including education, crime, the environment) was insurance companies making the medical decisions that doctors and patients should make. In addition, voters worried that older Americans would not be able to afford prescription drugs, that employers would reduce medical benefits, and that the number of people with no health insurance would rise.[3] Those concerns presaged the reality of U.S. health care as the next presidential election campaign geared up four years later.

Across a broad economic spectrum, people worried about their health care, and with good reason. In 2002, results of a nationwide survey developed by National Public Radio, the Kaiser Family Foundation, and Harvard's Kennedy School of Government revealed that one out of four middle-income families ($25,000–49,000 annual income) experienced problems paying medical bills (along with 38 percent of respondents with less than $25,000 annual income, versus 9 percent above $50,000). Close to half (44 percent) reported at least one problem with health-care payment, access, or quality. Moreover, they commonly perceived consequences of these problems to be serious. Among people within the middle-income range, one out of four identified health insurance as the reason for staying in a job longer than they would otherwise choose. Even without immediate problems, people worried. Nearly half of the survey respondents were very or somewhat worried about paying for medical care or prescription drugs, and half of those with insurance worried that in the future they would no longer be able to afford it. Baby boomers worried about daily care for an elderly parent, and about paying for needed health care if a family member became ill.[4]

By 2003, a report analyzing U.S. Census Bureau data confirmed Americans' concerns. As described in chapter 4, health insurance loomed as a problem of greater magnitude, in numbers alone, than the 43-plus million uninsured commonly reported. Including individuals without health insurance during any portion of a two-year span, the number jumped to nearly 82 million people—one-third of the population under sixty-five years of age lacking health insurance for all or part of 2002 and 2003. Nearly two-thirds of this group remained uninsured for six months or longer. In fourteen states, the uninsured proportion of the population exceeded one-third. Consistent with the survey cited above, lack of insurance resulted in serious consequences, including costly, avoidable hospital stays for patients who could not afford earlier doctors' visits and treatment—patients who grew sicker and more likely to die. Having even one uninsured family member jeopardized financial stability and security for all in that immediate family.[5]

In sum, economic recession brought home to the middle class, and middle-aged, just how crucial health insurance becomes when they face previously taken-for-granted doctor or hospital bills or the monthly tab for prescription drugs. During better economic times, a wider, less tattered blanket of job-related insurance coverage kept this reliance more hidden. Less apparent also during flush times is a fundamental American omission: a coherent and cohesive social principle supporting fair, equitable distribution of health care as everyone's right, regardless of ability to pay. President Bush touched fleetingly on the kernel of such a principle, at least for one segment of the population, in his 2003 State of the Union Address. Medicare, he asserted, reflects "the binding commitment of a caring society," a statement he repeated verbatim during the 2004 election campaign. At the risk of putting words in the presidential mouth, I articulate more fully that commitment: Medicare secures for all of the country's old and disabled access to health care and protection from the financial threat posed by illness or disability, with costs spread across that population.

Yet Bush's phrase stands disembodied from his policies and proposals, which can only undermine genuine social commitment. Rather than shore up this publicly financed health insurance program—a program popular with that public, albeit needing revisions—the Bush administration seeks to push Medicare recipients toward private, for-profit insurers whose ultimate commitment is to financial gain. The potential lure, early in 2003, was prescription drug coverage, to be available only through a private plan—a proposal that ignored the already failed experiment with private Medicare HMOs, that drew criticism from Republicans and Democrats alike, and that the administration quickly modified into a somewhat less radical (or less obviously radical) thrust toward privatization.

Furthermore, Bush's Medicare comment suggests the following question: Why not a caring commitment to people of any age, as reflected, at least in part, through the assurance of health care? That is, if a government program for the old and disabled represents society's best instincts, why not extend similar collective responsibility and protection across the entire population? This question is crucial, particularly given the efforts of the Bush administration and others to minimize government's role of ensuring the public's welfare. For instance, by cutting taxes that support the country's broad social safety net, by seeking to privatize Social Security and eviscerate other policies developed in response to the Great Depression, strong political forces continue to push in the direction the United States has been moving since the election of Ronald Reagan in 1980.[6]

At issue is the role of government on the one hand, and reliance on individual or family wealth on the other. One prominent health economist, Uwe Reinhardt of Princeton University, has addressed basic health-care principles as they reflect the country's social ethic. He focuses his comments in the *Journal of the American Medical Association* by asking: "As a matter of national policy, and to the extent that a nation's health system can make it possible, should the child of a poor American family have the same chance of avoiding preventable illness or of being cured from a given illness as does the child of a rich American family?"[7]

Unlike every other economically developed nation, the American answer remains no. This negative, Reinhardt argues, reflects a viewpoint held primarily by the more affluent, who wield the political power shaping social policy. Thus they can rest assured, and of course insured, knowing their own family members will obtain the best care and cures. Not only is this health-care status quo inefficient, demonstrated most dramatically by crowded emergency rooms and by a bloated administrative overhead built into American health care overall. It is unfair.

Interestingly, though in glancing reference, Reinhardt explicitly ties access to health care and its quality to principles of justice and fairness elaborated by the eminent political philosopher John Rawls, who died in 2002. Rawls's theoretical work is highly relevant to discussion of present and future directions for American health care, most pointedly to the distribution of limited services. Grossly simplified, Rawls develops an ethical framework for defining the individual rights, social relationships, and institutions of a society based on principles of justice.[8] To reach this determination, Rawls devised an illuminating thought experiment—he called it the "original position"—in which a group of people representing all generations of their family establish, from scratch, the society in which they will live. They must reach consensus through negotiation about basic principles underlying such social institutions as the government, economic system, and family, with all agreeing that the distribution of available goods and privileges is fair. The crucial characteristic of the group forging these principles, one that shapes the agreement it reaches, is that participants cannot know what their position within the society will be. They have no clue as to their sex, race, socioeconomic status, religion, personal aspirations, or abilities. Nor can they know their overall health—within a range allowing them to function as fully cooperating members of society throughout a lifetime—or their particular health problems. They are negotiating, in Rawls's conception, behind a "veil of ignorance" and will agree, therefore, only to principles that are fair to everyone, protecting people's essential interests whatever their individual circumstances and social position. Inequalities—for example, in taxation or use of health services—will be regulated and distributed in a way that raises the level of the least advantaged, since anyone in any family might turn out to belong to this group.

Rawls mentions medical care as one of several rights, or primary goods, to which everyone in the society will be entitled. Considering priorities and urgency among expenditures for competing needs (say, education, police and fire protection, the environment, foreign policy), he arrives at the general concept of a fixed minimum level of health care provided to individuals throughout life, along with societywide public health measures. Beyond these basics, there may be "widely divergent benefits individuals actually receive, depending on variable, unpredictable and temporary needs during their lifetime" (2001, 173), that is, the illnesses and accidents that unpredictably befall people. He cites as one example the primacy of treatment to restore good health and return citizens to active participation in society, over most cosmetic medicine; however, he does not "pursue further these difficult and complicated matters" (175). Such matters, more specific than core guidelines, will be determined through the society's legislative institutions.

Obviously, these few paragraphs cannot do justice to so rich and comprehensive a theory of justice, or to its difficult and complicated specifications. However, Rawls's basic framework does provide a context for assessing our health-care system, revealing a patchwork of programs and policies that exacerbate inefficiency and injustices. The economically better-off enjoy lopsided benefits, for instance, of employer-based, government-subsidized, private health insurance. Clearly, this not truly free market does not play by Rawls's rules. Far from a veil of ignorance, in fact, it perpetuates the antithesis: huge amounts of money for political lobbying and commercial marketing allow health-care-related corporations to profit while America's more wealthy individuals obtain an unfair portion of society's best health-care goods and services. Knowing full well their privileged position, many reject changes toward equalizing distribution of resources to improve conditions for the least advantaged, such as universal publicly financed health insurance.

Yet if positions in this country's social hierarchy seem clear, American health care is forcing, in its way, an at least partial veil of ignorance: no one can predict their own, or their parents', or their children's health and needs for care over a lifetime, which now often extends beyond ninety years. Employment, pensions, and insurance status are less certain than many people assumed throughout the 1990s economic boom. The vagaries of individual lives, in this day and age, include not only loss of job and income, but all versions of unpredictable illness and accident, as Rawls notes. People now risk experiencing chronic disabilities and dementias of old age, as well as virulent strains of a newly emerged virus, or even a newly emboldened terrorist. Moreover, with inequalities and inefficiencies reducing the quality of care for everyone, it is in everyone's interest to devise a system that more adequately guarantees fairness for all. Transposing concepts from Rawls, albeit in an exceedingly loose manner, Americans find themselves within a health-care realm akin in some manner to an original position of veiled representatives. The question before them: How can this society best reconfigure the way people obtain health care, especially delineating necessary limits on all that is medically possible, in order to reverse the inefficiency, unpredictability, and uncertainty that push everyone's health care into decline?

Pursuit of greater fairness in principle has not prevailed in a national health-care debate skewed toward interests of large pharmaceutical and private insurance corporations or other economic powers-that-be. In fact, it is important to recognize that the essential goal of universal health insurance can come in many forms, with varying consequences for the distribution and quality of care. Large private insurers are happy to support measures resulting in a population more fully insured by large private insurers—for example, reliance on tax incentives and medical savings accounts for individuals to purchase insurance, as the Bush administration advocates, and on a privatized Medicare for the old. With the 2003 Medicare law enticing private insurers back into the

Medicare arena through generous government subsidies, a déjà vu of marketing materialized in no time: free restaurant meals, media advertisements, promotional mailings. The very companies that discontinued Medicare HMOs during the 1990s, abandoning their members, seek once again to lure older Americans out of traditional Medicare, spurred on this time by the federal government's ideological and financial (taxpayers') encouragement. Just how many people will entrust their health insurance to commercial plans this time around remains uncertain. Yet according to one early analysis, "Wall Street investors are expecting a big payoff."[9]

The Republican administration's largesse to private industry may translate into satisfying profits for investors (assuming, that is, the opposite does not occur, that these companies, not realizing such gains, pull out of the Medicare market once again); however, this privatized route will create the same administrative waste and inequity of the previous Medicare HMO venture, which reflected well, in turn, the country's overall health insurance approach. In contrast, evidence already indicates that the most efficient system would also gain for American health care a system that is more fair and just. That system's insurance and payment structure eliminates the middlemen—materialized for the public in HMO bureaucrats authorizing or rejecting medical procedures—with their administrative overhead, executive salaries, marketing costs, and profit requirements. In California, for example, a state sponsored analysis compared ten alternative health insurance models aimed at increasing coverage throughout the state. An independent consulting firm reported in 2002 on each alternative's projected costs, services, access to care, and quality (including for vulnerable groups). The conclusions: by integrating current health-care spending into one state-run insurance program (MediCal, insurance programs targeting children, Workman's Compensation, in addition to Medicare and Veterans' Administration), thus significantly reducing overhead, and by negotiating lower prices for drugs and medical supplies, single-payer proposals provided the greatest cost savings. All California residents would receive coverage for comprehensive health services at no extra cost to the state.[10] Under this model, insurance would no longer be linked to employment, with all the uncertainties and inequity this dependence brings, nor would the insurer (the state government) abandon patients determined to be unprofitable, as private insurers have done with so many older Americans.

If enacted at the national level, such a system would replace existing public programs (such as all state-run Medicaid and Workman's Comp, Medicare, and veterans' and children's programs) and the myriad private plans with one publicly funded health insurance program, administered by the federal government as the single payer. The closest examples are Medicare (except Medicare HMOs), and Canada's health insurance program for all ages, administered by the provinces. Also called Medicare, the Canadian program insures all medically necessary services (mostly physician and general hospital care) to all citizens and residents. Patients maintain their choice of private doctors, who submit bills (mostly on an agreed fee-for-service basis) and receive payment from the government agency, as do hospitals and other providers. Private, investor-owned hospitals, agencies, and other facilities have little role in the Canadian system. Although some variations exist by province (for instance, long-term care), all provide prescription drug coverage to seniors.[11]

Opponents of a publicly funded national health insurance program have thwarted efforts reaching back nearly a hundred years. Defeat of the Clinton Health Security Act is only the most recent episode, coming half a century after the failure of President Truman, then later Nixon, to attain a similar goal. Even so, advocates of universal coverage, with the federal government as single payer, have not given up. In 2003 one prominent physicians' group formulated a proposal published in the *Journal of the American Medical Association,* coauthored by a former editor of the *New England Journal of Medicine,* and endorsed by nearly eight thousand additional physicians and medical students.[12] Describing their proposal as "in essence . . . an expanded and improved version of traditional Medicare" (Physicians' Working Group 2003, 798), the authors explain that it would insure every American for all necessary medical care. Coverage would eventually include prescription drugs (older Americans would be covered from the outset), along with mental health and dental services, and needed long-term care for the disabled of any age. Drawing on long-term-care programs in some Canadian provinces and in Germany, family caregiving would be supported and encouraged, when possible, with not-for-profit home-care agencies and residential-care facilities covered as well.

The physicians' group notes that private insurers in the United States currently spend 12 percent of premiums on overhead costs, compared to less than 3.2 percent on overhead for Medicare and for Canada's national health insurance program; 31 percent of all health-care spending in the United States goes to administrative costs, compared to 16.7 percent in Canada. The proposal outlines how its fundamental changes would initially contain and in future years lower overall health-care costs.[13] While affordability and cost containment are essential to any future health insurance program, even more compelling are the principles that give shape to this group's proposal. Most importantly, the program establishes comprehensive health care as a human right, with government responsible for ensuring access to care for all members of society. Neither corporate profit nor accumulation of personal wealth is a legitimate goal within the health-care system. Basic to the health-care right is patients' autonomy in choosing and changing their physician or other licensed health-care provider, and it is the patients and providers who make individual medical decisions, not corporate or government bureaucrats.

Unfortunately, in the wake of the Clinton administration's retreat from universal health insurance, this national goal largely vanished from public discourse. Legislators and politicians reverted quickly to attempting small steps, if any, toward incremental reforms—for instance, enrolling more low-income children and parents, offering temporary (though very expensive) insurance protection in case of job loss. This approach has resulted in business as usual, with new prescription drug coverage for Medicare finally emerging from congressional limbo dominated by a Republican majority during a Republican administration, defining lucrative rewards for the pharmaceutical and private insurance industries. Yet this usual business of the private marketplace proceeds in the face of a dire situation that one analyst calls the American "health care mess" requiring changes that represent, in the words of another, a great leap forward, a "giant leap of political will."[14]

Efforts short of such a leap have not succeeded in achieving a fully insured population. In fact, one sobering assessment of the decade since the Clintons' failed proposal demonstrates that American health care has gone from bad to worse on the most fundamental dimensions (insurance programs for low income Americans, problems of the uninsured, healthcare costs, patient's rights, quality of care). This analyst attributes the worsening conditions to the absence of an overall vision that would coordinate gradual, incremental health care reforms.[15] If perhaps this accurately depicts the subsequent Clinton years, an even more troubling reality may now prevail: that an overall vision does exist—centered around individuals as consumers within a private corporate health care marketplace that minimizes government involvement—pursued all the more forcefully during the second Bush administration.

Examining more narrowly health insurance and its lack, the Institute of Medicine—a private, nonprofit institution, part of the National Academy of Sciences, providing health policy advice to Congress and other policy makers—conducted a comprehensive evaluation. The Institute's Committee on the Consequences of Uninsurance concluded that incremental reforms will not solve the problems posed to all Americans by so many without health insurance. Nor will this national crisis be resolved state-by-state, even if the political will resides at that level. While individual states, such as Maine, may still initiate programs to provide universal coverage for state residents, prospects for success at the state level fade in light of economic dynamics nationwide, none more consequential than the Bush administration tax cuts, which not only diminish federal revenue but squeeze down state and local government resources as well.[16] In California, to cite a dramatic demonstration, the state lurches far from the single-payer analysis mentioned above: the actor and bodybuilder Arnold Schwarzenegger, a Republican elected as governor during the recall of Democrat Gray Davis, vowed to make drastic cuts in state spending on health care, and in the full gamut of social services and education, a threat reverberating locally throughout city and county fire and police departments, schools, and health services.

Rather than rely on incremental efforts or individual state programs, the Institute of Medicine committee's "clear and compelling overall recommendations" are that the president and Congress initiate immediate actions that will guarantee health insurance for everyone in the United States by 2010.[17] Toward that end, the committee delineates five key principles to guide further evaluation of potential health insurance structures:

- Health-care coverage should be *universal:* in this most basic and important principle, universal "means what it says. Everyone living in the United States should have health insurance."
- Health-care coverage should be *continuous,* not interrupted by gaps of time when a person is uninsured.
- Health-care coverage should be *affordable to individuals and families.*
- The health insurance strategy should be *affordable and sustainable for society.*

· Health insurance should *enhance health and well-being* by promoting access to high-quality care that is effective, efficient, safe, timely, patient-centered, and equitable.

To attain such coverage, the committee offers four simplified prototypes, ranging from least to most system change (including expanded public programs, required employer and/or individual insurance with premium subsidies and tax credits, publicly funded single payer) and notes their strengths and weaknesses. While the report suggests that the comprehensive change needed will likely combine the strongest elements of each prototype, it also concludes that any one of the four will more adequately reflect the five guiding principles than does "the current hodgepodge of insurance mechanisms." Consistent generally with Rawls's minimum level of health care for all in society, the insurance strategy would provide everyone with a basic benefit package (including preventive and screening services, prescription drugs, mental health care, outpatient, and hospital services). And, like the California analysis of ten insurance models cited above, the committee finds that the single-payer insurance structure, similar to Medicare, would provide the most simple and efficient strategy through significantly lowered administrative costs, absent the multiple intermediaries.

All Americans want the security of knowing good health care will be there when they need it. Important as the societal goal of universal health care remains—with services and costs fairly distributed—the actual need for care, like the experience of aging itself, returns the focus to individuals throughout a lifetime, with varying needs and life choices, strengths and vulnerabilities. The final section reviews concepts basic to allowing people to age in this country with care and support that are more fully and certainly secure.

REDEFINING AND REDESIGNING

Throughout *Our Parents, Ourselves,* I have focused on the presently old, especially the oldest, while raising questions for the greater number of people now at midlife. I have sketched personal stories and discussed health-care policies affecting these individuals. This final section encourages readers who are not yet old to put themselves into future stories, learning from our parents' generation the potential limitations and needs individuals experience, the strengths and resilience, and the way government policies could better provide support. Beyond immediate care decisions for an aged family member, the baby boom generations still have time to take seriously the concept—though overused in media and marketing—of redefining age. They have enough years ahead to develop environments and care systems that enhance options for purposeful activities and enjoyable living during late decades of life. They can envision national and local health policies as if negotiating or casting their vote in elections for a system that, given the unforeseen, brings greatest security and fairness all around.

THE MEDICAL QUESTION REVISITED

In chapter 3, discussion of prescription drugs distinguished the medical question of beneficial prescribing from the too often dominant question of a medication's cost. Here the medical question involves conclusions about health-care quality more broadly as people age, recognizing all the while that improvement remains constrained by expense built into American health care, especially its excessive administrative and drug costs. One certainty for aging baby boomers during the years ahead will be ever-expanding medical information about physical and cognitive health, for better and worse, and the public's increasing access to such information through the media and Internet. For individuals as for society, one challenge is to become more savvy about the continually evolving nature of medical knowledge and, therefore, about choosing medical interventions for which proven benefits outweigh risks. For instance, new understandings of heart disease may point in some identifiable cases to causes that no bypass surgery can circumvent. New insights about various cholesterols may alter prevailing wisdom about who can safely benefit from medications to lower the level of bad types and raise the good. Enough examples demonstrate that the preliminary promise of medical breakthroughs can go unfulfilled under greater scientific scrutiny, and that more treatment is not always better for patients. Likewise, longstanding medical approaches can prove to be unfounded, or at least surprisingly tentative. Still missing are systematic analyses and comparisons of many diagnostic and screening procedures, medications, and surgeries—information that should be the basis of decisions regarding medical interventions and other health-care needs.

Also certain is people's desire to benefit from the latest medical knowledge and technologies—for instance, in neurobiology, brain imaging, genomic medicine (potentially including prescription drugs tailored to individual genetic variations), and other expensive new treatments. Alluring as highly sophisticated medical solutions may seem, however, most health care for older adults does not require cutting-edge medical intervention. The more consistent need is for ongoing relationships with doctors who can determine, based on current medical knowledge, which tests and treatments are best suited to which patient, neither over- nor undertreating an individual's chronic or acute condition. Doctors need to develop, and Medicare to support, the foundation of primary and preventive care that maximize patients' cognitive and mental as well as physical health, including nonpharmacological interventions provided in coordination with nonphysician care providers (for instance, exercise, changes in social and physical environment, diet, stress reduction measures).[18] When appropriate, doctors also need the ability to prescribe affordable medications based on reliable scientific data about safety, efficacy, potential side effects, and interactions—not on drug manufacturers' product information, and not at unregulated manufacturer-determined prices, or for pharmaceutically defined disease.

Older Americans need not become Luddites. In fact, novel uses of advanced technology can assist individuals in their homes, gradually escalating over time to bolster independence in daily life. Community settings can also utilize technology in elder-accommodating ways—for instance, in banks, post offices, transportation, theaters, on city and park walkways. In homes and communities, architects and builders can more commonly incorporate transgenerational, or universal, design for people whose strength, abilities, eyesight, hearing, and even memory are limited for a variety of reasons—age, injury, pregnancy, disability. More broadly, to redefine aging requires awareness that much about health and well-being is not medical at all. Social networks and services, along with adequate financial means to support daily life and its inevitable disruptions by illness or injury, are of one piece with more straightforward health care. Defined more comprehensively, then, safeguarding health as people age requires physical and economic security, satisfying social activity and sensory stimulation, efforts to maintain physical mobility, and access to needed personal assistance and care.

IMMEDIATE NEEDS AND BEYOND

Current inadequacies of health care for older adults appear to be attracting increased attention within the medical world. Most prominent are concerns about health conditions common among the oldest and most vulnerable of the old. One report notes surprisingly little previous research on quality of care for older adults, and none on care for geriatric conditions that have profound impact on daily life; this first such study finds inadequate care for falls, mobility problems, incontinence, pressure sores, nutritional deficits, cognitive impairment, as well as end-of-life care.[19] While physicians score quite high on treatment of acute and more general illness among adults—stroke, heart failure, pneumonia, diabetes—they fail to provide a type of health care vulnerable elders need. To provide that care now, and for the much larger population of older adults in coming decades, requires newly trained doctors.[20] Moreover, beyond a set of common geriatric conditions, argues one group of medical educators, an even more important factor is "the process of providing individualized, integrated, humane care to old and failing patients . . . [care that is] longitudinal, proactive, coordinated."[21]

Whichever the emphasis, all agree that the systems of care available to older adults—starting with the very definition and organization of health services—require change, with a goal of allowing people with complex, multiple chronic illnesses and disabilities to live as independently as possible. Central to these changes are alterations in Medicare reimbursements and resource allocation that heavily favor acute care and medical procedures. Rather, incentives and support, including in the education of health professionals, would shift toward the nonacute, often time-consuming attention a growing number of older patients need. In sum, key components of high-quality care emerge:

- Multidisciplinary team-based assessment that identifies an individual's physical and mental problems early, monitors chronic conditions, and targets preventive measures to maintain abilities and slow declines

- Case-coordination of medical, psychological, and social services in ongoing care for chronic conditions and treatment of acute illness, including support for family caregivers and efforts to avert emergency room use and hospitalization when possible

- Continuous and comprehensive coordination and medical supervision throughout needed hospitalization, including programs to prevent such problems as delirium, and discharge planning that facilitates consistent follow-up care at home aimed at maintaining functional abilities and enjoyment of daily life[22]

· Attention to an individual's health-care goals and priorities, which may change with age toward enhancing the quality, rather than extending the length, of life

As discussed in chapter 2, no phenomenon of aging has been more apparent and troubling in recent years than the loss of mental abilities as dementia swallows patches of an individual's memory, language, reasoning, and judgment. Until research untangles the perplexing dynamics of mind and body, the interplay of dementias, depressions, and cardiovascular and neurological processes, optimal treatment will remain unknown. While scientists pursue greater understanding of cognitive health and threats to it—seeking interventions that prevent, reverse, or at least delay dementias—an ongoing and immediate challenge is to improve the environments and care of affected individuals.

People living near aged parents or friends who suffer substantial memory loss and dementia may find it difficult to maintain perspective on the heterogeneity of aging. Yet most women and men who live beyond their seventies manage quite well. Even among individuals with noticeable cognitive impairment, the speed and extent of mental decline varies, altering the distance in time and behaviors that separate initial trouble managing their lives from complete inability. Ideally, this variety of need would correspond to a variety of available assistance that supports, as much as possible, autonomy and choice within each individual's home or some form of group residential setting. At the same time, people living near aged parents and friends may become very aware that many of the oldest old cannot possibly manage on their own. Especially after their mideighties, individuals enjoy a far less ample and forgiving margin of error in maintaining their daily lives, and then the margin may vanish. Not only the margin for bathing and dressing, driving, shopping for food, and preparing meals, but also for managing bank accounts and credit cards; negotiating recorded phone menus with buttons to push and no human voice (including when calling the doctor); dealing with Medicare statements and supplements, taxes, house insurance and upkeep; or obtaining medications (not to mention taking them correctly).

Currently, long-term care for faltering individuals remains narrowly defined, if less hidden than in past years. The predominant image is the nursing home, a skilled nursing facility housing the most frail and mentally impaired of the old. Certainly, for the immediate future, long overdue measures that improve care, oversight, and regulation could help to create humane and needed residential settings for appropriately identified individuals, many of whom currently lack other acceptable options. More resources could support three-to-four-person care homes within the community, run by people wanting and able to provide their residents with personal, high-quality one-on-one attention. Regarding larger institutions, reform advocates know well the needs: lower staff-resident ratios allowing more individualized care and privacy; greater staff training; smaller subgroups with greater autonomy for residents and staff, rather than uniform, regimented, institutional routines and schedules; activities and settings that more resemble a small community, providing greater physical activity, social, visual, and mental stimulation; more appropriate use of medications; environments better designed and staff specifically trained to care for the large number of residents with dementia and other mental illness, while not treating all others as if similarly afflicted.[23]

Beyond skilled nursing facilities, development and oversight of assisted living for women and men able to maintain some degree of independence in daily life requires immediate attention, to cut short poor practices already identified and to realize the potential of such settings.[24] Availability of pleasant, well-run residences that provide high-quality personal care, meals, housekeeping, social activities—all calibrated for a range of individual needs—could not only mean a better life for residents who choose this option but might allay anxiety and fear about aging, more generally, in a population already losing bit by bit the ability to live independently. Whether older adults remain in their own home or move to assisted living, the spectrum of care and activities, along with access to skilled nursing if needed, could fulfill goals represented by life-care communities (see chapter 1)—but not only for the wealthy, as today.

For my own generation, more substantial redefinition of long-term care could create more enveloping and extended long-term well-being throughout later decades of life. Rather than settle for a final residential compromise or last-ditch medical intervention, today's middle-aged can define how they want to live during the years before age-related disabilities significantly cramp their style, within a setting of their choice where they can add greater assistance as needed. In fact, the sandwiched generation itself can expect redefinition. Ultimately, the top and bottom layers fall away, perhaps simultaneously. Just as parents die, care for them ended, children grow up and go off to college, jobs, lives of their own. The empty nest may feel emptier for a longer expanse of time while baby boom women and men are still relatively young and healthy. How then to refocus aging from a good end-of-life (see chapter 5) to a good rest-of-life, starting now? How to set up systems and resources that support individuals and families and networks of friends, including the help and health care they are likely to need at some indeterminate point?

An altered concept of long term will, by definition, begin at home. As suggested above, innovative devices and technologies can modify homes in ways that compensate for certain limitations on physical capacities and memory as individuals age. That is, homes would adapt, with age, to their residents. In addition, technology can help people avoid isolation and lack of stimulation as they become less able to get around—within their neighborhood or more distant locales. Already, older adults who learn computer skills navigate the Internet's boundless communication and informational avenues. In years to come, adults will have grown adept with computers and the Internet at a younger age, and the technology itself will have grown more enabling.

Although individuals vary in their desires for direct social contact, face-to-face interactions and relationships hold an irreplaceable value. To this end, neighborhoods and communities will remain a focus of attention for the long term. Beyond informal relationships among family and friends who live near each other, city and county services for older residents are often available, albeit generally sparse and underfunded. Among the most common are supplemental transportation and senior center recreation programs. Religious and ethnic communities may offer activities, as well as visitors to the old who are home alone. Some cities in states with large numbers of older residents have developed more extensive accommodations that attract older adults and support their ability to live independently, safely, and enjoyably. In Florida, for instance, with the country's largest proportion of older residents, the state provides assistance to cities that improve transportation, medical services, law enforcement, banking, and businesses in ways that benefit residents sixty-five and older.[25]

However, just as the ranks of older baby boomers begin to swell—with government budgets at all levels buckling in the economic downturn that followed the 1990s, in concert with the Bush administration's tax cuts—such programs may not survive and additional states and cities may not develop similar programs. Moreover, fundamental change for boomers' later decades of life will require a broader range of options and, for many people, more thorough and deliberate redesign of living-at-home and aging-in-place. My generation will need to consider a facet of life that experience with our parents has highlighted: How attached do we, as individuals, feel to our own place, perhaps a home of many years? How salient is our desire to live and die in a long familiar home, compared, for instance, to the pleasures of social activity and daily assistance a group residence can bring? And how can our communities honor and provide for our differing responses?

Models exist that suggest potential directions, materialized presently to varying degrees in theory and practice:

· Residents of a Maryland retirement community, population 2,500, establish a nonprofit cooperative to finance specified home health and preventive services, including respite and group support for members caring for a chronically ill partner. Annual dues also cover assistance with Medicare and supplemental insurance statements, nurses' consultations and home visits, medical and dental referrals, discounts on prescription drugs and long-term-care insurance.[26]

· Shared housing by two or more older individuals able to live independently provides companionship in place of isolation, as well as mutual help with daily tasks. Or a younger, healthier adult may live in the home of an older, less able individual, exchanging needed assistance for the cost of rent.[27]

· Intentional communities in various forms broaden companionship and mutual assistance. In one, individuals and families plan and create a cross-generational neighborhood, designed for the physically able and disabled, that includes communal space for recreation and meals. Among the twenty to thirty households, neighbors share tasks ranging from babysitting to personal care for the old, in some instances including end-of-life care at home.[28] In a very different setting, a group of middle-aged artists and writers, determined to remain actively involved in New York City life, seek to purchase a Manhattan apartment building. As individuals who work primarily on their own, requiring some degree of solitude, their goal is to maintain a continuum with their earlier lives while avoiding isolation and loneliness too common among aged city dwellers. In addition to approximately a hundred individual apartments with sliding-scale rent, they envision a community cultural center with several public rooms for meals, meetings, classes and lectures, art exhibits, and performances.[29]

· A university develops a nonprofit cooperative housing community for retired professors, offering a range of housing options and services, long-term health care, and opportunities for continued academic and professional activities.[30]

· A group of feminists purchases collectively a farm, aiming for self-sufficiency as they enter their older age.[31] More generally, expanding on women's support groups in their younger years—as feminists and mothers—and building on lifelong friendship patterns, midlife women are exploring a range of options with various financial and legal commitments, for two or more friends to live with and care for each other when older. Enough of a trend to merit a front-page *New York Times* report, the possibilities attract not only women with no male partner and/or no children, but also women aware of the demographic likelihood that in their older age they will otherwise be living alone.[32]

Such efforts require more than creative financing and legal agreements or changes in local zoning and building regulations. These long-term living and care arrangements depend also on shared social principles, in this instance that older adults should be able to shape their own lives and destiny. Of central importance, individuals are creating environments and services that they define and control. Rather than lose personal autonomy and choice for needed care, as is characteristic of residential-care facilities as well as formal care in an individual's own home, the aim is that older adults determine the place for living, the use of time, the amount and type of social interactions. Shared housing and intentional communities, in particular, create ways for older individuals to give and receive care among friends and neighbors, if not also family. Older women and men can establish what one ethicist describes as "voluntary mini-mutual aid societies," fulfilling a deliberate long-range plan for mutual support.[33] They gain security not only by shaping their own daily well-being but also by maintaining an ongoing sense of self and self-determination, consistent with earlier stages of their adult lives. And, as an additional gain for many individuals seeking alternative models for living their later years: they do not rely on or perpetuate the social inequality presently engrained in formal caregiving—predominantly by women and immigrants—and receiving.

246 CONCLUSIONS AND A LOOK AHEAD

Whatever the chosen place and style of daily life, much about people's later years will depend on their physical and mental health, and how well their best-laid plans allow for unpredictable changes. This fact of later life brings us back to health care in its more narrow sense. As I have argued throughout *Our Parents, Ourselves,* changes in the care older adults typically receive could greatly benefit today's old and then the large number of baby boomers now beginning to approach their sixties. Moreover, an extended, deliberate, and less fragile long term, as suggested in this chapter, could evolve more gradually and naturally, for many people, into care needed as they near the end of life. For instance, certain health services—home visits for assessment and care by a doctor, nurse, or physician's assistant, a physical therapist, a home health aide providing needed personal care—could become common practice, along the lines of neighborhood nurses available in parts of Canada and the United Kingdom. Reimbursed visits would no longer be limited to a few weeks following patients' hospitalization, as Medicare now covers, nor to those individuals wealthy enough to pay on their own.

For acute medical needs beyond home visits, special infirmaries or elder clinics particularly attuned to the old could provide appropriate and timely care.[34] Closer to life's end, greater attention could turn to determining whether treatment makes sense or misery for each individual. Health-care providers and patients alike would understand that, technically speaking, "there is nothing we can do" to prolong life is a phrase that rarely applies in today's medical world, but that eventually doing only strong palliative care to control pain and allow comfort can provide the greatest benefit of all. Recognizing that doctors now commonly refer the oldest old—people like my parents—to hospice care too late, if at all, a new standard of care could define the palliative approach more broadly, detached from a specifically defined length of time. An individual and family could more likely experience contentment with good, satisfying final years, culminating in a peaceful and acceptable death.

QUESTIONS REDEFINED

There are no right answers about care and living arrangements for the old, and for too many individuals at present there are not even good answers—not enough individual choice among a variety of good options, not enough economic support for those without substantial private wealth. In recent years, the most public questions about older Americans' health care have focused on how to structure and finance changes in Medicare, starting with prescription drugs—that is, the cost question. Barely three months after the Medicare drug benefit became law, Alan Greenspan, the Federal Reserve Board chairman, declared the country's need to reduce future Medicare and Social Security benefits, given unprecedented budget deficits of the Bush administration and the imminent arrival of sixty-five-year-old baby boomers. Certainly, cost is a real and pressing concern, central to policy decisions about what Medicare will cover (and whether to delay the age for eligibility, a question Greenspan also raised). Of equal importance should be knowledge about medical and other care that best maintains people's health and well-being. Government and pharmaceutical manufacturers have already entered a tug-of-war over which prescription medications will be covered, for what conditions—for instance, particular brand names or generics, expensive "me-too" formulations, the myriad off-label uses never approved by the FDA?

Beyond some drug coverage and currently covered hospital and technology-centered curative care, what of the ever more sophisticated and costly screening and diagnostic tests, surgeries, medical devices, and equipment? Historically, there have been no stated criteria or regulations that define "reasonable and necessary" care, which is the legal requirement for becoming a Medicare benefit. Rather, each policy decision relies heavily on the pull of powerful competing stakeholders who stand to gain or lose: drug and medical-device makers, employers providing health insurance, the private insurers, the medical profession. So, for example, Medicare recently (and quietly) added to its benefits three highly invasive and costly surgeries for advanced lung and heart disease. Yet what of services aimed at preventing disease and disability, enhancing the health over time of individuals living in their community?[35] Will Medicare direct resources into more extensive physical therapy and other rehabilitation for nonhospitalized patients, visiting nurses and home health aides, and finally, as needed toward the end of life, nursing and palliative care at home or in a suitable residential facility? Will Medicare pay for case-coordination (say, by a social worker or nurse) that could provide much needed integration of direct medical care with much needed follow-up on patients' medications and other treatments? Will benefits include expanded adult day health-care options essential to the quality of life for physically and mentally impaired individuals and their family caregivers, in communities throughout the country? Or will these services remain outside Medicare's domain, dependent largely on each person's economic means?

As if in caricature of the answers that American health care threatens to create, the early twenty-first century produced one private market solution to cost questions, at least for the very wealthy: luxury primary care, also known as concierge- or boutique-medicine.[36] Patients pay an annual fee ($3,000–5,000 up to $20,000) to assure themselves such medical attention as their own primary care physician available at all times by cell phone; easy scheduling of and no waiting at office appointments, which may last an hour; the physician's direct involvement with hospitalizations, which may also involve a private nurse (at some extra charge). This high-end privately paid capitation proceeds while the rest of the country experiences the various inadequacies that lower health-care quality, cited throughout the previous chapters: unaffordable health insurance, forcing the uninsured to rely on emergency room care, to everyone's detriment; unaffordable medications; rapidly rising out-of-pocket costs for the insured; limits on choice of doctors within commercial health plans; doctors refusing Medicare and Medicaid patients because of low reimbursement rates; fragmented and sometimes inappropriate or inadequate care for older adults, with many needed services dependent on individual and family resources (in money, as well as ability to perform time- and labor-intensive informal care).

If the United States is to divert progression toward these extremes of already troubling health-care disparities, the public, its elected representatives and candidates seeking office, health professionals, economists, and other policy makers need to address preliminary questions fundamental to the future shape of American health care. Why, for instance, are drugs so expensive here, especially compared to other countries? (And why can drug manufacturers withdraw their products from Canadian pharmacies that sell prescription medications to Americans at lower cost?) Why is there no affordable long-term care for people, including those with dementia, who need help daily at home but do not require skilled nursing? Why is there so little public discussion of end-of-life care, including physician-assisted suicide, in place of the Bush administration's unilateral attempts to eliminate any such option, including when voter-approved? Why can private insurers essentially avoid individuals with the greatest medical needs—that is, why is the United States the one economically developed country failing to spread risk and costs across society in order to provide health insurance for all of its residents?

Improving care for Americans over the age of sixty-five will not come cheaply. The era of small, simpler communities in which families naturally cared for elders who lived among them has long passed. Continuing to depend on informal caregiving by a family member—most commonly a wife, daughter, or daughter-in-law—is simply not feasible, nor is depending on individual or family wealth to pay for needed medical and personal care. A person's health is too important to be left at the mercy of market forces, rising or falling like any other commercial product. To meet the binding commitment to older Americans that President Bush cited in January 2003 and again in 2004—to become "a caring society"— requires political will as well as financing. It also requires society's resolve that the larger health-care system in which Medicare remains embedded not drag down health care for all. In grappling with critical policy decisions regarding limits and access, our challenge is to distribute fairly and pay for beneficial, often lifesaving interventions, as benefits within the basic coverage of a universal health insurance system. Eliminating the waste of competing private insurers, and the excessive profit for the pharmaceutical industry, could bring this country a considerable way toward the social commitment long displayed by other economically developed nations.

As suggested earlier, the pertinent questions involve nothing less than the role of government in assuring social and economic support, including health care, as people age, rather than leaving individuals to muster their own resources. Attempts to push Medicare into the for-profit commercial arena of private insurance companies, starting with prescription drugs, threaten to unravel a program that, on the whole, has successfully distributed publicly funded health care to all older and disabled Americans. From its inception Medicare has adhered to the premise of universal insurance coverage: to provide everyone with the same basic benefits while protecting individuals and families financially by spreading costs across the entire population from the most to least healthy, the most to least wealthy. Reliance instead on market dynamics has already left millions of recipients in the lurch, disenrolled by their Medicare HMO. The country's broader market version, a competition between private health-care insurers seeking profitable economic returns, has left tens of millions of younger adults and children un- or underinsured.

The baby boom generations presently have the most at stake—the most to risk, and potentially the most to gain. They have decades of life ahead, with a goal of healthy aging. This huge and, therefore, powerful segment of society has time also to acknowledge, advocate, and vote for health care as a right to which all of society's members are entitled, a right safeguarded and supported by their government. They can think first of their parents, then immediately of their own needs, formulating the central health-care question as would Rawls about this primary good, and as does the World Health Organization more specifically about long-term care: What does justice require?[37] Rather than a product marketed by competing insurance companies toward the goal of investor profit, health care would join other rights Americans enjoy— education through high school, protection from fire and crime, sanitary water from our taps—with services equitably distributed, its more reasonable costs spread across the society. Even as Medicare faces threats of privatization (as Social Security certainly does from the second Bush administration), it is hard for baby boomers to remember or imagine when turning sixty-five years old did not entitle people to government-run, publicly funded health insurance (along with Social Security income). Recreating for the moment our sandwiched-generation status, today's middle-aged can even think ultimately about our own children, so quickly grown. Certainly our children's generation should enjoy the security and well-being of living in a caring society, hardly able to imagine how assurance of high-quality health care for Americans of all ages, among everyone's equal and inalienable rights, could ever have been otherwise.

■ ■ ■

In the early morning hours of the third day after my mother died, our street's recycling day, I hear the rustling of bottles and cans. I know the sound from other dawns sleepless for other reasons. Lifting an edge of the window shades, I will find not Berkeley's official curbside recycling truck but a lone man, one of a small phalanx who know well the weekly schedule and routes and precede the large, noisy, oddly shaped truck that inches its way down this street every Tuesday sometime before noon. House by house, this week's early recycler moves down the sidewalk, filling his garbage-size bags and unwieldy shopping cart, sifting through the blue bins for cans, glass bottles—whatever earns him refunds. In this neighborhood and other hill routes, he gathers empty bottles from health drinks and from good wine, all lined up the previous evening alongside bundles of the past week's *New York Times*.

Berkeley remains a liberal outpost, a city of recyclers and supporters of other progressive causes. Yet it remains also a city of disparities—in these two tracks of ecological routines, in its children's schools, in the health status and mortality rates of its black, Hispanic, and white residents. Like other American cities, it is struggling with inadequate resources to maintain an at least adequate level of health care for its population. From my work with the Over 60 Health Center I know that behind the scenes, dynamics play out that community members never see—pressures affecting the hospital, for instance, and decisions that may make business sense but not reflect the best choice for patients' care.

On this morning, the recycler I see out my window looks familiar. He could be the man I observed just a few weeks before in the emergency room and then outside its entrance, the man waiting in the hospital wheelchair and needing a homeless shelter bed for that night. Or maybe not. Perhaps he is the man I will see next time, as I wait through hours to see a doctor and nurse, when the emergency is no longer a frail, aged parent but my husband, my son, myself.

Resources for Information and Referrals

The following organizations and public agencies provide information, referrals, and questions to ask when evaluating and choosing various support services, care at home, or residential options for older Americans.

GENERAL INFORMATION, INCLUDING LEGAL AND FINANCIAL

Eldercare Locator, 800-677-1116, www.eldercare.gov. A public service of the United States Department of Health & Human Services, Administration on Aging, to help locate elder services (nonprofit and public) in local communities throughout the country, including day-care programs, assisted living, and skilled nursing facilities.

Area Agency on Aging. See your telephone directory for local county listings.

Health Insurance Counseling and Advocacy Program, www.inlandagency.org/html/hicap_hom.htm. Information on Medicare coverage, prescription drug discounts, long-term care options.

American Association of Retired Persons (AARP), 800-424-3410, www.aarp.org; legal services network www.aarp.org/lsn.

National Academy of Elder Law Attorneys, www.naela.com. Information, education, networking, and assistance to people as they age.

State Medical Associations, www.ndmed.com/Resources/StateMedAssn.htm. Information on health care power of attorney and living will.

Employee Assistance Programs of many large employers maintain eldercare information and support programs. For federal government employees, www.opm.gov/ehs/eappage.asp.

American Health Care Association, National Center for Assisted Living, www.longtermcareliving.com. Guide to planning and paying for long-term care.

Alzheimer's Association, 800-272-3900, www.alz.org. Provides resources, services, research results, and advocacy. Offers Alzheimer's Association Safe Return programs. Call 800-438-4380 for caregiver support groups and education.

National Institute of Neurological Disorders and Stroke, 800-438-4380, www.ninds.nih.gov. Information on clinical studies.

National Institute on Aging, www.nia.nih.gov. Health and research information.

American Society of Consultant Pharmacists, www.ascp.com. Information on drugs and drug interactions.

NEWSLETTERS

Many subscription newsletters are published for laypeople. The following examples provide information related to aging and health care (I generally did not cite specific newsletters that provided similar information about topics discussed in this book).

Consumer Reports on Health (Consumers Union)
Focus on Healthy Aging (Mt. Sinai School of Medicine)
Health News (New England Journal of Medicine)
Mayo Clinic Health Letter
Public Citizen Health Research Group Health Letter
Wellness Letter (University of California, Berkeley)

FOR CAREGIVERS, INCLUDING FAMILIES

Family Caregiver Alliance: National Center on Caregiving, 800-445-8106, www.caregiver.org. Information, education, services, research, and advocacy.

National Alliance for Caregiving, www.caregiving.org. Support to family caregivers and the professionals who help them, plus education.

National Family Caregivers Association, 800-896-3650, www.nfcacares.org. Education, support, empowerment, advocacy.

FINDING A CARE MANAGER

Usually social workers or registered nurses who organize and supervise a range of care services for an older adult (maintain contact with physicians, arrange home care/day care/residential facility, respond to emergencies 24 hours, help with Medicare/Medicaid and long-term asset management). Fees range from $80 to $250 an hour, depending on services performed and other local and individual factors.

National Association of Professional Geriatric Care Managers, 520-821-8008, www.caremanager.org. Information and zip-code search for local private GCM.

END OF LIFE

National Hospice and Palliative Care Organization, www.nhpco.org.
National Hospice Helpline, 800-658-8898.
American Academy of Hospice and Palliative Medicine, www.aahpm.org.
Death With Dignity Alliance, www.dwda.org.
End-of-Life Choices (formerly the Hemlock Society), 800-247-7421, www.endoflifechoices.org.

Notes

1. Leiberman 1998.
2. See www.owl-national.org and the *Owl Observer* (print newsletter).
3. Kantrowitz 2000.
4. This book does not address additional legal and financial concerns and mechanisms essential during an individual's older age, at the end of life, or arrangements for body and soul after death. See appendix for relevant resources.
5. All knew I was writing about them and each gave permission at the outset of my project, before cognitive decline might thwart a consent process.
6. That the university sponsors this group and related services indicates the impact on the institution: nearly one-third of staff and faculty care for an aged family member (mostly parents), a statistic that translates also into a significant number of lost work days (S. Lustig, acting associate vice-chancellor, business and administrative services, private communication). For Alzheimer's disease alone, the yearly economic cost throughout the United States of workers' becoming family caregivers is an estimated $36.5 billion, including lost productivity and replacement costs but not caregivers' direct costs from lost income and expenses related to providing the care (Prigerson 2003).
7. City of Berkeley Health and Human Services Department 1999. Isaacs and Schroeder 2004 presents data tying racial and ethnic disparities in health to socioeconomic class.

CHAPTER 1. INDEPENDENCE IN DAILY LIFE

1. Cassel, Besdine, and Siegal 1999; also Fried et al. 1997; Guralnik 1996.
2. Hardy and Gill 2004.
3. Wenger et al. 2003.

4. Wenger et al. 2003; Fried 2003; Landefeld, Callahan, and Woolard (eds.) 2003; Stuck, Beck, and Egger 2004; Grumbach and Bodenheimer 2004; Holman 2004; Inouye et al. 1999; Rowe 1999.

5. Ashton et al. 2003; Fisher 2003.

6. Basic monthly cost averaged $2,200 in California (Newcomer and Maynard 2001).

7. Yaffe et al. 2002.

8. Harrington, Newcomer, and Fox 2001.

9. Pear 2000c.

10. Pear 2002b; 2002d.

11. Pear 2003f.

12. Bodenheimer 1999.

13. See the appendix for resources that can help identify appropriate residential facilities and home care, including suggested questions to ask; also, Hurley and Volicer 2002 on choosing a skilled nursing facility.

14. In 2000, a typical entry fee was around $100,000 with monthly fees of $2,500; in some types of CCRC, fees are lower, but members pay extra as needed for personal and medical services.

15. Goldstein 2001; Steinhauer 2001.

16. Snowden 2001.

17. During a subsequent hospitalization, perhaps in response to complaints about such restraints or threats of lawsuits over inadequate staffing, a "sitter" remained in the room of patients considered fall risks.

18. See www.rwjf.org/new/special/adultdayServicesSummary.html; see also figure 1.

19. Mattimore et al. 1997.

20. Ritchie and Lovestone 2002.

21. Yaffe et al. 2002.

22. Wenger et al. 2003; Fried 2003; Landefeld, Callahan, and Woolard (eds.) 2003.

23. Summarized in Levine, Boal, and Boling 2003.

24. Pear 2000a; Bodenheimer 1999.

25. Levine, Boal, and Boling 2003 outlines the types of home care available, as well as Medicare limits.

26. Levine, Boal, and Boling 2003, 1206.

27. For ongoing decline, Gill, Allore, and Guo 2003; for acute episodes, Hardy and Gill 2004.

28. Gill et al. 2002; Tinetti, Baker, and Gallo 2002; Binder et al. 2004.

29. Bassuk, Glass, and Berkman 1999; Rowe and Kahn 1997; Crimmins, Saito, and Reynolds 1997.

30. Fratiglioni et al. 2000.

31. Kaufman 1986 interviewees reflect such variations.

32. Balfour and Kaplan 2002; Koepsell et al. 2002; Isaacs and Schroeder 2004. Persistent disparities in health care and outcomes are documented in a growing number of studies, e.g., Rao et al. 2004 among Medicare recipients.

33. See www.owl-national.org brochures; *Owl Observer*.

34. Rimer 1999.

35. Schulz et al. 2003.
36. Arendell and Estes 1991.
37. Duenwald and Stamler 2004.
38. Miles and Parker 1997; Cassel, Besdine, and Siegal 1999. President Bush's proposed changes in Social Security could further threaten older women's financial circumstances in the years ahead.
39. Schulz et al. 2003; Rabow, Hauser, and Adams 2004.
40. Katz, Mohammed, and Langa 2000.
41. Butler 1996.
42. Butler 1996, 794.
43. Butler 1996, 795; also Cassel, Besdine, and Siegal 1999; Tinetti, Baker, and Gallo 2002; Gill et al. 2002, 2003; Hadler 2003.
44. Schulz and Beach 1999, 2219; also Yaffe et al. 2002, especially regarding decisions about nursing-home placement.
45. Prigerson 2003.
46. Friedrich 2002.
47. Survey 2000.
48. Schevitz 1999.
49. Baker et al. 2001.
50. McWilliams et al. 2003. Interestingly, during a time before the drug benefit was enacted, neither group increased its use of prescription medications on gaining Medicare coverage.
51. McWilliams et al. 2003.

CHAPTER 2. PATTERNS OF DECLINE

1. Ramachandrian 2000.
2. Myerhoff 1978, 18.
3. E.g., see Stern and Carstensen (eds.) 2002 National Institute on Aging summary of promising research directions; also Casserly 2004.
4. Burns and Zaudis 2002, 1965.
5. Grundman et al. 2004.
6. Boeve et al. 2003.
7. Ritchie and Lovestone 2002; Trinh et al. 2003.
8. Institute for the Study of Aging 2001.
9. Albert and Drachman 2000; Hurley and Volicer 2002; Kawas 2003 and Cummings 2004 summarize diagnosis and treatment of Alzheimer's.
10. Press 2004; National Parkinson's Foundation, www.parkinson.org.
11. Wilcock 2003.
12. Vermeer et al. 2003.
13. Casserly 2004; Blass and Ratan 2003; Vermeer et al. 2003; Ferrucci et al. 1996.
14. Ritchie and Lovestone 2002; Langa, Foster, and Larson 2004.
15. Mesulam 2003.
16. Margolis and Rabin 2002; Kawas 2003.
17. Grundman et al. 2004; Margolis and Rabin 2002; Elias et al. 2000; Brookmeyer and Kawas 1998.

18. Boeve et al. 2003. Certainly with the late onset of MCI an individual likely has fewer years ahead to develop full-blown dementia.

19. Burns and Zaudis 2002.

20. Vermeer et al. 2003.

21. Cummings 2004.

22. Snowden 2001.

23. Casserly 2004; also Vermeer et al. 2003; Jagust 2001; Ferrucci et al. 1996; Langa, Foster, and Larson 2004.

24. Colcombe et al. 2004.

25. Cohen 1998; Whalley 2001. Researchers in the developing countries of Asia, Africa, and Latin America are attempting to modify diagnostic tests for dementia to improve validity across cultures and educational levels.

26. E.g., Brookmeyer and Kawas 1998.

27. Casserly 2004.

28. Ritchie and Lovestone 2002; Lu et al. 2004.

29. Puca et al. 2001; Friedrich 2002; Kirkwood 2000; Hilts 1999; Angiers 1995.

30. Casserly 2004.

31. E.g., Carlson et al. 1999; Whalley 2001; Budson and Price 2005 reviews current knowledge about memory problems, including data from brain imaging techniques.

32. Raskind et al. 2004; Kawas 2003; Trinh et al. 2003; Sink, Holden, and Yaffe 2005 describes benefits of available medications as "modest at best" and "not particularly effective" and emphasizes a need to try stopping the drugs to assess whether an individual still appears to need them.

33. Schneider 2004a; AD2000 Collaborative Group 2004.

34. Aisen et al. 2003.

35. Reisberg et al. 2003; Tariot et al. 2004.

36. Wilcock 2003; Sink, Holden, and Yaffe 2005.

37. Boeve et al. 2003; Casserly 2004.

38. Wolfson et al. 2001.

39. Ritchie and Lovestone 2002; Hurley and Volicer 2002; Sink, Holden, and Yaffe 2005.

40. Teri et al. 2003.

41. Schulz and Beach 1999, during an average four and one-half year follow-up.

42. Schulz et al. 2003, 2004. In contrast to their high levels of depression and anxiety after the patient's institutionalization, caregivers showed considerable resilience after the care recipient's death. Depressive symptoms receded, and caregivers perceived the death as a relief for both themselves and the deceased family member; also Rabow, Hauser, and Adams 2004.

43. Cooney et al. 2004.

44. Rowe and Kahn 1999.

45. Lyness 2004; Cummings 2004. Consultation with a psychiatrist—particularly one with a geriatric specialization—can avert some problems.

46. Gallow and Leibowitz 1999; Pantilat and Steimle 2004.

47. Gallow and Leibowitz 1999; Pennix et al. 1999; Ciechanowski et al. 2004.

48. Snowden 2001; Ritchie and Lovestone 2002; Cummings 2004.

49. Ritchie and Lovestone 2002; Cassel 2002; Hurley and Volicer 2002; Teri et al. 2003; Ciechanowski et al. 2004.

50. Landes, Sperry, and Strauss 2001.

51. Landes, Sperry, and Strauss 2001.

52. When altering medications, it is best to add or eliminate one at a time, to identify beneficial and adverse effects. Yet the desire to do something that brings relief sooner rather than later commonly prevails.

53. Landes, Sperry, and Strauss 2001, 1704.

54. Unutzer et al. 2002; Bruce et al. 2004; Lin et al. 2003.

55. Ciechanowski et al. 2004.

56. Evans 2003.

57. Lyness 2004.

58. Calman 2004, 228.

59. Colcombe et al. 2004; Ball et al. 2002; Rowe 1999.

60. Lin et al. 2003. This study found that high-quality, coordinated depression care can help relieve arthritis pain and stiffness as well as a patient's depressive symptoms.

61. Bassuk, Glass, and Berkman 1999; Wilson et al. 2002; Ball et al. 2002; Berkman 2000; Fratiglioni et al. 2000.

62. Tinetti 2003; Tinetti, Williams, and Gill 2000; Satariano et al. 1996; Evans 2003. Among all Berkeley residents the two major reasons for hospitalization due to unintentional injury are falls (40 percent, mainly in people over 65 years) and adverse effects of a prescribed medication (34 percent spread across all ages); the third reason (at 10 percent) is motor vehicle injuries (City of Berkeley Heath and Human Services Department 2002).

63. Wald 2000.

64. Kleinfeld 2003; Evans 2003, a British gerontologist, discusses the fear of falling along with the dangers of actual falls, which he describes as "thoroughly unpleasant and undignified."

65. Gilsdorf 2004, 212.

66. Bischoff-Ferrari et al. 2004.

67. Tinetti et al. 1994; Tinetti 2003; Hardy and Gill 2004.

68. Gill 2002; Tinetti 2003; Tinetti, Baker, and Gallow 2002; Binder et al. 2004.

69. Day et al. 2002.

70. Feskanich, Willett, and Colditz 2002.

71. Wang, Collett, and Lau 2004 review of tai chi studies; Li et al. 2002; Gregg et al. 2003; Jette et al. 1999; Wolf et al. 1996.

72. Colcombe et al. 2004.

73. Whalley 2001 describes future, progressive home adaptations as "intelligent assisted living."

74. Jones 2001; Aisen et al. 2003; Casserly 2004.

75. Gustafson et al. 2003; Zandi et al. 2004; Wang et al. 2001. Being obese

or significantly overweight at age seventy appears to increase the likelihood that an individual will be diagnosed during the next ten to twenty years with Alzheimer's as well as various physical illnesses.

76. Rowe 1999; Casserly 2004; Colcombe et al. 2004. More generally, some gerontologists sound a voice of reason: regarding diet, they suggest people allow themselves moderate indulgences once or twice a week for each decade they have passed, so that by the age of seventy they can enjoy one or two each day (Rowe and Kahn 1999). For discussion of health-promoting measures after the age of seventy, see Knoops et al. 2004; Rimm and Stampfer 2004.

77. Institute for the Study of Aging 2001; Blass and Ratan 2003.

78. Brach et al. 2003.

79. Gregg et al. 2003; Gill, Allore, and Guo 2003.

80. Abbott et al. 2004; Wenve et al. 2004; Knoops et al. 2004.

81. Volz 2000; Institute for the Study of Aging 2001; Friedland et al. 2001; Belluck 2001; Verghese et al. 2003; Coyle 2003.

82. Gould et al. 1999; Spector 2001. Speculation even questions whether the middle-aged and younger may face cognitive risk from increasing reliance on digital memory devices. Early evidence suggests some loss of short-term memory skills, which might affect other mental abilities, for better or worse (Wilson 2001). Another line of research suggests that the myelination process, a sheathing of nerve fibers that completes cell growth, continues until approximately fifty-five years of age; researchers even speculate that this process may underlie certain changes in thought and behavior common during middle age (Gudrais 2001), although the mellowing and new perspective they cite as evidence do not explain so many midlife crises.

83. Friedland et al. 2001.

84. Verghese et al. 2003.

85. E.g., see Rowe and Kahn 1997, 1999; Rowe 1999.

86. Institute for the Study of Aging 2001.

87. Solomon et al. 2002.

88. Fries 1980, 2002.

89. Fried et al. 1991, 1997; Crimmins, Saito, and Reynolds 1997; Crimmins, Reynolds, and Saito 1999.

90. Manton and Gu 2001; Schoeni, Freedman, and Wallace 2001; see also Freedman, Martin, and Schoeni 2002 review article.

91. Daviglus et al. 2003.

92. Schoeni, Freedman, and Wallace 2001; Rao et al. 2004.

93. Jasny and Roberts (eds.) 2003.

94. Hurley and Volicer 2002.

95. Olshansky et al. 1991; Rubenstein 1996; Lewontin 2001.

96. Rowe and Kahn 1999.

97. Olshansky et al. 1991, 207. See also Olshansky and Carnes 2001.

98. Kirkwood 2000, 17; also Feskens, Havekes, and Kalmijn 1994; Hilts 1999; Puca et al. 2001; Olshansky and Carnes 2001.

99. Nuland 1993.

100. Kaufman 1986, 12; see also Myerhoff 1978.

101. Isaacs and Schroeder 2004; Hadler 2003; Rao et al. 2004; Lantz et al. 1998.

CHAPTER 3. THE PHARMACEUTICAL AGE

1. Davis et al. 1999; Stolberg 2000a; GAO 2002; Altman and Parks-Thomas 2002.

2. Willcox, Himmelstein, and Woolhandler 1994; Zahn et al. 2001; Goulding 2004.

3. Evans 2003; see chapter 2.

4. Zahn et al. 2001.

5. Goulding 2004.

6. Avorn 2001; Rochon and Gurwitz 1999.

7. Avorn 2001.

8. Philips, Christenfeld, and Glynn 1998; Stolberg 1999.

9. Hampton 2004.

10. Gurwitz et al. 2003.

11. Juurlink et al. 2003.

12. For an economist's discussion of this question see Reinhardt 2004.

13. Kovacs et al. 2003.

14. Kolata 2004.

15. Federman et al. 2001.

16. Kawas 2003.

17. Tamblyn et al. 2001; Soumerai and Ross-Degnan 1999; Tseng et al. 2004.

18. Rector 2000.

19. Altman 2004; Angell 2004.

20. Voelker 2003.

21. Harris 2003a.

22. Becker and Pear 2004.

23. Taylor 2004; Angell 2004; Pear 2004d; Harris 2004c.

24. Pear 2000d, 2001, 2002a; Thomas 2003.

25. Pear 2004a.

26. Physicians' Working Group 2003; Kennedy 2004; Families USA 2004b; profitability summarized in Angell 2004.

27. Gross, Schondolmeyer, and Retzman 2004.

28. Families USA 2004a. During 2003 the fastest price rises were for

Combivent (chronic asthma): 13.2 × inflation
Alphagan (glaucoma): 10.3 ×
Evista (osteoporosis): 10.3 ×
Diovan (high blood pressure): 8.6 ×
Detrol LA (overactive bladder): 8.5 ×
Xalatan (glaucoma): 6.8 ×

29. Mitka 2003; Weisbrot 2000; for a review of studies demonstrating the

success of these approaches during the last two decades, see Wazana 2000; Blumenthal 2004. The various strategies discussed in this chapter reach back even further, as documented in an early, classic critique, *Pills, Profits, and Politics,* coauthored by M. Silverman and P. R. Lee (Berkeley and Los Angeles: University of California Press, 1974).

30. Harris 2004b.

31. Mitka 2003; Elliot and Ives 2004.

32. GAO 2002; also Bodenheimer 2001.

33. Petersen 2003; Pear 2002e.

34. Stolberg and Gerth 2000b.

35. ALLHAT 2002.

36. Cannon et al. 2004.

37. Topol and Falk 2004, 640.

38. Harris 2004a; Pear 2003c.

39. Kolata 2003; Gilsdorf 2004.

40. Angell 2004; Stolberg and Gerth 2000a; see also Croghan and Pittman 2004.

41. Angell 2004; Scherer 2004; Dukes 2002 notes that other countries, which regulate prices, employ various formulas to determine fair return.

42. Pear 2003b.

43. Angell 2004; Stolberg and Gerth 2000a; Editors 2002a; Scherer 2004.

44. See www.pbs.org/wgbh/pages/frontline/shows/prescription; also Harris 2004e.

45. Stolberg 2000b.

46. Kolata and Andrews 2001.

47. Petersen and Berenson 2003.

48. Psaty et al. 2004, 2629; Fontanarosa, Drummond, and De Angelis 2004.

49. Editors 2003b; also Public Citizen Health Research Group 2003.

50. Jenkins et al. 2003.

51. Petersen 2001, C1, C5.

52. Although Merck's full-page newspaper explanation claimed that the company undertook these new studies out of concern for patients' safety, the primary purpose was to determine whether Vioxx would prevent colon polyps, which can be precursors of cancer. Topol 2004, 1708 summarizes the unsettling Vioxx history since its 1999 approval. An original critic of the new drug as unsafe, with minimal added benefit, if any, Topol asks in frustration, "If Merck would not initiate an appropriate trial and the FDA did not ask them to do so, how would the truth ever be known?" See also Editors 2004c; Maxwell and Webb 2005.

53. Juni 2004, 2025; Horton 2004b, 1995; also Topol 2004; Berenson et al. 2004; Editors 2004c.

54. Graham et al. 2005. The lead author is an FDA drug-safety investigator who attempted to alert agency officials, other researchers, and the public about the dangers of Vioxx and similar medications.

55. Psaty et al. 2004, 2629. Likewise, for many Americans the health-care system works well if they are not sick. Also Strom 2004; Fontanarosa, Drummond, and De Angelis 2004, 2649.

56. Currently, a pattern of previously unknown side effects is appearing as new antipsychotic medications, increasingly prescribed for agitation in dementia, gain more widespread use (Goode 2003). The new evidence will require, at least, a reevaluation of benefits and risks for this older patient population. Regarding an antiseizure drug, the Health Research Group reports widespread promotion to doctors of off-label use, including instructions to sales staff, "We need to be holding [the doctors'] hand and whispering in their ear: Neurontin for pain, Neurontin for everything" (Public Citizen Health Research Group 2004).

57. Lasser et al. 2002.

58. Fontanarosa, Drummond, and De Angelis 2004; Psaty et al. 2004; Topol 2005. Beyond limited resources and pharmaceutical industry influence, the FDA's postmarketing surveillance brings an inherent conflict of interest: the agency must seek to prove itself wrong in having approved a drug that was, in fact, unsafe. A new FDA advisory board, announced in February 2005, does not eliminate this basic conflict.

59. Grady et al. 2002; Hulley et al. 2002.

60. Manson et al. 2003; Hodis et al. 2003.

61. Chlebowski et al. 2003.

62. Anderson et al. 2003.

63. Hays et al. 2003.

64. Chlebowski et al. 2004.

65. Cauley et al. 2003, 1729.

66. Rapp et al. 2003; Shumaker et al. 2003; J. Mitchell et al. 2003.

67. Shumaker et al. 2003.

68. Wassertheil-Smoller et al. 2003; Yaffe 2003; see chapter 2.

69. WHI Steering Committee 2004; Shumaker et al. 2004; Schneider 2004b; Hulley and Grady 2004. In addition, increased risk of blood clots in deep veins and lungs was reported for estrogen only and in combination with progestin (Smith et al. 2004; Cushman et al. 2004).

70. Petersen 2002.

71. Toner 1999.

72. Mello, Studdert, and Brennan 2004; Harris 2003b.

73. Pear 1999.

74. Although AARP bristled at the intrusion of such pretenders, this organization of older Americans ultimately joined the drug and insurance industries as a key supporter of the 2003 Medicare prescription drug bill. With strong ties to the insurance industry (including revenue from Medigap policies and as manager of pharmacy benefits), AARP orchestrated its own media blitz to advocate passage, then explain its actions to members and the wider public. Tens of thousands of members resigned in protest. (See chapter 4 for an example of industry-funded consumer advocacy groups regarding medications for a particular illness.)

75. Pear and Oppel 2002.

76. Defined initially as yearly individual drug costs above $5,000, the catastrophic level is expected to rise much faster than older Americans' incomes during the program's first seven years to $9,000, along with increased premiums and deductions (Kennedy 2004).

77. Madrick 2003; Pear 2004b; Kennedy 2004; Altman 2004; Pear 2005; see Iglehart 2004 for analysis of the politics of this extremely close vote. The Medicare administrator, Thomas Scully, had already resigned, moving through the revolving door to become a lobbyist for major drug companies, pharmaceutical benefit managers, and other Medicare-affected clients (Pear 2004e).

78. Pear 2004f; Pear 2003h.

79. Tseng et al. 2004; Tamblyn et al. 2001.

80. Pear and Freudenheim 2004. How the new drug benefit can work for nursing-home residents, many suffering cognitive impairment as well as immobility, remains a mystery, based as it is on consumers' comparing and choosing among several plans using retail pharmacies. Currently, skilled nursing facilities obtain drugs through specialized long-term-care pharmacies, with most residents covered by Medicare and Medicaid (Pear 2004g).

81. Families USA 2004a, 1.

82. See Dukes 2002, the final article of a series on the global pharmaceutical industry; also Scherer 2004. In the United States, similar supply-demand dynamics arise with proliferating medical technologies, such as the various imaging methods (CT and PET scans, MRI, etc.).

83. Angell 2004. Richard Horton, editor of *Lancet,* provides a scathing depiction of the pharmaceutical industry's self-promoting cycle of research, education, and marketing in a review of S. Krimsky's *Science in the private interest* (Horton 2004a).

84. See Union of Concerned Scientists, www2.ucsusa.org. Just days later, a clear instance emerged into public view. The secretary of Health and Human Services, Tommy Thompson, admitted that his department rewrote a report documenting profound racial and ethnic disparities in health care, omitting and presenting false data and altering the report's conclusions in order to convey a more positive conclusion than the actual findings demonstrate. Or as he put it, "There was a mistake made" (Pear 2004c; see Bloch 2004 and Steinbrook 2004a for physicians' response to this instance of manipulating and imposing politics on government science). Soon after that, yet another instance, this time an unusual FDA ruling: a high-level administrator rejected an FDA scientific advisory panel's unanimous recommendation that emergency contraception (a product called Plan B) be sold in pharmacies over-the-counter, without a doctor's prescription. More than five thousand scientists have signed the UCS statement.

85. Editors 2004a.

86. Blackburn 2004, 1380.

87. Reinhardt 2004; AD2000 Collaborative Group 2004; Editors 2004b; Steinbrook 2004c; Meier 2004a, 2004b; Maxwell and Webb 2005. Rennie 2004 reviews recent events leading to the journal editors' announcement, including revelation of hidden drug manufacturers' data about suicide risk for children and teenagers prescribed SSRI-type antidepressants; International Committee of Medical Journal Editors 2004 (also published in other member journals). A more general proposal for revamping medical research, "to achieve a coordinated, safe, and more efficient and effective [national] enterprise," including informed public participation, appears in *JAMA* (Crowley et al. 2004).

As noted in chapter 1, rather than increase government regulation and oversight, the Bush administration championed informed consumers' choosing among competing skilled nursing facilities as the way to improve quality and lower costs. No similar free-market argument prevails about increasing data provided to consumers choosing medications.

88. Safran et al. 2002.

CHAPTER 4. HEALTH-CARE RATIONING

1. Croghan and Pittman 2004. Throughout the developing world, in contrast, pandemics that afflict and kill vast populations, including huge numbers of children, comprise the orphan diseases presenting no prospect for a drug manufacturer's financial gain (e.g., Dukes 2002).

2. Steinbrook 2004b.

3. Huskamp et al. 2003; Thomas 2003.

4. Huskamp et al. 2003; Thomas 2003; Goldman, Joyce, and Escarce 2004.

5. Ashton et al. 2003; Fisher 2003.

6. Freudenheim 1999; also Kassirer 1998.

7. Pear 2004a.

8. Himmelstein et al. 1999.

9. Correa 2001, C2. With oncologists administering extremely expensive intravenous chemotherapy in their office, their particular battle with drug manufacturers and insurers over this significant source of income is a complicated ongoing story in itself. The amount Medicare will pay under the new drug benefit is already a focus of dispute (Harris 2004d).

10. Pear 2000b; Mariner 2004 discusses subsequent judicial decisions that further define and limit liability of managed-care organizations.

11. Pear 1998b.

12. St. John 2000.

13. Pear 2003d.

14. Pear 2003d. See also Steinhauer 2000.

15. Phillips et al. 2004.

16. Pear 1998a; Pear 2003a. Also in 2003, congressional negotiators struggling with Medicare legislation were "seriously considering" requiring a patient's co-payments for the home health care that is covered; such out-of-pocket expense for recipients was eliminated in 1972 as a way to encourage care at home rather than in more costly hospitals or skilled nursing facilities. Although this requirement did not survive the political compromising, potential policy directions for the future—in reality a return to the past—remain clear (Pear 2003g). Medicare covers only short-term, strictly defined transitional stays in a skilled nursing facility following a hospitalization, and minimal nurse or physical therapist visits at home. Many home health-care agencies refuse such patients because of the government's low reimbursement rates, the same dynamic described in chapter 1 with regard to residential care facilities.

17. Outpatient Services Trialists 2004.

18. Manion 1998, 1068; also Kassirer 1998.

19. Needleman et al. 2002.

20. Aiken et al. 2002; Aiken et al. 2003.

21. Manion 1999, 1362; see also Pantilat, Albers, and Wachter 1999; Rabow, Hauser, and Adams 2004.

22. E.g., Drazen 2003; see chapter 5.

23. Prendergast and Puntillo 2002, 2736.

24. While a troubling history of experimenting and learning upon these poor patients also characterizes many such settings, the answer is not to eliminate needed services.

25. Institute of Medicine 2004.

26. Levit et al. 2003, 2004; Pear 2004a; Strunk and Ginsburg 2003.

27. McGlynn et al. 2003; Kerr et al. 2004.

28. Robinson 2004.

29. Web site, coveringtheuninsured.org; for the insured, a health insurance association full-page ad promised that managed-care companies were taking steps sounding much like, and perhaps intended to preempt, proposed congressional patient's rights legislation.

30. Institute of Medicine 2004.

31. Families USA 2003; report available from www.familiesusa.org, 2003.

32. Report available from www.familiesusa.org, 2004. Even the usual yearly census statistics were rising, up to a record 45.0 million uninsured throughout 2003, including 12.1 million people in families earning $50,000 or more. In fact, this income level accounted for about 90 percent of the increase in people uninsured during the last ten years (Freudenheim 2004d).

33. Freudenheim 2003; www.familiesusa.org 2003.

34. Steinbrook 2004b.

35. See www.kff.org Kaiser/Hewitt 2004. Nearly half raised retirees' deductibles and/or co-payments or expected to do so in 2005.

36. Freudenheim 2004b.

37. Baker et al. 2001; Porter 2004; Freudenheim 2004e.

38. Egan 2003.

39. Harris 2003b.

40. Pear 2003e.

41. Harris 2003b.

42. Mello, Studdert, and Brenan 2004.

43. Anand 2003; Regalado 2003; Wysocki 2003.

44. Abelson and Petersen 2003; Deyo, Nachemson, and Mirza 2004; Kolata 2004.

45. Goodwin 1999.

46. Editors 1993, 1.

47. Kuttner 1998, 1559.

48. Naylor et al. 1999.

49. Retchin et al. 1997; Outpatient Service Trialists 2004; Binder et al. 2004.

50. Ware et al. 1996.

51. Asch et al. 2000; Tseng et al. 2004 reports specifically on patients reducing their medications after exceeding Medicare HMO coverage cap.

52. Landon, Zaslavsky, and Bernard 2004.

53. Baker 1999.

54. Schwartz 1998.

55. E.g., Walter and Covinsky 2001.

56. Callahan, ter Meulen, and Topinkova 1995; Callahan 1998; see also Gillick 1994; Hadler 2003, and chapter 5.

57. Wenger et al. 2003; Fried 2003.

58. Gillick 1994.

59. See also Lunney et al. 2003; Hadler 2003, and chapter 5.

60. S. Mitchell et al. 2003.

61. Gillick 2000, 209; see also Hurley and Volicer 2002; Morrison and Meier 2004.

62. S. Mitchell et al. 2003, 78.

63. E.g., Walter and Covinsky 2001.

64. Pear 2002c.

65. Landefeld, Callahan, and Woolard (eds.) 2003.

66. Janofsky 2004; Rowe 1999.

67. Rhymes et al. 2000; see also Morrison and Siu 2000; Prendergast and Puntillo 2002. Quill 2004 presents another such case, his own father (see chapter 5).

CHAPTER 5. END OF LIFE

1. Actual elder abuse (physical, emotional, financial) is a serious problem, whether at home or in a care facility. Lachs and Pillemer 2004 suggests measures doctors and other health professionals can use for screening, diagnosis, and intervention.

2. E.g., Gillick 1994; Goodwin 1999; also personal communications.

3. E.g., Singer, Martin, and Kelner 1999.

4. Helft, Siegler, and Lantos 2000; in the younger population, defining and determining death, especially "brain death," are central to organ donation for transplants.

5. Prendergast and Puntillo 2002.

6. Brody 1997.

7. SUPPORT 1995; Prendergast and Puntillo 2002.

8. Fried et al. 2002; also Singer, Martin, and Kelner 1999; SUPPORT 1995.

9. Gillick 1994; Lunney et al. 2003; Gill, Allore, and Guo 2003; Hadler 2003.

10. Pantilat and Steimle 2004.

11. Gillick 2000, 206; also S. Mitchell et al. 2003; Morrison and Meier 2004.

12. Hurley and Volicer 2002.

13. Gillick 2004.

14. Lynn et al. 1997; SUPPORT 1995; Prendergast and Puntillo 2002; Teno et al. 2004.

15. E.g., S. Mitchell et al. 2003 study of feeding tube use in nursing homes, see chapter 4.

16. Gillick 2004; states differ in standard forms available (e.g., from a state medical association).

17. Singer, Martin, and Kelner 1999; Lynn 2001; Gillick 2004.

18. Von Guten, Ferris, and Emanuel 2000; SUPPORT 1995; Groopman 2002; Rabow, Hauser, and Adams 2004; Morrison and Meier 2004. Lawyers more commonly help clients prepare written directives, though usually with little expertise in ferreting out individuals' wishes about the crucial medical issues.

19. Rocker and Curtis 2003.

20. Sprung et al. 2003.

21. Fisher 2003.

22. Schneiderman et al. 2003.

23. Cook et al. 2003.

24. Drazen 2003, 1109.

25. Wenger et al. 2003; Fried 2003.

26. Prendergast and Puntillo 2002, 2736.

27. Van der Heide et al. 2003, 349.

28. For examples, see Rabow, Hauser, and Adams 2004, including doctor-initiated family meetings; Morrison and Meier 2004; Pantilat and Steimle 2004; Weissman 2004. For results, see SUPPORT 1995.

29. Gillick 2004, 8; also Morrison and Meier 2004; Pantilat and Steimle 2004.

30. An approach consistent with recent reports, e.g., Morrison and Meier 2004.

31. Meier and Morrison 2002, 1088; see also Rabow, Hauser, and Adams 2004.

32. Morrison and Meier 2004; also Pantilat and Steimle 2004. Publication of these two articles just weeks apart in the two most prominent American medical journals suggests some momentum toward improved palliative care at the end of life. Weissman 2004 explores the transition from life-prolonging to palliative care during terminal illness, particularly when a crisis threatens life more immediately.

33. On dialysis, see Cohen, Germain, and Poppel 2003.

34. Gillick 2000; Prigerson 2003; Mitchell, Kiely, and Hammel 2004; Mitchell et al. 2004.

35. E.g., McClain, Rosenfeld, and Breitbart 2003.

36. Rabow, Hauser, and Adams 2004.

37. Lamberg 2002; see appendix.

38. The term "hospice" derives from medieval times, describing a place where travelers who were tired and sick could rest, often tended by a religious order of monks; the first U.S. hospice opened in 1974 in New Haven, Connecticut.

39. Teno et al. 2004.

40. Quill 2004.

41. Larsen and Tobin 2000.

42. Lynn 2001; Lunney et al. 2003; Gill 2004; Hadler 2003.

43. Mitchell, Kiely, and Hammel 2004; Mitchell et al. 2004.

44. Dean 2003, 2380.

45. E.g., views expressed in Moyers 2000, PBS special on death and dying.

46. The Death with Dignity Alliance (a national organization combining the efforts of Death with Dignity National Center, Oregon Death with Dignity Le-

gal Defense and Education Center, and Compassion in Dying Federation) calls this process assisted death or administration of life-ending medication.

47. Quill 1991, 693.

48. Meier et al. 2003.

49. Ganzini et al. 2003; Jacobs 2003.

50. Ganzini et al. 2000.

51. Bascom and Tolle 2002.

52. Ganzini et al. 2002; Steinbrook 2002.

53. Ganzini et al. 2000.

54. Sullivan, Hedberg, and Fleming 2000; Bascom and Tolle 2002.

55. Bascom and Tolle 2002; Ganzini et al. 2002.

56. Burt 1997; Steinbrook 2002.

57. Orentlicher and Caplan 2000; Angell 1999; Steinbrook 2002.

58. Angell 1999, 1924.

59. Steinbrook 2002, 463.

60. Liptak 2004; Greenhouse 2005. A similar cast of characters and principles focuses on a doctor's right to recommend marijuana to patients as a medical treatment. In 1996, after California voters approved a medical marijuana initiative, the DEA threatened to revoke the prescribing license of any doctor who recommended marijuana for medical treatment. The Court of Appeals for the Ninth Circuit ruled this federal policy in violation of free speech and state authority over medical practice. Ashcroft's Department of Justice appealed to the Supreme Court, which in October 2003 let stand the Appeals Court ruling.

61. Ganzini et al. 2002; Black and Pearlman 2001; Meier et al. 2003.

62. Meier et al. 2003.

63. The Death with Dignity Alliance characterizes the relevant patient competence as "You can understand the nature of your condition, the treatment alternatives available, the likely outcomes of treatment versus non-treatment, and can accept responsibility for your decisions" (www.dwda.org).

64. E.g., Humphry 1996.

65. Nuland 2000, 584.

66. Orentlicher 1997, 1239. Van der Heide, van Delden, and van der Wal 2004 discusses complex and still evolving legislation allowing a doctor's assistance.

67. Onwuteaka-Philipsen et al. 2003. Interestingly, van der Heide, van Delden, and van der Wal 2004 notes more frequent assistance *without* a patient's explicit request in countries where a physician's assistance is illegal.

68. The remaining third of deaths are sudden and unexpected, van der Heide et al. 2003.

69. Lynn et al. 1997, 97; see also Nuland 1993; Dean 2003.

70. Wenger et al. 2003; Fried 2003.

71. Landefeld, Callahan, and Woolard (eds.) 2003; Thomas et al. 2003; Wenger et al. 2003; Rabow, Hauser, and Adams 2004.

72. Lynn 2001; see also Morrison and Meier 2004; Lunney et al. 2003; Gillick 1994.

73. Meier and Morrison 2002, 1088.

74. E.g., Teno et al. 2004.

75. Nuland 1993, 249.

76. See also the Gawande 2003 profile of the famed surgeon Francis D. Moore. Oncologists brandishing chemotherapy represent another such specialty; also Groopman 2002; Hadler 2003.

77. Calman 2004, 232.

78. Quill 2004, 2032.

79. Black and Pearlman 2001. Lynn 2004 presents a comprehensive overview of current end-of-life policies and issues, along with policy recommendations aimed at improving care systems.

CHAPTER 6. CONCLUSIONS AND A LOOK AHEAD

1. Institute of Medicine 2004.

2. Crenshaw 2000; Himmelstein et al. 2005. Most of these people were middle class, with some health insurance, but not enough to cover their share of health-care costs. Job loss or reduced hours did figure prominently in this explosive rise.

3. Broder 1999.

4. Report (2002) available at www.npr.org.

5. See www.familiesusa.org 2004; Institute of Medicine 2004.

6. Madrick 2003.

7. Reinhardt 1997, 1446. Isaacs and Schroeder 2004 also emphasizes the unjust link between Americans' health and their socioeconomic status (closely entangled with race).

8. Rawls 2001.

9. Freudenheim 2004c, C10.

10. Elements of three single-payer proposals were incorporated into a bill still working its way through the state legislature in 2005 (www.healthcare options.ca.gov).

11. Detsky and Naylor 2003.

12. Physicians' Working Group 2003.

13. See also Woolhandler, Campbell, and Himmelstein 2003; McCormick et al. 2004 reports that 63.5 percent of Massachusetts doctors surveyed think a single-payer system would provide the best care for the most people, compared to managed care or traditional fee-for-service.

14. Fein 2003; Bindman and Haggstrom 2003.

15. Budetti 2004. His comprehensive vision would incorporate universal coverage, cost containment, quality improvement, and subsidies for low-income Americans. Budetti employs the analogy of Yogi Berra's observation: "If you don't know where you are going, you will wind up somewhere else," adding that regarding health care, the United States continues to "stumble toward somewhere else, and it is probably not a place we should want to go" (2005). I suggest that the current problem is that George Bush does know where he wants to take the country, and it definitely is not a place we should want to go.

16. Riley and Kilbreth 2004; Freudenheim 2004a.

17. Institute of Medicine 2004.

18. Rowe 1999.

19. Wenger et al. 2003.

20. Landefeld, Callahan, and Woolard (eds.) 2003; Holman 2004.

21. Mold and Green 2003, 595. Also Stuck, Beck, and Egger 2004; Fletcher et al. 2004, regarding proactive preventive assessments through home visits.

22. See Inouye et al. 1999 for description of a successful program to prevent delirium; Phillips et al. 2004 for review of discharge-planning and case-coordination studies.

23. E.g., Rimer 1998; Winzelberg 2003.

24. Steinhauer 2001.

25. Canedy 2002.

26. Retirees 2000 describes the Heritage Harbor Health Group.

27. In Berkeley and Oakland, for example, the Gray Panthers established a home-share matching service, operated by a nonprofit fair housing organization.

28. Durrett and McCamant 1994.

29. Gornick 1999.

30. Fiore 1999 describes the University of Arizona community.

31. Fiore 1999.

32. Gross 2004; also Duenwald and Stamler 2004.

33. Fiore 1999.

34. Gillick 1994. With universal health care in this American future, however, there would be less need to find ways of sparing aged individuals the lengthy ordeal they currently experience all too often at today's overcrowded emergency rooms.

35. Gillick 2004, Tunis 2004 on lung-volume reduction surgery, implantable cardioverter-defibrillators and left ventricular assist devices; Rowe 1999.

36. Brennan 2002.

37. Editors 2003a.

References

Abbott RD, LR White, GW Ross, et al. 2004. Walking and dementia in physically capable elderly men. *JAMA* 292:1447–53.

Abelson R, and M Petersen. 2003. An operation to ease back pain bolsters the bottom line, too. *New York Times* (12/31/03) A1.

AD2000 Collaborative Group. 2004. Long-term doneqezil treatment in 565 patients with Alzheimer's disease. *Lancet* 363:2105–15.

Aiken LH, SP Clarke, RB Cheung, et al. 2003. Educational levels of hospital nurses and surgical patient mortality. *JAMA* 290:1617–23.

Aiken LH, SP Clarke, DM Sloane, et al. 2002. Hospital nurse staffing and patient mortality, nurse burnout, and job dissatisfaction. *JAMA* 288:1987–93.

Aisen PS, KA Schafer, M Grundman, et al. 2003. Effects of rofecoxib or naproxen vs placebo on Alzheimer Disease progression. *JAMA* 289:2819–26.

Albert MS, and DA Drachman. 2000. Alzheimer's Disease: what is it, how many people have it, and why do we need to know? *Neurology* 55:166–68.

ALLHAT Officers. 2002. Major outcomes in high-risk hypertensive patients randomized to angiotensive-converting enzymes inhibitor or calcium channel blocker vs. diuretic. *JAMA* 288:2981–97.

Altman D. 2004. The new Medicare prescription-drug legislation. *NEJM* 350:9–10.

Altman S, and C Parks-Thomas. 2002. Controlling spending for prescription drugs. *NEJM* 346:855–56.

Anand G. 2003. The big secret in health care: rationing is here. *Wall Street Journal* (9/12/03) A1.

Anderson GL, HL Judd, AM Kaunitz, et al. 2003. Effects of estrogen plus progestin on gynecologic cancers and associated diagnostic procedures. *JAMA* 290:1739–48.

Angell M. 1999. Care for the dying—Congressional mischief. *NEJM* 341:923–24.

———. 2004. The truth about the drug companies. *New York Review of Books* (7/15/04) 52–58 (article appears in different form in *The truth about the drug companies: how they deceive us and what to do about it* [New York: Random House]).

Angiers N. 1995. If you're really ancient, you may be better off. *New York Times* (6/11/95) Science 1.

Arendell T, and CL Estes. 1991. Older women in the post-Reagan era. *Int J Health Serv* 21:59–73.

Asch SM, EM Sloss, C Hogan, et al. 2000. Measuring underuse of necessary care among elderly Medicare beneficiaries using inpatient and outpatient claims. *JAMA* 284:2325–33.

Ashton CM, J Souchek, NJ Petersen, et al. 2003. Hospital use and survival among veterans affairs beneficiaries. *NEJM* 349:1637–46.

Avorn J. 2001. Improving drug use in elderly patients. *JAMA* 286:2866–68.

Baker DW, JJ Sudano, JM Albert, et al. 2001. Lack of health insurance and decline in overall health in late middle age. *NEJM* 345:1106–12.

Baker LC. 1999. Association of managed care market share and health expenditures for FFS Medicare patients. *JAMA* 281:432–47.

Balfour JL, and GA Kaplan. 2002. Neighborhood environment and loss of physical function in older adults: evidence from the Alameda County study. *Am J Epidem* 155:507–15.

Ball K, DB Berch, KF Helmers, et al. 2002. Effects of cognitive training interventions with older adults. *JAMA* 288:2271–81.

Bascom P, and SW Tolle. 2002. Responding to requests for physician-assisted suicide. *JAMA* 288:91–98.

Bassuk S, TA Glass, and LF Berkman. 1999. Social disengagement and incident cognitive decline in community-dwelling elderly persons. *Ann Intern Med* 131:165–73.

Becker E, and R Pear. 2004. Trade agreement may undercut importing of inexpensive drugs. *New York Times* (7/12/04) A1.

Belluck P. 2001. Nuns offer clues to Alzheimer's and aging. *New York Times* (5/7/01) A1.

Berenson A, G Harris, B Meier, et al. 2004. Despite warnings, drug giant took long path to Vioxx recall. *New York Times* (12/14/04)A1.

Berkman LF. 2000. Which influences cognitive function: living alone or being alone? *Lancet* 355:1291–92.

Binder EF, M Brown, DR Sinacore, et al. 2004. Effects of extended outpatient rehabilitation after hip fracture. *JAMA* 292:837–46.

Bindman AB, and DA Haggstrom. 2003. Small steps or a giant leap for the uninsured? *JAMA* 290:816–818.

Bischoff-Ferrari HA, B Dawson-Hughes, WC Willett, et al. 2004. Effect of vitamin D on falls: a meta-analysis. *JAMA* 291:1999–2006.

Black AL, and RA Pearlman. 2001. Desire for physician-assisted suicide: requests for a better death? *Lancet* 358:344–45.

Blackburn E. 2004. Bioethics and the political distortion of biomedical science. *NEJM* 350:1379–80.

Blass JP, and RR Ratan. 2003. "Silent" strokes and dementia (editorial). *NEJM* 348:1277–78.

Bloch MG. 2004. Health care disparities—science, politics, and race. *NEJM* 350:1568–70.

Blumenthal D. 2004. Doctors and drug companies. *NEJM* 351:1885–90.

Bodenheimer T. 1999. Long-term care for frail elderly people—the On Lok model. *NEJM* 341:1324–28.

———. 2001. Affordable prescriptions for the elderly. *JAMA* 286:1762–63.

Boeve B, J McCormick, G Smith, et al. 2003. Mild cognitive impairment in the oldest old. *Neurology* 60:477–80.

Brach J, S Fitzgerald, AB Newman, et al. 2003. Physical activity and functional status in community-dwelling older women. *Arch Intern Med* 163:2565–71.

Brennan TA. 2002. Luxury primary care—market innovation or threat to access? *NEJM* 346:1165–68.

Broder D. 1999. Voters yearn for honest president. *San Francisco Examiner* (11/7/99) A6.

Brody H. 1997. Medical futility: a useful concept? In Zucker MB, and HD Zucker, eds. *Medical futility and the evaluation of life-sustaining interventions.* Cambridge: Cambridge University Press.

Brookmeyer R, and C Kawas. 1998. Projections of Alzheimer's Disease in the United States and public health impact of delaying disease onset. *Am J Public Health* 88:1337–42.

Bruce ML, TR TenHave, CF Reynolds III, et al. 2004. Reducing suicidal ideation and depressive symptoms in depressed older primary care patients. *JAMA* 291:1081–91.

Budetti PP. 2004. 10 years beyond the Health Security Act failure. *JAMA* 292:2000–06.

Budson AE, and BH Price. 2005. Memory dysfunction. *NEJM* 352:692–99.

Burns A, and M Zaudis. 2002. Mild cognitive impairment in older people. *Lancet* 360:1963–65.

Burt RA. 1997. The Supreme Court speaks. *NEJM* 337:1234–46.

Butler RN. 1996. On behalf of older women. *NEJM* 334:794–96.

Callahan D. 1998. *False hopes: why America's quest for perfect health is a recipe for failure.* New York: Simon & Schuster.

Callahan D, RHJ ter Meulen, and E. Topinkova. 1995. *A world growing old: the coming health care challenges.* Washington DC: Georgetown University Press.

Calman NS. 2004. So tired of life. *Health Aff* 24:228–32.

Canedy D. 2002. Florida redoubles efforts for the elderly. *New York Times* (5/5/02) A1.

Cannon CP, E Braunwald, CH Hill, et al. 2004. Intensive versus moderate lipid lowering with statins after acute coronary syndromes. *JAMA* 350:1495–1511.

Carlson MC, LP Fried, QL Xue, et al. 1999. Association between executive attention and physical functional performance in community-dwelling older women. *J Gerontol: Soc Sci* 54:S262–70.

Cassel CK. 2002. Use it or lose it. *JAMA* 288:2333–35.

Cassel CK, RW Besdine, and LC Siegel. 1999. Restructuring Medicare for the next century: what will beneficiaries really need? *Health Aff* 18:118–131.

Casserly I. 2004. Convergence of atherosclerosis and Alzheimer's disease: inflammation, cholesterol, and misfolded proteins. *Lancet* 363:1139–46.

Cauley JA, J Robbins, Z Chen, et al. 2003. Effects of estrogen plus progestin on risk of fracture and bone mineral density. *JAMA* 290:1729–38.

Chlebowski RT, SL Hendrix, RD Langer, et al. 2003. Influence of estrogen plus progestin on breast cancer and mammography in healthy postmenopausal women. *JAMA* 289:3243–53.

Chlebowski RT, J Wactawski-Wende, C Ritenbaugh, et al. 2004. Estrogen plus progestin and colorectal cancer in postmenopausal women. *NEJM* 350:991–1004.

Ciechanowski P, E Wagner, K Schmaling, et al. 2004. Community-integrated home-based depression treatment in older adults. *JAMA* 291:1569–77.

City of Berkeley Health and Human Services Department. 1999. *Health status report*. Berkeley, California.

———. 2002. *Health status report: mortality and hospitalizations*. Berkeley.

Cohen L. 1998. *No aging in India: Alzheimer's, the bad family, and other modern things*. Berkeley and Los Angeles: University of California Press.

Cohen LM, MJ Germain, and DM Poppel. 2003. Practical considerations in dialysis withdrawal. *JAMA* 289:2113–19.

Colcombe SJ, AF Kramer, KI Erickson, et al. 2004. Cardiovascular fitness, cortical plasticity, and aging. *PNAS* 101:3316–21.

Cook D, G Rocker, J Marshall, et al. 2003. Withdrawal of mechanical ventilation in anticipation of death in the intensive care unit. *NEJM* 349:1123–32.

Cooney LM, GJ Kennedy, KA Hawkins, et al. 2004. Who can stay at home? *Arch Intern Med* 164:357–60.

Correa T. 2001. A doctor says no to his HMO. *Fresno Bee* (3/38/01) C1.

Coyle JT. 2003. Use it or lose it—Do effortful mental activities protect against dementia? *NEJM* 348:2489–90.

Crenshaw A. 2000. Study cites medical bills for many bankruptcies. *Washington Post* (4/25/00) E1.

Crimmins EM, SL Reynolds, and Y Saito. 1999. Trends in health and ability to work among the older working-age population. *J Gerontol* 54B:S33–40.

Crimmins EM, Y Saito, and SL Reynolds. 1997. Further evidence on recent trends in the prevalence and incidence of disability among older Americans from two sources: The LSOA and NHIS. *J Gerontol: Soc Sci* 52: S59–S71.

Croghan TW, and PM Pittman. 2004. The medicine cabinet: what's in it, why, and can we change the contents? *Health Aff* 23:23.

Crowley WF, L Sherwood, P Salber, et al. 2004. Clinical research in the United States at a crossroads. *JAMA* 291:1120–26.

Cummings JL. 2004. Alzheimer's Disease. *NEJM* 351:56–67.

Cushman J, LH Kuller, R Prentice, et al. 2004. Estrogen plus progestin and risk of venous thrombosis. *JAMA* 292:1573–80.

Daviglus JM, K Liu, A Pirzada, et al. 2003. Favorable cardiovascular risk profile in middle age and health-related quality of life in older age. *Arch Intern Med* 163:2460–68.

Davis M, J Poisal, G Charles, et al. 1999. Prescription drug coverage, utilization, and spending among Medicare beneficiaries. *Health Aff* 18:231–43.

Day L, B Fildes, I Gordon, et al. 2002. Randomised factorial trial of falls prevention among older people living in their own home. *BMJ* 325:128–31.

Dean C. 2003. Grams. *JAMA* 290:2380.

Detsky AS, and CD Naylor. 2003. Canada's health care system—reform delayed. *NEJM* 349:804–10.

Deyo RA, A Nachemson, and S Mirza. 2004. Spinal-fusion surgery—the case for restraint. *NEJM* 350:722–26.

Drazen JM. 2003. Decisions at the end of life. *NEJM* 349:1109–10.

Duenwald M, and B Stamler 2004. On their own, in the same boat. *New York Times* (4/13/04) Retirement Suppl, 1.

Dukes MNG. 2002. Accountability of the pharmaceutical industry. *Lancet* 360:1682–84.

Durrett C, and K McCamant. 1994. *Co-housing: a contemporary approach to housing ourselves.* Berkeley: Ten Speed Press.

Editors. 1993. Do doctors short-change old people? *Lancet* 342:1–2.

———. 2002a. Countering delays in introduction of generic drugs. *Lancet* 359:181.

———. 2002b. A way forward for U.S. health care? *Lancet* 360:1709.

———. 2003a. The coming crisis of longterm care. *Lancet* 361:1755.

———. 2003b. The statin wars: why AstraZeneca must retreat. *Lancet* 362:1341.

———. 2004a. Keeping ideology and bureaucracy out of science. *Lancet* 363:501.

———. 2004b. AD 2000: Donepezil in Alzheimer's disease. *Lancet* 363:2100–2101.

———. 2004c. Vioxx: an unequal partnership between safety and efficacy. *Lancet* 364:1287.

Egan T. 2003. A prescription plan hailed as a model is budget casualty. *New York Times* (3/5/03) A1.

Elias MF, A Beiser, P Wolf, et al. 2000. The preclinical phase of Alzheimer's Disease. *Arch Neurol* 57:808–13.

Elliott S, and N Ives. 2004. Selling prescription drugs to the consumer. *New York Times* (10/12/04) C1.

Evans JG. 2003. Drugs and falls in later life. *Lancet* 361:448.

Families USA. 2003. Going without health insurance: nearly 1 in 3 non-elderly Americans. www.familiesusa.org (publication no. 03-103).

———. 2004a. Sticker shock: rising prescription drug prices for seniors. www.familiesusa.org (publication no. 04-103).

———. 2004b. One in three: non-elderly Americans without health insurance. www.familiesusa.org (publication no. 04-104).

Federman AD, AS Adams, D Ross-Degnan, et al. 2001. Supplemental insurance and use of effective cardiovascular drugs among elderly Medicare beneficiaries with coronary heart disease. *JAMA* 286:1732–39.

Fein R. 2003. Universal health insurance—Let the debate resume. *JAMA* 290:818–20.

Ferrucci L, JM Guralnik, ME Salive, et al. 1996. Cognitive impairment and risk of stroke in the older population. *J Am Geriatr Soc* 44:237–41.

Feskanich D, W Willett, and G Colditz. 2002. Walking and leisure-time activity and risk of hip fracture in postmenopausal women. *JAMA* 288:2300–06.

Feskens EJ, LLM Havekes, and S Kalmijn. 1994. A polipoprotein e4 allele and cognitive decline in elderly men. *BMJ* 309:1202–04.

Fiore RN. 1999. Caring for ourselves: peer care in autonomous aging. In Walker MV, ed. *Mother time: women, aging, and ethics.* Lanham MD: Rowman & Littlefield.

Fisher ES. 2003. Medical care—Is more always better? *NEJM* 349:1665–67.

Fletcher AE, GM Price, ESW Ng, et al. 2004 Population-based multidimensional assessment of older people in UK geriatric practice: a cluster-randomised factorial trial. *Lancet* 364:1667–77.

Fontanarosa PB, R Drummond, and CD De Angelis. 2004. Postmarketing surveillance—lack of vigilance, lack of trust. *JAMA* 292:2647–50.

Fratiglioni L, H Wang, K Ericsson, et al. 2000. Influence of social network on occurrence of dementia: a community-based longitudinal study. *Lancet* 355:1315–19.

Freedman VA, LG Martin, and RF Schoeni. 2002. Recent trends in disability and functioning among older adults in the United States. *JAMA* 288:3137–46.

Freudenheim M. 1999. Big HMO to give decisions on care back to doctors. *New York Times* (11/28/99) A1.

———. 2003. Employees paying ever-bigger share for health care. *New York Times* (9/10/03) A1.

———. 2004a. Broader health coverage may depend on less. *New York Times* (1/20/04) C1.

———. 2004b. Companies limit health coverage of many retirees. *New York Times* (2/3/04) A1.

———. 2004c. Using new Medicare billions, HMO's again court elderly. *New York Times* (3/9/04) A1.

———. 2004d. Record level of Americans not insured on health. *New York Times* (8/27/04) C1.

———. 2004e. Cost of insuring workers' health increases 11.2%. *New York Times* (9/10/04) C1.

Fried LP, M Freedman, TE Endres, et al. 1997. Building communities that promote successful aging. *West J Med* 167:219.

Fried LP, SJ Herdman, DE Kuhn, et al. 1991. Preclinical disability. *J Aging Health* 3:285–99.

Fried LS. 2003. Establishing benchmarks for quality care for an aging population: caring for vulnerable older adults. *Ann Intern Med* 139:784–86.

Fried TR, EH Bradley, VR Towle, et al. 2002. Understanding the treatment preferences of seriously ill patients. *NEJM* 346:1061–66.

Friedland R, T Fritsch, KA Smythe, et al. 2001. Patients with Alzheimer's Disease have reduced activities in midlife compared with healthy control-group members. *Proc Natl Acad Sci* 98:3440–45.

Friedrich MJ. 2002. Biological secrets of exceptional old age. *JAMA* 288:2247–53.

Fries JF. 1980. Aging, natural death, and the compression of morbidity. *NEJM* 303:130–35.

———. 2002. Reducing disability in older age. *JAMA* 288:N3164–5.

Frontline (PBS). 2003. Dangerous prescription (viewed 11/13/03). www.pbs .org/wgbh/pages/frontline/shows/prescription.

Gallow JJ, and BD Leibowitz. 1999. The epidemiology of late life mental disorders in the community. *Psychiatr Serv* 50:1158–66.

Ganzini L, ER Goy, LL Miller, et al. 2003. Nurses' experiences with hospice patients who refuse food and fluids to hasten death. *NEJM* 349:359–65.

Ganzini L, TA Harvath, A Jackson, et al. 2002. Experiences of Oregon nurses and social workers with hospice patients who requested assistance with suicide. *NEJM* 347:582–88.

Ganzini L, HD Nelson, TA Schmidt, et al. 2000. Physicians' experience with the Oregon Death with Dignity Act. *NEJM* 342:557–63.

Gawande A. 2003. Desperate measures. *New Yorker* (5/5/03) 70–81.

Gill MR. 2004. Advance care planning. *NEJM* 350:7–8.

Gill TM, H Allore, and Z Guo. 2003. Restricted activity and functional decline among community-living older persons. *Arch Intern Med* 163:1317–22.

Gill TM, D Baker, M Gottshalk, et al. 2002. A program to prevent functional decline in physically frail elderly persons who live at home. *NEJM* 347:1068–74.

Gillick MR. 1994. *Choosing medical care in old age.* Cambridge MA: Harvard University Press.

———. 2000. Rethinking the role of tube feeding in patients with advanced dementia. *NEJM* 342:206–9.

———. 2004. Medicare coverage for technological innovations—time for new criteria? *NEJM* 350:2199–2203.

Gilsdorf JR. 2004. As drug marketing pays off, my mother pays up. *Health Aff* 23:208–12.

Goldman DP, GF Joyce, and JJ Escarce. 2004. Pharmacy benefits and the use of drugs by the chronically ill. *JAMA* 291:2344–50.

Goldstein A. 2001. Better than a nursing home? www.time.com vol 158; no 6 (8/13/01).

Goode E. 2003. Leading drugs for psychosis come under new scrutiny. *New York Times* (5/20/03) A1.

Goodwin J. 1999. Geriatrics and the limits of modern medicine. *NEJM* 340:1283–85.

Gornick V. 1999. Alive in New York until the last minute. *Nation* (5/24/99) 22–23.

Gould E., AJ Reeves, MS Graziano, et al. 1999. Neurogenesis in the neocortex of adult primates. *Science* 86:548–52.

Goulding MR. 2004. Inappropriate medication prescribing for elderly ambulatory care patients. *Arch Intern Med* 164:305–12.

Government Accounting Office [GAO]. 2002. Prescription drugs: FDA oversight of direct-to-consumer advertising has limitations. www.gao.gov/new .items/do3177.pdf.

Grady D, D Herrington, V Bittner, et al. 2002. Cardiovascular disease outcomes during 6.8 years of hormone therapy. *JAMA* 288:40–57.

Graham D, D Campen, R Hui, et al. 2005. Risk of acute myocardial infarction and sudden cardiac death in patients treated with Cox-2 selective and non-selective non-steroidal anti-inflammatory drugs: nested case-control study. *Lancet* 365:475–81.

Greenhouse L. 2005. Justices accept case weighing assisted suicide. *New York Times* (2/23/05) A1.

Gregg EW, JA Cauley, K Stone, et al. 2003. Relationship of changes in physical activity and mortality among older women. *JAMA* 289:2379–86.

Groopman J. 2002. Dying words. *New Yorker* (10/28/02) 62–70.

Gross DJ, SW Schondolmeyer, and SO Retzman. 2004. Trends in manufacturer prices of brand name prescription drugs used by older Americans, 2000 through 2003. AARP Public Policy Institute publication ID: 2004–06.

Gross J. 2004. Older women team up to face future together. *New York Times* (2/27/04) A1.

Grumbach K, and T Bodenheimer. 2004. Can health care teams improve primary care practice? *JAMA* 291:1246–51.

Grundman M, RC Petersen, SH Ferris, et al. 2004. Mild cognitive impairment can be distinguished from Alzheimer Disease and normal aging for clinical trials. *Arch Neurol* 61:59–66.

Gudrais E. 2001. The brain at midlife. *Harvard Magazine* (May–June 2000) 9–10.

Guralnik JM. 1996. Assessing the impact of comorbidity in the older population. *Annals Epidemiol* 6:376–80.

Guralnik JM, LP Fried, and ME Salive. 1996. Disability as a public health outcome in the aging population. *Annu Rev Public Health* 17:25–46.

Gurwitz JH, TS Field, LR Harrold, et al. 2003. Incidence and preventability of adverse drug events among older persons in the ambulatory setting. *JAMA* 289:1107–16.

Gustafson D, E Rothenberg, K Blennow, et al. 2003. An 18-year follow-up of overweight and risk of Alzheimer Disease. *Arch Intern Med* 163:1524–28.

Hadler N. 2003. A ripe old age. *Arch Intern Med* 163:1261–62.

Hampton T. 2004. Similar drug names a risky prescription. *JAMA* 291:1948–49.

Hardy SE, and TM Gill. 2004. Recovery from disability among community-dwelling older persons. *JAMA* 291:1596–1602.

Harrington C, R Newcomer, and P Fox. 2001. Long-term care for older Californians. *California Policy Research Center Brief: Strategic Planning on Aging* no 9 (May 2001).

Harris G. 2003a. U.S. moves to halt import of drugs from Canada. *New York Times* (9/10/03) C2.

————. 2003b. Drug makers resist state efforts to cut Medicaid expenses. *New York Times* (12/18/03) A1.

————. 2004a. 2 cancer drugs, no comparative data. *New York Times* (2/26/04) C1.

————. 2004b. As doctor writes prescription, drug company writes a check. *New York Times* (6/27/04) A1.

————. 2004c. Guilty plea seen for drug maker. *New York Times* (7/16/04) A1.

————. 2004d. Proposal would slash what Medicare pays for cancer drugs. *New York Times* (7/27/04) C1.

————. 2004e. At FDA, strong drug ties and less monitoring. *New York Times* (12/6/04) A1.

Hays J, Ockene JK, RL Brunner, et al. 2003. Effects of estrogen plus progestin on health-related quality of life. *NEJM* 348:1839–54.

Helft PR, M Siegler, and J Lantos. 2000. The rise and fall of the futility movement. *NEJM* 343:293–96.

Hilts PJ. 1999. Life at 100 is surprisingly healthy. *New York Times* (6/1/99) A1.

Himmelstein DU, E Warren, D Thorne, et al. 2005. Illness and injury as contributors to bankruptcy. *Health Aff* www.healthaffairs.org (accessed 2/2/05).

Himmelstein DU, S Woolhandler, I Hellander, et al. 1999. Quality of care in investor-owned vs. not-for-profit HMOs. *JAMA* 282:159–63.

Hodis HN, WJ Mack, SP Azen, et al. 2003. Hormone therapy and the progression of coronary-artery atherosclerosis in postmenopausal women. *NEJM* 349:535–45.

Holman H. 2004. Chronic disease—the need for a new clinical education. *JAMA* 292:1057–59.

Horton R. 2004a. The dawn of McScience. *New York Review of Books* (3/11/04) 7–9.

————. 2004b. Vioxx, the implosion of Merck, and aftershocks at the FDA. *Lancet* 364:1995–96.

Hulley S, C Furberg, E Barrett-Connor, et al. 2002. Noncardiovascular disease outcomes during 6.8 years of hormone therapy. *JAMA* 288:58–66.

Hulley SB, and D Grady. 2004. The WHI estrogen-alone trial—do things look any better? *JAMA* 291:1769–71.

Humphry D. 1996. *Final exit: the practicalities of self-deliverance and assisted suicide for the dying.* New York: Dell.

Hurley AC, and L Volicer. 2002. Alzheimer Disease. *JAMA* 288:2324–31.

Huskamp H, PA Deverka, AM Epstein, et al. 2003. The effect of incentive-based formularies on prescription-drug utilization and spending. *NEJM* 349:2224–32.

Iglehart JK. 2004. The new Medicare prescription drug benefit—a pure power play. *NEJM* 350:826–33.

Inouye SK, ST Bogardus, PA Charpentier, et al. 1999. A multicomponent intervention to prevent delirium in hospitalized older patients. *NEJM* 340:669–76.

Institute for the Study of Aging. 2001. *Achieving and maintaining cognitive vitality with aging: a workshop report.* New York: International Longevity Center www.ilcusa.irg/publications; www.aging-institute.org.

Institute of Medicine. 2004. Insuring America's health: principles and recommendations. www.iom.org.edu/uninsured.

International Committee of Medical Journal Editors. 2004. Clinical trial registration. *JAMA* 292:1363–64.

Isaacs SL, and SA Schroeder. 2004. Class—the ignored determinant of the nation's health. *NEJM* 351:1137–42.

Jacobs S. 2003. Death by voluntary dehydration—What the caregivers say. *NEJM* 349:325–26.

Jagust W. 2001. Untangling vascular dementia. *Lancet* 358:2097–98.

Janofsky M. 2004. Costs and savings in Medicare change on wheelchairs. *New York Times* (1/30/04) A10.

Jasny BR, and L Roberts, eds. Are we there yet? *Science* 302:587–608.

Jenkins JA, CW Kendall, A Marchie, et al. 2003. Effects of dietary portfolio of cholesterol-lowering foods vs. lovastatin on serum lipids and C-reactive protein. *JAMA* 290:502–12.

Jette, AM, M Lachman, MM Giorgetti, et al. 1999. Exercise—it's never too late. *Am J Public Health* 89:66–72.

Jones RW. 2001. Inflammation and Alzheimer's disease. *Lancet* 358:436–37.

Juni P, L Nartey, S Reichenbach, et al. 2004. Risk of cardiovascular event and rofecoxib: cumulative meta-analysis. *Lancet* 364:2021–2029.

Juurlink DN, M Mamdani, A Kopp, et al. 2003. Drug-drug interactions among elderly patients hospitalized for drug toxicity. *JAMA* 289:1652–58.

Kaiser/Hewitt 2004. Survey on retiree health benefits. www.kff.org/medicare (accessed 12/14/04).

Kantrowitz B. 2000. The new middle age: a boomer's guide to health, wealth and happiness. *Newsweek* (4/3/00) 57.

Kassirer J. 1998. Doctor discontent. *NEJM* 339:1543–54.

Katz SJ, K Mohammed, and KM Langa. 2000. Gender disparities in the receipt of home care for elderly people in the United States. *JAMA* 284:3022–27.

Kaufman SR. 1986. *The ageless self: sources of meaning in late life.* Madison: University of Wisconsin Press.

Kawas CH. 2003. Early Alzheimer's Disease. *NEJM* 349:1056–63.

Kennedy T. 2004. Dramatic improvement or death spiral. *NEJM* 350:747–49.

Kerr EA, EA McGlynn, J Adams, et al. 2004. Profiling the quality of care in twelve communities: results from the CQI study. *Health Aff* 23:247–56.

Kirkwood TB. 2000. Evolution of aging: how genetic factors affect the end of life. *Generations* (Spring 2000) 12–18.

Kleinfeld NR. 2003. For elderly, fear of falls is a risk in itself. *New York Times* (3/5/03) A1.

Knoops KT, LC deGroot, D Kromhout, et al. 2004. Mediterranean diet, lifestyle factors, and 10-year mortality in elderly European men and women: the HALE project. *JAMA* 292:1433–39.

Koepsell T, L McCloskey, M Wolf, et al. 2002. Crosswalk markings and the risk of pedestrian–motor vehicle collisions in older pedestrians. *JAMA* 288:2136–43.

Kolata G. 2003. Bone diagnosis gives new data but no answers. *New York Times* (9/28/03) A1.

———. 2004. With costs rising, treating back pain often seems futile. *New York Times* (2/9/04) A1.

Kolata G, and EL Andrews. 2001. Anticholesterol drug pulled after link with 31 deaths. *New York Times* (8/9/01) C1.

Kovacs FM, V Abraira, A Pena, et al. 2003. Effect of firmness of mattress on chronic non-specific back pain: a randomized, double-blind controlled, multicentre trial. *Lancet* 362:1599–1604.

Kuttner R. 1998. Must good HMOs go bad? *NEJM* 338:1558–63, 1635–39.

Lachs MS, and K Pillemer. 2004. Elder abuse. *Lancet* 364:1263–72.

Lamberg L. 2002. "Palliative care" means "active care." *JAMA* 288:943–44.

Landefeld CS, CM Callahan, and N Woolard, eds. 2003. Improving geriatrics training: training internists in the care of older adults (suppl). *Ann Intern Med* 139:607–34.

Landes AM, SD Sperry, and ME Strauss. 2001. Apathy in Alzheimer's Disease. *J Am Geriatr Soc* 49:1700–1707.

Landon BE, AM Zaslavsky, and SL Bernard. 2004. Comparison of performance of traditional Medicare vs Medicare managed care. *JAMA* 291:1744–52.

Langa KM, NL Foster, and EB Larson. 2004. Mixed dementia. *JAMA* 292:2901–08.

Lantz PM, JS House, JM Lepkowski, et al. 1998. Socioeconomic factors, health behaviors, and mortality: results from a nationally representative prospective study of US adults. *JAMA* 279:1703–08.

Larsen DG, and DR Tobin. 2000. End of life conversations. *JAMA* 284:1573–78.

Lasser KE, PD Allen, S Woolhandler, et al. 2002. Timing of new black warnings and withdrawals for prescription medications. *JAMA* 287:2215–20.

Leiberman T. 1998. Hunger in America. *Nation* (3/30/98) 11–16.

Levine SA, J Boal, and PA Boling. 2003. Home care. *JAMA* 290:1203–07.

Levit K, C Smith, C Cowan, et al. 2003. Trends in health care spending, 2001. *Health Aff* 22:154–64.

———. 2004. Health spending rebound continues in 2002. *Health Aff* 23:147–56.

Lewontin R. 2001. After the genome, what then? *New York Review of Books* (7/9/01) 36.

Li F, KJ Fisher, P Harmer, et al. 2002. Delineating the impact of tai chi training on physical function among the elderly. *Am J Prev Med* 23:92–97.

Lin HB, W Katon, M VonDorff, et al. 2003. Effect of improving depression care on pain and functional outcomes in older adults with arthritis. *JAMA* 290:2428–34.

Liptak A. 2004. Ruling upholds law authorizing assisted suicide. *New York Times* (5/27/04) A1.

Lu T, Y Pan, S-Y Kao, et al. 2004. Gene regulation and DNA damage in the ageing human brain. *Nature* 429:883–91.

Lunney JR, J Lynn, DJ Foley, et al. 2003. Patterns of functional decline at the end of life. *JAMA* 289:2387–92.

Lyness JM. 2004. Treatment of depressive conditions in later life. *JAMA* 291:1626–27.

Lynn J. 2001. Serving patients who may die soon. *JAMA* 285:925–32.

———. 2004. *Sick to death and not going to take it anymore!* Berkeley and Los Angeles: University of California Press.

Lynn J, JM Teno, RS Phillips, et al. 1997. Perceptions by family members of the dying experience of older and seriously ill patients. *Ann Intern Med* 126:97–106.

Madrick J. 2003. Health for sale. *New York Review of Books* (12/18/03) 71–74.

Manion FA. 1998. Should we accept mediocrity? *NEJM* 338:1067–69.

———. 1999. Whither continuity of care? *NEJM* 340:1362–63.

Manson JE, J Hsia, KC Johnson, et al. 2003. Estrogen plus progestin and the risk of coronary heart disease. *NEJM* 349:523–34.

Manton KG, and X Gu. 2001. Changes in the prevention of chronic disability in the United States black and non-black population above age 65 from 1982–99. *Proc Natl Acad Sci* 98:6354–59.

Margolis S, and PV Rabin. 2002. *Memory.* Baltimore MD: Johns Hopkins Medical Institutes.

Mariner WK. 2004. The Supreme Court's limitation of managed-care liability. *NEJM* 351:1347–51.

Mattimore TJ, NS Wenger, NA Desbiens, et al. 1997. Surrogate and physician understanding of patients' preferences for living permanently in a nursing home. *J Am Geriatr Soc* 45:818–24.

Maxwell RJ, and DJ Webb. 2005. Cox-2 selective inhibitors—important lessons learned. *Lancet* 365:449–51.

McClain CS, B Rosenfeld, and W Breitbart. 2003. Effect of spiritual well-being on end-of-life despair in terminally-ill cancer patients. *Lancet* 361: 1603–07.

McCormick D, DU Himmelstein, S Woolhandler, et al. 2004. Single-payer national health insurance: physicians' views. *Arch Intern Med* 164:300–304.

McGlynn EA, SM Asch, J Adams, et al. 2003. The quality of health care delivered to adults in the U.S. *NEJM* 348:2635–45.

McWilliams JM, AM Zaslavsky, E Meara, et al. 2003. Impact of Medicare coverage on basic clinical services for previously uninsured adults. *JAMA* 290:757–64.

Meier B. 2004a. Group is said to seek full drug-trial disclosure. *New York Times* (6/15/04) A1.

———. 2004b. A.M.A. urges disclosure on drug trials. *New York Times* (6/17/04) C1.

Meier DE, C Emmons, A Litke, et al. 2003. Characteristics of patients requesting and receiving physician-assisted death. *Arch Intern Med* 163:1537–42.

Meier DE, and RS Morrison. 2002. Autonomy reconsidered. *NEJM* 346:1087–88.

Mello MM, DM Studdert, and TA Brennan. 2004. The pharmaceutical industry versus Medicaid—limits on state initiatives to control prescription-drug costs. *NEJM* 350:608–12.

Mesulam MM. 2003. Primary progressive aphasia—a language-based dementia. *NEJM* 349:1535–42.

Miles S, and K Parker. 1997. Men, women, and health insurance. *NEJM* 336:218–20.

Mitchell JL, KJ Cruickshanks, BE Klein, et al. 2003. Postmenopausal hormone therapy and its association with cognitive impairment. *Arch Intern Med* 163:2485–90.

Mitchell SL, DK Kiely, and MB Hamel. 2004. Dying with advanced dementia in the nursing home. *Arch Intern Med* 164:321–26.

Mitchell SL, DK Kiely, MB Hamel, et al. 2004. Estimating prognosis for nursing home residents with advanced dementia. *JAMA* 291:2734–40.

Mitchell SL, JM Teno, J Roy, et al. 2003. Clinical and organizational factors associated with feeding tube use among nursing home residents with advanced cognitive impairment. *JAMA* 290:73–80.

Mitka M. 2003. Survey suggesting that prescription drug ads help public met with skepticism. *JAMA* 289:827–28.

Mold JW, and LA Green. 2003. General internists and family physicians: partners in geriatric medicine? *Ann Intern Med* 139:594–95.

Morrison RS, and DE Meier. 2004. Palliative care. *NEJM* 350:2582–90.

Morrison RS, and AL Siu. 2000. Survival in end-stage dementia following acute illness. *JAMA* 283:47–52.

Moyers B. 2000. On our own terms. Public Broadcasting Corporation video #10473–76.

Myerhoff B. 1978. *Number our days*. New York: Simon & Schuster.

National study of adult day services, 2001–2002. 2002. www.rwjf.org/news/special/adultdayServicesStudy (accessed 9/4/03).

Naylor MD, D Brooten, R Campbell, et al. 1999. Comprehensive discharge planning and home follow-up of hospitalized elders. *JAMA* 281:613–20.

Needleman J, P Buerhaus, S Mattke, et al. 2002. Nursing staff levels and the quality of care in hospitals. *NEJM* 346:1715–22.

Newcomer R, and R Maynard. 2001. Residential care for older Californians. *California Policy Research Center Brief: Strategic Planning on Aging* no 10.

Newhouse JP. 2000. Switching health plans to obtain drug coverage. *JAMA* 283:2161–62.

Nuland S. 1993. *How we die*. New York: Random House.

———. 2000. Physician-assisted suicide and euthanasia in practice. *NEJM* 342:583–85.

Olshansky SJ, and BA Carnes. 2001. *The quest for immortality*. New York: WW Norton.

Olshansky SJ, MA Rudberg, BA Carnes, et al. 1991. Trading off longer life for worsening health. *J Aging Health* 3:194–216.

Onwuteaka-Philipsen BD, A van der Heide, D Koper, et al. 2003. Euthanasia and other end-of life decisions in the Netherlands in 1990, 1995, and 2001. *Lancet* 362:395–99.

Orentlicher D. 1997. The Supreme Court and physician-assisted suicide. *NEJM* 337:1236–39.

Orentlicher D, and A Caplan. 2000. The Pain Relief Promotion Act of 1999: a serious threat to palliative care. *JAMA* 283:255–58.

Outpatient Service Trialists. 2004. Rehabilitation therapy services for stroke patients living at home: systematic review of randomised trials. *Lancet* 363:352–56.

Pantilat SZ, A Alpers, and RM Wachter. 1999. A new doctor in the house. *JAMA* 282:171–74.

Pantilat SZ, and AE Steimle. 2004. Palliative care for patients with heart failure. *JAMA* 291:2476–82.

Pear R. 1998a. Home-care denial in Medicare is ruled improper. *New York Times* (2/15/98) A1.

———. 1998b. Hospitals told not to delay emergency room treatment. *New York Times* (12/1/98) A1.

———. 1999. Clinton lays out plan to overhaul Medicare system. *New York Times* (6/30/99) A1.

———. 2000a. Medicare spending for care at home plunges by 45%. *New York Times* (4/21/00) A1.

———. 2000b. Justice Souter takes on a health care taboo. *New York Times* (6/18/00) A1.

———. 2000c. U.S. recommending strict new rules at nursing homes. *New York Times* (7/23/00) A1.

———. 2000d. Rise in health care costs rests largely on drug prices. *New York Times* (11/14/00) A1.

———. 2001. Spending on prescription drugs increases by almost 19%. *New York Times* (5/8/01) A1.

———. 2002a. Propelled by drug and hospital costs, health spending surged in 2000. *New York Times* (1/8/02) A16.

———. 2002b. Nine in ten nursing homes lack adequate staff, study finds. *New York Times* (2/18/02) A1.

———. 2002c. Medicare is now covering treatment for Alzheimer's. *New York Times* (3/31/02) A1.

———. 2002d. U.S. begins issuing consumer data on nursing homes. *New York Times* (4/25/02) A1.

———. 2002e. Investigators find repeated deception in ads for drugs. *New York Times* (12/4/02) A1.

———. 2003a. Bush pushes plan to curb appeals in Medicare cases. *New York Times* (3/16/03) A1.

———. 2003b. U.S. limiting costs of drugs for Medicare. *New York Times* (4/21/03) A1.

———. 2003c. Congress weighs drug comparisons. *New York Times* (8/24/03) A1.

———. 2003d. Emergency rooms get eased rules on patient care. *New York Times* (9/3/03) A1.

———. 2003e. Rising costs prompt states to reduce Medicaid further. *New York Times* (9/23/03) A16.

———. 2003f. Proposed rule would ease stance on feeding at nursing homes. *New York Times* (9/25/03) A19.

———. 2003g. House and senate weigh co-payment for care at home. *New York Times* (10/14/03) A14.

———. 2003h. New Medicare plan for drug benefits prohibits insurance. *New York Times* (12/7/03) A1.

———. 2004a. Health spending at a record level. *New York Times* (1/9/04) A1.

———. 2004b. Bush's aides see higher price tag for drug benefit. *New York Times* (1/30/04) A1.

———. 2004c. Taking spin out of report that made bad into good. *New York Times* (2/22/04) A16.

———. 2004d. Investigators say drug makers repeatedly overcharge. *New York Times* (6/30/04) A17.

———. 2004e. Inquiry confirms top Medicare official threatened actuary over cost of drug benefits. *New York Times* (7/7/04) A17.

———. 2004f. Drug law is seen causing big drop in retiree plans. *New York Times* (7/14/04) A1.

———. 2004g. New Medicare drug plan is raising difficult issues for nursing home patients. *New York Times* (12/5/04) A24.

———. 2005. Estimate revives fight on Medicare costs. *New York Times* (2/20/05) A16.

Pear R, and M Freudenheim. 2004. Drug discounts beginning today, but sign-ups lag. *New York Times* (6/1/04) A1.

Pear R, and RA Oppel, Jr. 2002. Election gives industry new influence. *New York Times* (11/21/02) A1.

Pennix BJ, S Leveille, L Ferrucci, et al. 1999. Exploring the effect of depression on physical disability. *Am J Public Health* 89:1346–52.

Petersen M. 2001. Doubts are raised on the safety of two popular arthritis drugs. *New York Times* (5/22/01) C1.

———. 2002. Madison avenue plays growing role in the business of drug research. *New York Times* (11/22/02) A1.

———. 2003. Who's minding the drugstore? *New York Times* (6/29/03) Section 3:1.

Petersen M, and A Berenson. 2003. Papers indicate that Bayer knew of dangers of its cholesterol drug. *New York Times* (2/22/03) A1.

Philips D, N Christenfeld, and LM Glynn. 1998. Increase in United States prescription error deaths between 1983 and 1993. *Lancet* 351:634–44.

Phillips CO, SM Wright, DE Kern, et al. 2004. Comprehensive discharge planning with postdischarge support for older patients with congestive heart failure. *JAMA* 291:1358–67.

Physicians' Working Group for Single-Payer National Health Insurance. 2003. Proposal of the physicians' working group for single-payer national health insurance. *JAMA* 290:798–805.

Porter E. 2004. Cost of benefits cited as factor in slump in jobs. *New York Times* (8/19/04) A1.

Prendergast TJ, and KA Puntillo. 2002. Withdrawal of life support. *JAMA* 288:2732–40.

Press D. 2004. Parkinson's dementia—a first step? *NEJM* 351:2547–49.

Prigerson HG. 2003. Costs to society of family caregiving for patients with end-stage Alzheimer's Disease. *NEJM* 349:1891–92.

Psaty BM, CD Furberg, WA Ray, et al. 2004. Potential for conflict of interest in the evaluation of suspected adverse drug reaction. *JAMA* 292:2622–31.

Public Citizen Health Research Group. 2003. DO NOT USE! *Health Letter* 19:3–5.

———. 2004. Medizine: drug ads masquerading as news. *Health Letter* 20:12.

Puca A, MJ Daly, SJ Brewster, et al. 2001. A genetic scan for linkage to human exceptional longevity identifies a locus on chromosome 4. *Proc Natl Acad Sci* 98:1505–8.

Quill TE. 1991. Death and dignity: a case of individualized decision-making. *NEJM* 324:692–94.

———. 2004. Dying and decision making—evolution of end-of-life options. *NEJM* 350:2029–32.

Rabow MW, JM Hauser, and J Adams. 2004. Supporting family caregivers at the end of life. *JAMA* 291:483–91.

Rafkin HS, and T Rainey. 1997. Experience in the critical care setting. In Zucker MB, and HD Zucker, eds., *Medical futility and the evaluation of life-sustaining interventions.* Cambridge: Cambridge University Press.

Ramachandrian VS. 2000. Memory and the brain: new lessons from old symptoms. In Schacter DL, and E Scarry, eds., *Memory, brain, and belief.* Cambridge MA: Harvard University Press.

Rao SV, KA Schulman, LH Curtis, et al. 2004. Socioeconomic status and outcome following acute myocardial infarction in elderly patients. *Arch Intern Med* 164:1128–33.

Rapp SR, MA Espeland, SA Shumaker, et al. 2003. Effect of estrogen plus progestin on global cognitive function in postmenopausal women. *JAMA* 289:2663–72.

Raskind M, ER Peskind, L Truyen, et al. 2004. The cognitive benefits of galantamine are sustained for at least 36 months. *Arch Neurol* 61:252–56.

Rawls J. 2001. *Justice as fairness.* Cambridge MA: Harvard University Press.

Rector T. 2000. Exhaustion of drug benefits and disenrollment of Medicare beneficiaries from managed care organizations. *JAMA* 283:2163–67.

Regalado A. 2003. To sell pricey drug, Lilly fuels a debate over rationing. *Wall Street Journal* (9/18/03) A1.

Reinhardt UE. 1997. Wanted: a clearly articulated social ethic for American health care. *JAMA* 278:1446–47.

———. 2004. An information infrastructure for the pharmaceutical market. *Health Aff* 23:107–12.

Reisberg B, R Doody, A Stoffler, et al. 2003. Memantine in moderate-to-severe Alzheimer's Disease. *NEJM* 348:1333–41.

Rennie D. 2004. Trial registration. *JAMA* 292:1359–62.

Retchin SM, RS Brown, SC Yeh, et al. 1997. Outcomes of stroke patients in Medicare fee-for-service and managed care. *JAMA* 278:119–24.

Retirees pioneer a health program just for them. 2000. *San Francisco Chronicle* (8/7/00) A1.

Rhymes JA, LB McCullough, RJ Luchi, et al. 2000. Withdrawing very low-burden interventions in chronically ill patients. *JAMA* 283:1061–67.

Riley T, and E Kilbreth. 2004. Health coverage in the states—Maine's plan for universal access. *NEJM* 350:330–32.

Rimer S. 1998. Seattle's elderly find a home for living, not dying. *New York Times* (11/22/98) A1.

———. 1999. Caring for elderly kin can be costly, study finds. *New York Times* (11/27/99) A1.

Rimm EB, and MJ Stampfer. 2004. Diet, lifestyle, and longevity—the next steps? *JAMA* 292:1490–92.

Ritchie K, and S Lovestone. 2002. The dementias. *Lancet* 360:1759–66.

Robinson JC. 2004. Reinvention of health insurance in the consumer era. *JAMA* 291:1880–86.

Rochon PA, and JH Gurwitz. 1999. Prescribing for seniors: neither too much nor too little. *JAMA* 282:113–15.

Rocker GM, and JR Curtis. 2003. Caring for the dying in the intensive care unit. *JAMA* 290:820–22.

Rowe JW. 1999. Geriatrics, prevention, and the remodeling of Medicare. *NEJM* 340:720–21.

Rowe JW, and RL Kahn. 1997. Successful aging. *Gerontologist* 37:433–40.

———. 1999. *Successful aging.* New York: Dell.

Rubenstein LZ. 1996. Update on preventive medicine for older people. *Generations* (Winter 1996–97) 47–53.

Safran DG, P Newman, C Shoen, et al. 2002. Prescription drug coverage and seniors: how well are states closing the gaps? *Health Aff* www.healthaffairs .org:W253–W268.

Satariano WA, GN DeLovenze, D Reed, et al. 1996. Imbalance in an older population: an epidemiological analysis. *J Aging Health* 8:334–58.

Scherer FM. 2004. The pharmaceutical industry—prices and progress. *NEJM* 351:927–32.

Schevitz T. 1999. For many, retiring early ailments win. *San Francisco Chronicle* (9/7/99) A17.

Schneider LS. 2004a. AD2000: Donepezil in Alzheimer's disease. *Lancet* 363:2100–2101.

———. 2004b. Estrogen and dementia. *JAMA* 291:3005–07.

Schneiderman LJ, T Gilmer, HD Teetzel, et al. 2003. Effect of ethics consultations on nonbeneficial life-sustaining treatments in the intensive care setting. *JAMA* 290:1166–72.

Schoeni RF, VA Freedman, and RB Wallace. 2001. Persistent, consistent, widespread, and robust? Another look at recent trends in old-age disability. *J Gerontol: Soc Sci* 56B:S206–18.

Schulz R, and SR Beach. 1999. Caregiving as a risk factor for mortality. *JAMA* 282:2215–19.

Schulz R, SH Belle, SJ Czaja, et al. 2004. Long-term care placement of dementia patients and caregiver health and well-being. *JAMA* 292:961–67.

Schulz R, AB Mendelsohn, WE Haley, et al. 2003. End-of-life care and the effects of bereavement on family caregivers of persons with dementia. *NEJM* 349:1936–42.

Schwartz WB. 1998. *Life without disease*. Berkeley and Los Angeles: University of California Press.

Shumaker SA, C Legault, L Kuller, et al. 2004. Conjugated equine estrogens and incidence of probable dementia and mild cognitive impairment in postmenopausal women. *JAMA* 291:2947–58.

Shumaker SA, C Legault, SR Rapp, et al. 2003. Estrogen plus progestin and the incidence of dementia and mild cognitive impairment in postmenopausal women. *JAMA* 289:2651–62.

Singer PA, DK Martin, and M Kelner. 1999. Quality end-of-life care: patients' perspective. *JAMA* 281:163–68.

Sink KM, KF Holden, and K Yaffe. 2005. Pharmacological treatment of neuropsychiatric symptoms of dementia. *JAMA* 293:596–608.

Smith NL, SR Heckbert, RN Lemaitre, et al. 2004. Esterified estrogens and conjugated equine estrogens and the risk of venous thrombosis. *JAMA* 292:1581–87.

Snowden D. 2001. *Aging with grace*. New York: Bantam.

Solomon PR, F Adams, A Silver, et al. 2002. Ginkgo biloba for memory enhancement: a randomized controlled trial. *JAMA* 287:835–40.

Soumerai SB, and D Ross-Degnan. 1999. Inadequate prescription-drug coverage for Medicare enrollees—A call to action. *NEJM* 340:722–27.

Spector M. 2001. Rethinking the brain. *New Yorker* (7/23/01) 42–53.

Sprung CL, SL Cohen, P Sjokvist, et al. 2003. End-of-life practices in European intensive care units. *JAMA* 290:790–97.

St. John K. 2000. Critical condition. *San Francisco Chronicle* (11/20/00) A1.

Steinbrook R. 2002. Physician-assisted suicide in Oregon—an uncertain future. *NEJM* 346:460–64.

———. 2004a. Disparities in health care—from politics to policy. *NEJM* 350:1486–88.

———. 2004b. The cost of admission—tiered copayments for hospital use. *NEJM* 350:2539–42.

———. 2004c. Public registration of clinical trials. *NEJM* 351:315–17.

Steinhauer J. 2000. Emergency room, to many, remains the doctor's office. *New York Times* (10/25/00) A1.

———. 2001. As assisted living centers grow, calls for standards and oversight. *New York Times* (2/12/01) A1.

Stern PS, and LL Carstensen, eds. 2002. *The aging mind: opportunities in cognitive research*. Washington DC: National Academy Press.

Stolberg SG. 1999. The boom in medications brings rise in fatal risks. *New York Times* (6/3/99) A1.

———. 2000a. Drug plan sounds great, but who gets to set prices? *New York Times* (7/9/00) A1.

———. 2000b. FDA warns of overuse of two new drugs against flu. *New York Times* (1/13/00) A1.

Stolberg SG, and J Gerth. 2000a. How companies stall generics and keep themselves healthy. *New York Times* (7/23/00) A1.

—. 2000b. High-tech stealth being used to sway doctor prescriptions. *New York Times* (11/16/00) A1.

Strom BL. 2004. Potential for conflict of interest in the evaluation of suspected adverse drug reaction: a counterpoint. *JAMA* 292:2643–45.

Strunk B, and PB Ginsburg. 2003. Tracking health care costs: trends stabilize but remain high in 2002. *Health Aff* 22:12–23.

Stuck AE, JC Beck, and M Egger. 2004. Preventing disability in elderly people. *Lancet* 364:1641–42.

Sullivan AD, K Hedberg, and DW Fleming. 2000. Legalized physician-assisted suicide in Oregon—the 2nd year. *NEJM* 342:598–64.

SUPPORT. 1995. A controlled trial to improve care for seriously ill hospitalized patients. *JAMA* 274:1591–98.

Survey finds boomer women not preparing for golden years. 2000. *Berkeley Voice* (7/21/00) 1.

Tamblyn R, R Laprise, JA Hanley, et al. 2001. Adverse events associated with prescription drug cost-sharing among poor and elderly persons. *JAMA* 285:421–29.

Tariot PN, MR Farlow, GT Grossberg, et al. 2004. Memantine treatment in patients with moderate to severe Alzheimer Disease already receiving donepezil. *JAMA* 291:317–24.

Taylor B. 2004. Giveaway drugs: good intentions, bad design. *Health Aff* 23:213–17.

Teno JM, BR Clarridge, V Casey, et al. 2004. Family perspectives on end-of-life care at the last place of care. *JAMA* 291:88–93.

Teri L, LE Gibbons, SM McCurry, et al. 2003. Exercise plus behavioral management in patients with Alzheimer Disease. *JAMA* 290:2015–22.

Thomas CP. 2003. Incentive-based formularies. *NEJM* 349:2186–88.

Thomas DC, RM Leipzig, LG Smith, et al. 2003. Improving geriatrics training in internal medicine residency programs. *Ann Intern Med* 139:628–34.

Tinetti ME. 2003. Preventing falls in elderly persons. *NEJM* 348:42–47.

Tinetti ME, DI Baker, G McAvay, et al. 1994. A multifactorial intervention to reduce the risk of falling among elderly people living in the community. *NEJM* 331:821–27.

Tinetti ME, ND Baker, and WT Gallo. 2002. Evaluation of restorative care vs. usual care for older adults receiving an acute episode of home care. *JAMA* 287:2098–2105.

Tinetti, ME, CS Williams, and TM Gill. 2000. Health, functional, and psychological outcomes among older persons with chronic dizziness. *J Amer Geriatric Soc* 48:417–21.

Toner R. 1999. Drawing up plans to pay for pills for the elderly. *New York Times* (5/10/99) A1.

Topol EJ. 2004. Failing the public health—rofecoxib, Merck, and the FDA. *NEJM* 351:1707–09.

—. 2005. Arthritis medicines and cardiovascular event—"house of coxibs." *JAMA* 293:366–68.

Topol EJ, and GW Falk. 2004. A coxib a day won't keep the doctor away. *Lancet* 364:639–40.

Trinh N, J Hoblyn, S Mohanty, et al. 2003. Efficacy of cholinesterase inhibitors in the treatment of neuropsychological symptoms and functional impairment in Alzheimer's Disease. *JAMA* 289:210–16.

Tseng CW, RH Brook, E Keeler. 2004. Cost-lowering strategies used by Medicare beneficiaries who exceed drug benefit caps and have a gap in drug coverage. *JAMA* 292:952–60.

Tunis SR. 2004. Why Medicare has not established criteria for coverage decisions. *NEJM* 350:2196–98.

Union of Concerned Scientists. 2004. Scientific integrity in policymaking—executive summary. www2.ucsusa.org.

Unutzer J, W Katon, CM Callahan, et al. 2002. Collaborative care management of late-life depression in the primary care setting: a randomized controlled trial. *JAMA* 288:2836–45.

van der Heide A, L Dellens, K Faisst, et al. 2003. End-of-life decision-making in six European countries: descriptive study. *Lancet* 361:345–50.

van der Heide A, J van Delden, and G van der Wal. 2004. Doctor-assisted dying: what difference does legalisation make? *Lancet* 364:24–25.

Verghese J, RB Lipton, MJ Katz, et al. 2003. Leisure activities and the risk of dementia in the elderly. *NEJM* 348:2508–16.

Vermeer SE, ND Prins, T den Heijer, et al. 2003. Silent brain infarcts and the risk of dementia and cognitive decline. *NEJM* 348:1215–22.

Voelker R. 2003. Northern Rxposure. *JAMA* 290:2921.

Volz J. 2000. Successful aging: the second fifty. *Monitor on Psychology* 31:24–35.

Von Guten CF, FD Ferris, and LL Emanuel. 2000. Ensuring competency in end-of-life care. *JAMA* 284:3051–57.

Wald ML. 2000. Accidental deaths on rise as the population ages fast. *New York Times* (4/26/00) A18.

Walter LC, and KE Covinsky. 2001. Cancer screening in elderly patients. *JAMA* 285:2750–56.

Wang C, JP Collet, and J Lau. 2004. The effect of tai chi on health outcomes in patients with chronic conditions. *Arch Intern Med* 164:493–501.

Wang H-X, A Wahlin, H Basun, et al. 2001. Vitamin B12 and folate in relation to development of Alzheimer's Disease. *Neurology* 56:1188–94.

Ware J, MS Bayliss, WH Rogers, et al. 1996. Differences in 4-year health outcomes for elderly and poor, chronically ill patients treated in HMO and FFS systems. *JAMA* 276:1039–47.

Wassertheil-Smoller S, SL Hendrix, M Limacher, et al. 2003. Effect of estrogen plus progestin on stroke in postmenopausal women. *JAMA* 289:2673–84.

Wazana A. 2000. Physicians and the pharmaceutical industry. *JAMA* 283:373–80.

Weisbrot M. 2000. Rx for Medicare. *San Francisco Chronicle* (2/13/00) A1.

Weissman DE. 2004. Decision making at a time of crisis near the end of life. *JAMA* 292:1738–43.

Wenger NS, DH Solomon, CP Roth, et al. 2003. The quality of medical care provided to vulnerable community-dwelling older patients. *Ann Intern Med* 139:740–47.

Wenve J, JH Kang, JE Manson, et al. 2004. Physical activity, including walking, and cognitive function in older women. *JAMA* 292:1454–61.

Whalley L. 2001. *The aging brain*. New York: Columbia University Press.

Wilcock GK. 2003. Dementia with Lewy Bodies. *Lancet* 362:1689–90.

Willcox SM, DU Himmelstein, and S Woolhandler. 1994. Inappropriate drug prescribing for the community-dwelling elderly. *JAMA* 272:292–96.

Wilson D. 2001. Some losing it, bit by bit. *Los Angeles Times* (7/17/01) A1.

Wilson RS, CF Mendes de Leon, LL Barnes, et al. 2002. Participation in cognitively stimulating activities and risk of incident Alzheimer's Disease. *JAMA* 287:742–48.

Winzelberg G. 2003. The quest for nursing home quality. *Arch Intern Med* 163:2552–56.

Wolf SL, HX Barnhart, NG Kutner, et al. 1996. Reducing frailty and falls in older persons: an investigation of t'ai chi and computerized balance training. *J Am Geriatr Soc* 44:489–97.

Wolfson C, DB Wolfson, M Asgharian, et al. 2001. A reevaluation of the duration of survival after onset of dementia. *NEJM* 344:111–16.

Women's Health Initiative [WHI] Steering Committee. 2004. Effects of conjugated equine estrogen in postmenopausal women with hysterectomy. *JAMA* 291:1701–12.

Woolhandler S, T Campbell, and DU Himmelstein. 2003. Costs of health care administration in the United States and Canada. *NEJM* 349:768–75.

Wysocki B. 2003. At one hospital, a stark solution for allocating care. *Wall Street Journal* (9/23/03) A1.

Yaffe K. 2003. Hormone therapy and the brain. *JAMA* 289:2717–19.

Yaffe K, P Fox, R Newcomer, et al. 2002. Patient and caregiver characteristics and nursing home placement in patients with dementia. *JAMA* 287:2090–97.

Zahn C, J Sangl, AS Bierman, et al. 2001. Potentially inappropriate medication use in the community-dwelling elderly. *JAMA* 286:2823–29.

Zandi PP, JC Anthony, AS Khachaturian, et al. 2004. Reduced risk of Alzheimer Disease in users of antioxidant vitamin supplements. *Arch Neurol* 61:82–88.

Index

Compositor:	Sheridan Books, Inc.
Text:	10/13 Sabon
Display:	Akzidenz Grotesk
Indexer:	Patricia Deminna
Printer and binder:	Sheridan Books, Inc.